Alex Berman
Michael A. Flannery

America's Botanico-Medical Movements
Vox Populi

Pre-publication
REVIEWS,
COMMENTARIES,
EVALUATIONS . . .

"**A**s the current movement toward herbal medicine continues its momentum and as public policy debates 'nutritional supplements,' Alex Berman and Michael Flannery offer us a learned perspective about the first mass movement in American history, a movement that uncannily mimics our age. Against the excesses of medicine's emphasis on minerals, especially the infamous calomel with its mercury base, the unlikely instigator of an herbal medicine corrective was Samuel Thomson (1769-1843), whose background was more in farming than medicine. Preaching the clarion call for nature's remedies, Thomson's name transforms into an episode known as Thomsonism. Alex Berman teams with Michael Flannery to produce a medical perspective that modern medicine should not ignore. Whereas we may not have the equivalent of calomel, the cumulative mistrust of synthetics and medical technology results in a vox populi return to nature's remedies just as there was disillusionment with early nineteenth-century medicine. Judgments about what are scientific facts and what superstitious lore are eschewed in favor of a scholarly narrative, easily read, fascinatingly presented."

John M. Riddle
Alumni Distinguished Professor,
Department of History,
North Carolina State University,
Raleigh

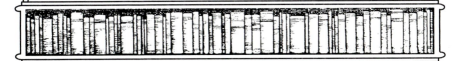

More pre-publication
REVIEWS, COMMENTARIES, EVALUATIONS . . .

"**A**merica's Botanico-Medical Movements is an engaging exploration of the therapeutic ancestors of today's alternative healers. Berman and Flannery provide a thoroughly researched and documented history of the American botanico-medical movements. No other book ties together so well the pharmaceutical and medical aspects of sectarian medicine in the United States. This is an important book in the history of American pharmacy."

Gregory J. Higby, PhD
Director,
American Institute
of the History of Pharmacy

"**W**ith the current fascination on the part of both scholars and the general public with the potential botanical healing properties of plants and herbs, the appearance of Berman and Flannery's significant examination of the background over the past two centuries of this part of medical science is most welcomed. Based on Berman's 1950's dissertation and updated by Flannery's current research on botanical healing, this volume is the key resource for anyone interested in the origins, growth, decline, and reemergence of this important part of health care.

The authors thoroughly describe the reasons for the emergence of nineteenth-century American botanical sects such as the Thomsonians, physio-medicals, and eclectics, and how many segments of the public eagerly welcomed their therapeutic approach rather than rely on the extremely harsh, potentially deadly therapeutics used by the traditional nineteenth-century physicians. Later chapters discuss the destructive competition between the botanical healing sects and their outspoken leaders, and their failure to adapt to the new medical scientific world of the twentieth century, leading to their virtual disappearance in the 1930s. The concluding chapter does an outstanding job of explaining the reemergence, beginning in the 1960s, of botanical healing in the United States and why both mainstream and alternative medicine have chosen to include botanical healing as part of their therapeutic regimens. Based extensively on primary documentation, this book presents the fascinating history of the individuals and national movements that created the impetus for botanical healing, from the Jeffersonian era, through Jacksonian democracy, up to the current research on botanical healing."

Jonathon Erlen, PhD
Assistant Professor,
Department of Health Sciences
Administration,
Graduate School of Public Health,
University of Pittsburgh,
Pennsylvania

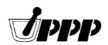

Pharmaceutical Products Press
An Imprint of The Haworth Press, Inc.

America's Botanico-Medical Movements
Vox Populi

PHARMACEUTICAL PRODUCTS PRESS

Pharmaceutical Heritage:
Pharmaceutical Care Through History

Mickey C. Smith, PhD
Dennis B. Worthen, PhD
Senior Editors

Laboratory on the Nile: A History of the Wellcome Tropical Research Laboratories by Patrick F. D'Arcy

America's Botanico-Medical Movements: Vox Populi by Alex Berman and Michael A. Flannery

Medicines for the Union Army: The United States Army Laboratories During the Civil War by George Winston Smith

Pharmaceutical Education in the Queen City: 150 Years of Service, 1850-2000 by Michael A. Flannery and Dennis B. Worthen

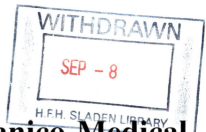
America's Botanico-Medical Movements
Movements
Vox Populi

Alex Berman
Michael A. Flannery

Pharmaceutical Products Press®
An Imprint of the Haworth Press, Inc.
New York • London • Oxford

Published by

Pharmaceutical Heritage Editions, a series from Pharmaceutical Products Press®, an imprint of The Haworth Press, Inc., 10 Alice Street, Binghamton, NY 13904-1580

Cover design by Jennifer M. Gaska.

Library of Congress Cataloging-in-Publication Data

Berman, Alex, 1914-
    America's botanico-medical movements : vox populi / Alex Berman, Michael A. Flannery.
      p. ; cm.
    Includes bibliographical references and index.
    ISBN 0-7890-0899-8 (alk. paper) — ISBN 0-7890-1235-9 (alk. paper)
    1. Medicine, Botanic—United States—History. 2. Materia medica—United States—History.
I. Title: Vox populi. II. Flannery, Michael A., 1953- III. Title.
    [DNLM: 1. Berman, Alex, 1914- 2. Medicine, Herbal—History—United States. 3. History of Medicine, 19th Cent.—United States. 4. History of Medicine, 20th Cent.—United States. 5. Materia Medica—United States. 6. Plants, Medicinal—United States. WB 925 B516a 2000]
RV5 .B47 2000
615′.32′0973—dc21

                                                                00-033660

For
Hortense Berman
and
Dona Flannery,
with deep gratitude for their devotion and inspiration . . .

ABOUT THE AUTHORS

Alex Berman, PhD, was Professor Emeritus of history and historical studies in pharmacy at the University of Cincinnati. He earned his PhD in the history of pharmacy, medicine, and science at the University of Wisconsin in 1954. Prior to obtaining his doctorate he worked as a community and hospital pharmacist and served in World War II as a military pharmacist. Dr. Berman taught at several universities. In addition to his influential articles on American botanics, he wrote extensively on the history of French pharmacy. His work was supported by a Guggenheim Fellowship (1958-1959) and grants from the National Science Foundation and the National Library of Medicine. Dr. Berman was also the recipient of the prestigious Kremers Award given for excellence in the history of pharmacy in the United States by the American Institute of the History of Pharmacy.

Michael A. Flannery, MA, MLS, is Associate Director for Historical Collections at the University of Alabama at Birmingham. Mr. Flannery earned his MA in history from California State University, Dominguez Hills, and his MLS from the University of Kentucky. He has taught the history of pharmacy at the University of Cincinnati and teaches the history of medicine at UAB. He is the author of numerous articles on the history of pharmacy and medical botany and is the author of a book-length biography of perhaps America's most noted medical botanist, *John Uri Lloyd: The Great American Eclectic.*

In Memoriam

Sadly, as this book was being prepared for press, Alex Berman passed away on June 29, 2000. Although he will be greatly missed, all those who read and find some value in the present work will form a lasting tribute to this man who spent the better part of his scholarly career delineating the botanico-medical movement in America. I think for Alex on one level and myself on another, there is something of George Eliot's *The Choir Invisible* in this work:

> Oh, may I join the choir invisible
> Of those immortal dead who live again
> In minds made better by their presence.

Alex has joined that "choir invisible" but he will not be forgotten, for surely my mind was made better by his presence. May this be true for the reader.

Michael A. Flannery
July 7, 2000

For God has lodged the fund of common
sense in the mass of the assembled multitude . . .
and it was on the appeal to that assembly, and
its decisions, that the ancients established the
maxim, so often in their mouth, *vox populi,*
vox Dei.

Samuel Robinson
A Course of Fifteen Lectures
on Medical Botany, 1829

CONTENTS

PART II: THE BOTANICO-MEDICAL REVOLT, DECLINE, AND REVIVAL

Chapter 4. The Thomsonians   69

Chapter 5. The Neo-Thomsonians   95

Chapter 6. The Eclectics   115

RESOURCES

Foreword

For old hands and new, understanding the medical botanical movement in America means starting with the scholarship of Alex Berman, former Emeritus Professor at the University of Cincinnati. Beginning in the 1950s, Professor Berman was the preeminent authority in medical botanical history, providing students and scholars with a wealth of information and interpretation on this significant piece of medical history. His dissertation, "The Impact of the Nineteenth Century Botanico-Medical Movement on American Pharmacy and Medicine," completed in 1954, remains one of the most frequently cited in American medical historiography. That this work as well as his numerous articles published between 1951 and 1980 have stood the test of time is not surprising to those who knew Professor Berman. He was a meticulous scholar and a man of great personal charm who knew the historian's craft and remained active for more than twenty years after his retirement.

I first became acquainted with Professor Berman's scholarship thirty years ago. His dissertation and articles formed the bedrock of my early work and remain so today. The true test of a person's historical scholarship is its ability to stand the test of time—from one generation's history to the needs of another. For those of my generation who have carried on the historian's craft, and who soon will be handing it off to a newer generation of scholars, the work of Alex Berman has been accurate in both the macro and micro worlds—a true compass.

This work, based on Professor Berman's 1954 dissertation, was accomplished with the assistance of Michael Flannery, former director of the Lloyd Library and Museum, utilizing the library's unique collections in a manner that brings added significance to Berman's original work. Flannery is no novice to scholarship, having written a superb biography of John Uri Lloyd, one of America's preeminent industrial pharmacists and co-founder of the library that bears his name.

This publication is to be welcomed by medical historians everywhere. It not only gives recognition to a man whose life's work has long been held forth as an exemplary model in the field of medical scholarship, but, equally significant, it provides scholars and lay readers with easy access to one of the classic works of American historiography.

John S. Haller Jr.
Professor of History
Southern Illinois University, Carbondale

Preface

THE SIGNIFICANCE
OF THE BOTANICO-MEDICAL MOVEMENTS

The botanico-medical movement, as defined in this book, refers to an organized effort begun by Samuel Thomson as early as 1790 to challenge medical orthodoxy. By calling for a vegetable materia medica of chiefly indigenous North American plants in distinction to the exotic vegetable *and* mineral preparations of the medical establishment, Thomson's botanical system was the inception of a movement that would last well into the twentieth century. Drawing upon the spirit of Jacksonian democracy early in the nineteenth century, a continuing populist strain throughout the mid- to late 1800s, and a real need for primary medical care in a predominantly rural America, this effort would grow—albeit in various and distinct guises—and continue to maintain some influence over health care until the closure of the Eclectic Medical College (prior to 1910, the Eclectic Medical Institute) of Cincinnati in 1939.

Yet at the dawn of the twenty-first century, botanical medicine is very much with us. Anyone who walks into an American supermarket or pharmacy and sees the vast array of herbal products that are taking up more and more of the retail shelving space knows that there is renewed interest in botanical remedies and "natural" health maintenance regimens. Indeed, the current popularity of natural and holistic health programs promoted by such notable figures as Drs. Andrew Weil and James A. Duke (including celebrity endorsements for various herb products on TV and radio) suggests that a new and energetic botanico-medical movement has arisen Phoenix-like from the ashes of its predecessor. Today, as before, it exists beyond the pale of medical orthodoxy, falling under the rubric of "alternative" or "complementary" medicine. This is a significant development and one examined at some length in this book. This fact underscores historian William

G. Rothstein's observation that "[o]f all the forms of American medical care not associated with professional medicine, none has had so long, so successful, or so tenacious a history as botanical medicine."[1]

Thus, *America's Botanico-Medical Movements* describes the growth, development, and influence of an extremely important group of health care proponents that has taken on various manifestations but, even up to present, has represented a persistent voice of opposition to mainstream medicine in America. Sometimes that voice was clear and resonant, but, more often than not, the botanics failed to speak in unison, as personal animosities, private ambitions, hidden agendas, and collective jealousies degenerated into a cacophony of invectives and accusations directed as frequently against one another as against the regular medical community. The botanico-medical movements have been unique to the United States, and today, as yesterday, they display the colorful individualism and entrepreneurial spirit so often associated with the American character.

One final word is in order regarding our treatment of the botanical sectarians in this book. In essence, the principle of Ockham's razor works as well in history as in philosophy—i.e., "entities are not to be multiplied beyond necessity." Although it is true that the nineteenth century saw a proliferation of botanical groups, from self-styled herbalists to Thomsonians, neo-Thomsonians, and eclectics, America, broadly speaking, has been witness to essentially two botanico-medical movements. The first, which occurred with Samuel Thomson around 1790, continued throughout the nineteenth century in an unbroken continuum, with a number of sects developing within the context of Jacksonian democratic ideals, and concluded with the final closure of the Eclectic Medical College of Cincinnati in 1939. The second movement, although sharing some general parallels with the first, grew largely out of the counterculture of the 1960s and then gained considerable momentum in the 1980s and 1990s, as the public became increasingly dissatisfied with the costs and side effects associated with conventional treatments. Because these movements have their own distinctive roots and are self-contained historically, we will often discuss each botanico-medical movement within its respective phases in the singular. Yet the title of the book itself refers to the broad sweep of botanico-medical movements in both its historic and current phases. The reader will find the bulk of this book devoted to the first phase of botanicism, a prolonged movement covering nearly 150 years. The second phase is discussed at length in Chapter 7 and covers a movement whose growth is relatively recent and whose future is both unclear and uncertain.

Thus, Alex Berman began writing on this subject before the second movement had even emerged. The historiography of American botanicism is almost exclusively concerned with the first botanico-medical movement, for which Berman played an important and seminal role.

HISTORIOGRAPHICAL REVIEW—
THE BERMAN LEGACY

In 1951 Alex Berman published the first of a number of seminal works exploring the botanico-medical movement. In "The Thomsonian Movement and Its Relation to American Pharmacy and Medicine," Berman gave to the scholarly community its first objective account of Samuel Thomson (1769-1843) and his rather heterogeneous grassroots health crusaders. A few years later, in his "Neo-Thomsonianism in the United States," Berman investigated a group founded by Thomson's rebellious protégé, Alva Curtis (1797-1881), that ultimately dubbed itself physio-medicalism. Moving from Thomson and his progeny, he then published a third article, this time discussing "Wooster Beach and the Early Eclectics."[2] This by no means exhausts Berman's contributions to the botanico-medical movement (see Bibliography), but it was primarily through these three articles that he captured the attention of the scholarly community.

More than thirty years later, Norman Gevitz acknowledged the significance of this body of work by calling it "the first extended scholarly portrait of the history of an unorthodox group. Relying heavily upon original sources," he continued, "Berman independently and critically examined the arguments and practices of Thomson and his followers and those of his opponents, considered in the medical and social context of the period. He offered a variety of explanations for the growth of Thomsonianism, detailed its internal struggles, and looked at its transformation from a self-help movement to a professionally oriented alternative to orthodox medicine. Berman's three articles constitute a model for other historians to emulate."[3]

And emulate they did. Historians soon followed Berman's lead in studying the American botanics. Referring to those sectarians who broke with Samuel Thomson over issues of education and the development of their botanic theory and practice as "neo-Thomsonians," Berman coined a term that was picked up by subsequent scholars and applied in their own historical work.[4] More important, Berman's work caused American medical historians generally to include the botanics in their discussions of nineteenth-century medical practice.

Interestingly, one of the first in-depth examinations of the botanico-medical movement to follow Berman came in Joseph F. Kett's *The Formation of the American Medical Profession* (1968). Despite the recasting of familiar themes, *The Formation of the American Medical Profession* was not entirely a mere repetition of Berman's earlier work.[5] Kett departed from him at some critical junctures. For example, although Kett placed the Thomsonians within the context of Jacksonian egalitarianism, he viewed them as an extension of the "colonial domestic practitioner" that differed, he believed, only in Thomson's special claims for a cure-all theory of medicine.[6] This is not on its face incorrect. There were broad connections between the two, a matter that will form the starting point for this book. Nonetheless, the distinctive features of Thomsonian practice, in both its promotional and organizational aspects, are too different—too uniquely *American*—to consider it a mere variation on colonial domestic practice. Kett ascribed the demise of the Thomsonian movement to the end of Jacksonian egalitarianism, an assertion that is also broadly correct but incomplete.

Kett's other significant thesis was that the regular medical profession had sown the "seeds of stability" by mid-nineteenth century and that by 1860 its regulatory foundations had been firmly established. Kett's themes will be examined in Chapter 7 of this book.

William G. Rothstein's *American Physicians in the Nineteenth Century* (1972) offered even more extended discussion of the nineteenth-century botanico-medical movement. Rothstein viewed the regulars themselves as but one variation on a variety of sectarian and sectarian-like practices contending for professional dominance in the nineteenth century.[7] Lacking a scientific consensus of acceptable practice, regular medicine was, with varying degrees, as sectarian as Thomsonianism, neo-Thomsonianism, eclecticism, mesmerism, magnetism, hydropathy, homeopathy, or any other *ism* or *opathy* then current in medical fashion. Rothstein's point echoes Abraham Flexner's astute observation that "[p]rior to the placing of medicine on a scientific basis, sectarianism was, of course, inevitable. Every one started with some sort of preconceived notion; and from a logical point of view, one preconception is as good as another."[8] Moreover, Rothstein's book carried forward Berman's observation that the botanics were engaged in an ardent "struggle for scientific respectability."

Berman's work pointed the way, but until now it remained scattered in a number of different journals. Berman's most thorough treatment of this diverse and complex medical movement was his PhD dissertation, which was presented as "The Impact of the Nineteenth-Century Botanico-Medical Movement on American Pharmacy and Medicine" in 1954 at the University of Wisconsin, Madison, under the direction of famed pharmaceutical historian George Urdang (1882-1960).

Perhaps because of its scattered and diffused nature, Berman's contributions have sometimes been missed by historians. Lamar Riley Murphy, for example, credited Kett and Rothstein with attributing "Thomsonian success to contemporary medical inefficacy and the democratic temper of the times,"[9] despite the fact that Berman had already dealt with these issues at considerable length in both his dissertation and his articles.[10] Different, but with similar effect, was John Harley Warner's demonstration that in the 1870s and 1880s bloodletting "had been virtually discarded from practice."[11] With Berman's earlier investigation into the decline of bloodletting in the medical profession, a strange sense of déjà vu hangs over Warner's analysis of this heroic therapy. When Warner's essay "From Specificity to Universalism in Medical Therapeutics: Transformation in the 19th-Century United States" replaced Berman's "The Heroic Approach in 19th-Century Therapeutics" in *Sickness and Health in America: Readings in the History of Medicine and Public Health* (1997), it was clear that Berman's work was being supplanted by younger scholars.[12]

Yet Berman's influence was, and *is,* not over. Besides the books already mentioned, others have written articles examining various aspects of the botanico-medical movement and have cited Berman's earlier studies.[13] None, however, have established themselves as authoritatively as has John S. Haller Jr., whose recent series of publications has made him the leading scholar of nineteenth-century sectarian

American medicine. Haller's *Medical Protestants: The Eclectics in American Medicine, 1825-1939* (1994) is the fullest and most objective account of American eclecticism available.[14] Likewise, Haller's study of physio-medicalism a few years later offered new and valuable insights into this sectarian group.[15] Haller's work continues. His recent study of the Eclectic Medical Institute, *A Profile in Alternative Medicine* (1999), provides a unique and detailed look at a leading sectarian medical school.[16] In addition, his book on Samuel Thomson and his followers offers a fresh and vivid picture of these colorful sectarians. Haller's dedication of *The People's Doctors* to Alex Berman brings the historiography full circle.[17]

A NOTE ON METHODOLOGY

This book is divided into two parts: the first covers the larger historical context of heroic therapeutics, the botanical reaction against it within the rising tide of Jacksonian egalitarianism, the state of the medical profession as seen through its educational institutions and statutory regulations, and the utilization of a vegetable materia medica from both regular and sectarian perspectives; the second focuses in detail upon each of the major botanical groups that have impacted American pharmaco-medical practice, from the Thomsonians of the 1830s to the herbal movement of the 1990s. Although the broad flow of the narrative is chronological, it must be remembered that many of the activities of the nineteenth-century botanics were both concomitant and, at times, complicated. This sometimes forces a topical approach that ties in with general development of the movement itself. As an example, C. S. Rafinesque is discussed in depth (pp. 59-64) *after* William Procter's critique of John Kost's *Elements of Materia Medica and Therapeutics* (1858) and John King's *American Eclectic Dispensatory* (1854 and 1859) as well as William Cook's dispensatory (all of which occurred well after Rafinesque's death in 1840) because Rafinesque's writings were used by botanic propagandists into the 1890s, and his influence, in fact, transcends his own times. The chronological and topical mix of this book reflects two overriding facts about American botanicism: its activities are rarely simple, and its overall influences are often interconnected within both the movement itself and the larger scientific and professional communities in which it resides.

As difficult as the subject can be, the present publication represents the fruition of work begun over forty years ago. Just as historians have been shaped and influenced by Berman's early publications, so too has this co-author. I came to this study having examined the life of eclecticism's most renowned figure, John Uri Lloyd. This and other studies related to nineteenth-century botanicism have formed the basis for my joining Berman in carrying his original work forward in the present book (see Bibliography). In this sense, *America's Botanico-Medical Movements* represents much more than an exercise in nostalgic reverence, for it was Berman who pointed the way toward my own historical interests. Although the Berman dissertation forms the basis for the present work, considerable updating has occurred; this is, in every sense of the term, a *new* book in form and substance. In short, this book represents the collaboration of mentor and protégé.

As a pharmacist and professor of pharmaceutical history, however, Berman brings special strengths and insights to our understanding of these peculiarly American practitioners. My interest in medical botany, too, suggests a specifically *pharmaceutical* emphasis. Our hope is that this book provides an overview of the botanical movements treated as an integrated whole. Although Haller paints an intricate portrait of the entire subject and its participants, the present book offers a broad landscape of the movements (old and new) in all of their various components, with particular emphasis upon their impact on American pharmacy up to the present.

Michael A. Flannery

Acknowledgments

We would like to thank Series Editors Drs. Mickey C. Smith and Dennis B. Worthen for their support in this project. Special appreciation goes to Dennis for transforming an idea into a book. Without his persistence, this fruitful collaboration might never have taken place. Also, thanks go to Dr. John S. Haller Jr., of Southern Illinois University, who read earlier versions of this manuscript and became a scholarly scout helping us to fix our compass points along numerous stages of this fascinating journey. Additionally, special thanks go to Dr. James A. Ramage, Professor of history at Northern Kentucky University, who provided a fresh perspective and helped us along the historical trail by adhering to John Erskine's wise counsel: "We have not really budged a step until we take up residence in someone else's point of view." Finally, we wish to express our appreciation to the staffs of the Lloyd Library and Museum (Akram S. Pari, Catalog Librarian; Library Assistants Mary Lee Schmidt and Rose Marie Weckenmann; Cataloging Assistant Cheryl Calhoun; Serials Cataloger Betsy Kruthoffer; and Library Aide Annie Schmidt) and the Historical Collections of the University of Alabama at Birmingham (Tim Pennycuff, Assistant Director; Stefanie Babinsack, Museum Curator; Donnelly Lancaster, Archivist; Katie Oomens, Historical Collections Unit Specialist; and Jason McCracken, Student Assistant). The former provided invaluable assistance in transcription, photography, and information retrieval; the latter provided essential support by handling, with their usual professionalism and skill, a hundred would-be distractions during the critical editorial phase of this book.

PART I:
BACKGROUND
OF THE BOTANICO-MEDICAL
MOVEMENT

I am stating only what everybody knows to be true, when I say that the general confidence which has heretofore existed in the science and art of medicine, as this science has been studied, and as this art has been practiced, has within the last few years been violently shaken and disturbed, and is now greatly lessened and impaired. The hold which medicine has so long had upon the popular mind is loosened; there is a wide-spread skepticism as to its power of curing diseases, and men are everywhere to be found who deny its pretensions as a science, and reject the benefits and blessings which it proffers them as an art.

Elisha Bartlett
*An Inquiry into the Degree of Certainty
in Medicine; and into the Nature
and Extent of its Power over Disease*
Philadelphia, 1848, p. 9

Chapter 1

The Therapeutic Factor

The growth of an organized botanico-medical movement had roots in colonial healing practices transplanted from England. The masses had become suspicious of a medical establishment that offered high fees and lofty degrees instead of comfort and cures. Thus, the rise of nineteenth-century medical sects in America was in many ways more of a reaction *against* regular medical practice than merely a movement of advocacy of botanicals in therapeutics. Indeed, as will be seen, regulars already possessed a substantial vegetable materia medica. If the number and variety of botanicals in the physicians armamentarium were the only issues facing the medical community of the early 1800s, sectarians would never have arisen. More complex factors were involved, and they come into sharper focus by examining the therapeutic contention that grew between physicians who believed they had to aggressively intervene and actively subdue disease entities with long-used mineral agents and those physicians who questioned the wisdom of this time-honored approach to the healing art.

THE COLONIAL ROOTS OF BOTANICISM

It may come as a surprise that the first medical book ever published in America, *The English Physician* (Boston, 1708), attributed to Nicholas Culpeper (1616-1654), but probably in reality the work of Nicholas Boone (1679-1738), was not the work of the regular medical community, but of an herbalist. From a modern perspective, one is liable to ask why that matters, but in late eighteenth-century Western medicine, one's professional affiliation was about *all* that mattered. Medical practitioners could not convincingly invoke any particular claim to scientific respectability (a subject that will be addressed in greater detail in this book), but they could lay claim to the authority of credentials. Until sound and verifiable paradigms for the etiology of disease were established during the last quarter of the nineteenth century, "quality" and standard of care was a nebulous thing. Reassured by little more than the physician's word, patients were generally unimpressed by expensive, university-trained physicians sporting degrees and connections with learned societies.

In this kind of environment, departure from orthodox medical care was practiced by some and welcomed by many. This was particularly true in England, where as early as 1543 Henry VIII had given herbalists special legal protections from prosecution by the medical elite, a matter of some consternation to orthodox medical practitioners. In the eighteenth century, the Royal College of Physicians of London lost further ground in the courts when William Rose's unauthorized medical "advising" was upheld in a celebrated trial that effectively cost the regular physicians their monopoly to prescribe medicines.[1] With the regular practitioners' credibility in question and their power limited, self-styled healers proliferated on the English scene. Much of the blame rested with the orthodox physicians themselves. The problem was that many "well-trained" medical men relied on theory alone, offering only costly exotic preparations to cure diseases made even more frightening and mysterious by their recondite nosology, while a host of folk practitioners plied their healing art armed with a broad knowledge of familiar English botanicals and an instinct for keen observation at the bedside. The great political theorist-philosopher Thomas Hobbes (1588-1679) expressed the sentiment of many when he said, "I would rather have the advice to take physick from an experienced old woman that had been at many peoples' bedsides than from the learnedst [sic] but unexperienced [sic] physician."[2]

Amidst this atmosphere of public suspicion of mainstream practitioners, it is no wonder that colonists chose to reprint, not a treatise from the learned elite, but a humble herbal by a man widely regarded as the people's physician. Historian David Cowen has called Culpeper's work "noteworthy as a giant step by which a homely version of classical medicine crossed the Atlantic,"[3] and Culpeper was no exception to the rule. If the records of a typical English entrepreneur in the Atlantic drug trade in the early 1700s are any indication, his dealings with a wide assortment of New England clerics, merchant apothecaries, and itinerant healers show a strong preference for botanical simples, elixirs, and cordials, not only recommended in the published herbals of the venerable empiric Culpeper, but also touted in the popular works of William Salmon (1644-1713).[4] This transplantation of domestic healing set the stage for a botanico-medical movement that would take on a peculiar life of its own in America. By the time of independence, one thing was very evident on the American health care scene: if the people had grown suspicious of the medical elite, they were even more wary of their assorted therapeutic prestidigitations. This was a fact of more-than-fleeting significance.

THE HEROIC APPROACH— "A STRANGE MISHMASH INDEED"

The therapeutic mayhem perpetrated by American physicians during the first decades of the nineteenth century is painful but commonplace knowledge. "It is fortunate in that day," wrote an elderly doctor in 1878, "that we had a hardy, well developed race of men and women, possessing sufficient tenacity of life to not only resist the disease, but the remedies used to combat it." As an afterthought, he added, "Should this practice again prevail with the badly developed race we now have, the percentage of deaths would be largely increased, and few would come safely out of the hands of the doctors."[5] A more recent investigator has called the therapeutics of the period "a strange mishmash indeed."[6]

The worst features of this early nineteenth-century therapy quickly became the target of violent attack by rising American botanico-medical groups, providing them with powerful means for making converts and, indeed, constituting for them a fundamental raison d'être. It should be emphasized that the savagery of orthodox practice was frequently matched by the barbarity of early heterodox botanicism, as will be demonstrated in succeeding pages.

William Cullen (1710-1790), of Edinburgh, and his pupil Benjamin Rush (1745-1813), of Philadelphia, were probably most influential in promoting the heroic medication employed during this period. Rush's ruthless application of his theory of disease was characterized by a contemporary critic as "one of the great discoveries . . . which have contributed to the depopulation of the earth."[7]

Hooker devoted a portion of an essay published in 1857 to an analysis of Cullen's influence on therapy.[8] He concluded that Cullen's writings (notably his *Materia Medica* [1772] and his *Practice of Physic* [1784]) imparted to contemporary medical practice "a more definite and decided character." Remedies such as calomel, antimony, emetics, purgatives, opiates, as well as bleeding, etc., although previously employed with some restraint, suddenly became more frequently used, and with some abandon. Cullen criticized Stahl, Boerhaave, Sydenham, Van Swieten, Lieutaud, and others for timidity in therapeutics and for too much trust in the curative powers of nature. According to Hooker, this so-called "active" medication reached its high point in the first quarter of the nineteenth century. Although not solely introduced by Cullen, he did begin the era of active therapeutic intervention, an approach that was consummated by those who followed him. Nowhere was this more clearly demonstrated than in the use of mercury. Following Cullen's advice, use of this substance rose to new heights, as it was applied indiscriminately by his successors in the treatment of inflammations and fevers and a variety of ill-defined and vaguely understood ailments. Finally, by 1857, Hooker concluded, "During the past twenty-five or thirty years, the reign of active medication has been manifestly declining."[9]

The evidence seems to indicate that what we call "active" medication today reached a culminating point later than "somewhere in the first quarter" of the nineteenth century, and that its decline between 1825 and 1857 was considerably slower than implied in the previous statements.[10] Vestiges of the heroic approach persisted as late as 1878, as exemplified by the practices of George B. Wood (1797-1879) and his nephew, H. C. Wood (1841-1920), the influential Philadelphia professors. In his article "The Heroic Treatment of Idiopathic Peritonitis," H. C. Wood remembered his uncle, Dr. George B. Wood, claiming to have cured every case of adult peritonitis by bleeding the patient from the arm and applying leeches on the adbomen. The nephew proudly followed in his uncle's footsteps by bleeding his patients profusely and added, "I take my stand on the old theory that calomel has power to modify inflammatory action." H. C. Wood went on in praise of blistering in cases of peritonitis. Recalling that his uncle applied an abdominal blistering poultice of ten by ten inches, nephew Wood routinely ordered a blister eight by ten inches.[11] So much for therapeutic moderation.

Because of the prestige and influence of Benjamin Rush, blood-letting persisted for several decades in the United States. Rush advocated profuse bleeding during the Philadelphia yellow fever epidemic of 1793, which, he maintained, was a highly successful therapeutic measure.[12] Moreover, Dr. Rush prescribed "frequent and copious" bloodletting for "madness" and considered it effective in "fevers." He also approved the technique used by Dr. Physick in 1795 "in a case of dislocated humerus of two months' continuance. The Doctor bled this patient until he fainted and then reduced his shoulder in less than a minute with a very small exertion force."[13] That Dr. Rush had to overcome a great deal of opposition to his bloodletting therapy is evident from his writings: "In contemplating the prejudices against bloodletting which prevail so generally in our country, I have been led to ascribe them to a cause wholly political," he insisted. For Rush, the reluctance to rely upon bloodletting was the product of British error, ignorance, and prejudice."[14]

Rush, of course, had no monopoly on monistic pathology. His friend Dr. Edward Miller (1760-1812), whose theory of disease causation resembled the one much later advanced by Broussais in France, made constant use of his lancet. Others were John Esten Cooke (1785-1853), whose obsession with the liver caused him and his pupils to inundate the Mississippi valley with calomel; Dr. J. A. Gallup (d. 1849), who viewed disease as sthenic and inflammatory, bled without mercy; and Drs. Miner and Tully—Gallup's contemporaries, who had exactly opposite notions of what constituted disease—condemned bloodletting and pushed calomel and opium to extremes. These gentlemen were subjected to a searching and devastating criticism by Elisha Bartlett in 1844.[15]

The unfortunate reliance of many regular or allopathic[16] physicians on calomel and bloodletting therapy helped the Thomsonians to win support among sections of the populace. Moreover, the advent of Asiatic cholera in 1832 offered an opportunity for Thomsonian practitioners to boast of their alleged cures and to jeer at the helplessness of the traditional doctors.[17]

While increasing numbers of regular practitioners were gradually losing faith in the efficacy of calomel medication, many of the professors at the Transylvania Medical School at Lexington, Kentucky, continued to prescribe inordinate amounts of this remedy. Thus, for example, Professor J. E. Cooke was proud of the fact that "there were few towns and no counties east of the Mississippi and south of the Ohio which did not have a Transylvania graduate following successfully his teaching in the use of calomel."[18] Cooke described a case of cholera that he treated by giving a tablespoon of calomel every six hours, with the patient "continuing to live contrary to all expectations." After consuming from thirteen to seventeen tablespoons of the drug, however, the patient finally gave up the ghost.[19]

Daniel Drake, taken aback at the goings-on at Transylvania Medical School during the cholera epidemic, wrote, "It would appear, however, that some of our friends in Lexington have administered this drug [calomel] in quantities which are unprecedented as the mortality which they sought to avert. . . . We have understood on pretty good authority that some patients swallowed not less than a quarter of a pound in two or three days."[20]

The Thomsonians were quick to use such incidents in making converts, and *The Thomsonian Recorder* praised Dr. Drake for his critical attitude: "We rejoice in that candor by which Professor Drake so often distinguishes himself. He has been so addicted to making truth the grand object of his habitual pursuit." Then warming up, the editorial continued by calling upon the people to oppose "the extravagant and dangerous measures" of the "Mineral Faculty" and resist being "calomelized." Calling calomel the regulars' "kill-all" remedy, the editorial made its case for Thomson's botanical cures.[21]

Dr. Charles Caldwell, described by W. F. Norwood as "perhaps the most spectacular character to adorn the Transylvania Medical Faculty," cautioned, in a fit of panic, that removing calomel from the armamentarium would be as disasterous as striking iron from the mechanic's toolbox.[22] Caldwell was moved by the growing uneasiness among physicians regarding the efficacy of calomel and called the claims of calomel abuse one of "the slanderous imputations of the present day," further insisting, "I could name habitual railers against the employment of that remedy, who administer it frequently in their own practice, in doses from thirty to one hundred grains!—and at times in still larger ones!"[23]

Some eight years later, in 1844, T. D. Mitchell, also of Transylvania Medical School, openly accused many of his colleagues of killing their patients with lethal doses of calomel.[24] "The English writers who have quoted some accounts of large doses of calomel as employed in India and in this country," stated Mitchell, "have yet to learn what is meant by large doses." Mitchell was scornful of early experimental pharmacologist Robert Christison who was only able "to cite the use of this medicine to no greater extent than *840 grains in eight days.*" "What will he say," asked Mitchell, "*of table spoonful doses every hour,* until the patient held, somewhere between the mouth and rectum, a *pound* of the article? That such doses have been given, is just as susceptible of proof as the fact that calomel is employed at all. I have known it to be prescribed in tea spoonful doses, as if it were calcined magnesia."[25]

One writer, Alexander Means, admitted that calomel had been misused at times; he conceded that it was a powerful remedy, but he indignantly questioned whether physicians should "consent to cower at the outcry of blind prejudice, or ignorant and interested empiricism, and, before the eyes of the living myriads whom it has rescued from the jaws of the grave, deliberately pronounce the blistering curse of Science upon its head, and consign it to the reproach and maledictions of posterity?"[26] Means left no doubt as to where he stood on the question. For him, mercury was "THE MASTODON IN HARNESS," a remedy "to do the work of an age in a year."[27]

The editors of the *New Orleans Medical Journal* referred to Means' article as a "most spirited defense of this once omnipotent, but now much abused medicine." They assured their readers that only "the ignorant steam doctors, whose business it is to pander to the whims and prejudices of the unprofessional community," denied the value of mercurial preparations, and that there was no danger of these remedies becoming obsolete.[28]

The justification for "active" medication was often rationalized on the grounds that powerful methods were very efficacious if employed judiciously, and this is illustrated in the treatment advocated for pulmonary consumption by Dr. Charles W. Wilder, in 1843, before the Massachusetts Medical Society.[29] "Effective means are not wanting when the principle of action is once established. The lancet, the leech, the cupping-glass, the Spanish fly, Croton oil, tartarized antimony, ipecacuanha and mercury, are instruments of power and of great utility when skillfully used. Much, however, depends on the time and manner of their use."[30]

EARLY THOMSONIANS AND ECLECTICS

By the middle 1830s, the followers of Thomson constituted a formidable bloc of medical practitioners. We have no way of knowing their precise numbers, but the evidence indicates that at that time they were considerable. In the meantime, a rival botanic group under the leadership of Wooster Beach had sprung up in 1829, styling itself the Reformed Medical Society of the United States, the nucleus of the later eclectic movement.

For sheer fanaticism and aggressiveness, the Thomsonians[31] were probably unmatched by any medical sect in the country. The heroic treatment of the regular physicians was denounced in emotional prose and verse. Converts to the cause were offered allegedly safe "courses"[32] of treatment, consisting of frequent lobelia emetics,[33] scalding capsicum and herb teas, medicated enemas, and parboiling steam baths—in short, a process of internal and external scouring.

Whereas the Thomsonians built their therapeutics around a distinctive, monistic pathology of their own, the early eclectics accepted the prevailing approach to disease causation and the concepts of "phlogosis" and "antiphlogistics,"[34] never questioning, at this time, the correctness of heroic thinking. Similar to the regulars, they felt it necessary to make a "profound impression" on the patient. Where they differed from orthodox physicians was in attempting to substitute less lethal remedies, usually vegetable, to accomplish the same ends.

Instead of bloodletting, the early eclectics advocated cording the limbs. By this method, even syncope could be produced without loss of blood. The blood then could be slowly returned from the corded extremities into the general circulation. Many early followers of Beach believed that strong cathartics and diuretics could also be used to achieve the antiphlogistic effects of bloodletting.

Similarly, podophyllin or leptandra were used by the "Beachites" in place of the proscribed calomel, allegedly to induce biliary secretion. Since the regulars often considered salivation and involvement of the gums desirable in mercury therapy, the eclectics attempted to produce these conditions by using iris.

According to Fyfe, "the doctrine of substitution was the bane of the new school."[35] To illustrate further, the heroic purging of the regulars was aped by the eclectics in their use of gamboge, scammony, and colocynth; instead of using tartar emetic as a nauseant expectorant for respiratory disorders, the Beachites used lobelia and sanguinaria but, at the same time, were reluctant to part with the traditional ipecac of the "calomel doctors." Similar to the regulars, they believed in strong counterirritants and blistering, substituting, however, vegetable irritating plasters for tartar emetic ointment and plaster, but retaining cantharides; in the case of "stimulant expectorants," they could think of no substitutes, and so continued to use the orthodox remedies—squill, senega, and tolu. As Fyfe so aptly puts it, "The doctrine of substitution ramified in every direction, and in some cases it was so slight that there was no real difference."[36]

We cannot say with assurance which system at this time offered the most favorable chances of survival to the unfortunate patient who perforce had to choose between the violent ministrations of the regular physicians and the roughshod treatment of the sectarian botanics, although it is quite likely that the botanic practitioner gave the patient a better fighting chance during the time when heroic treatment was in vogue.[37]

One regular physician, Dr. John Dawson, admitted in 1841 before a state medical convention that during a local epidemic of "fever," the Thomsonians had effected cures, while the regulars had been unsuccessful. This admission is interesting because it demonstrates so clearly the grossly empirical state of prevailing medical practice. It is also one of the rare instances in which a hostile, orthodox doctor conceded that Thomsonian treatment had proven efficacious. Dr. Dawson's report of an epidemic "winter" fever in his native Green County noted that the "Steam Doctors" used medicinal infusions of "mucilaginous drinks" and the "water of the sub-acid fruits," which "were found to be of service throughout the whole course of the disease."[38]

THE DECLINE OF HEROIC THERAPY

By 1860, the worst features of the heroic practice had disappeared. To be sure, traces of the old therapeutics persisted; and the abuse of calomel was still widespread at the time of the Civil War, and even after.[39] By and large, however, physicians no longer thought it necessary to resort to the violent methods mentioned previously. The old heroic treatments were described in an 1860 issue of *The Medical and Surgical Reporter* as "matters of history," and current therapeutic regimens called for nutrition where bleeding was once employed, and the general tendency was to "build up" by "sustaining and stimulating," rather than depleting, the patient.[40]

One would like to regard the improvement in therapeutics at this time as being part of the general scientific advance. The facts indicate, however, that scientific considerations played a minor role in demolishing the old heroic practice, and what was called "rational" medication in 1860 was brought about largely by irrational factors.[41] Contributing also to the abandonment of the old curative measures was the constant barrage of criticism hurled at the regulars by Thomsonian and other sectarian practitioners.

In 1871, the eminent Henry I. Bowditch pleaded in vain for judicious revival of bloodletting.[42] Deprecating its former indiscriminate use, Bowditch pointed out certain cases in which venesection could prove to be of value.[43] "The bleeders have now been so effectually silenced," he announced, "that we have virtually thrown aside, as worse than worthless, one of the most valuable of all the therapeutic means which the long experience of the ages has taught us."[44]

Four years later, Dr. Samuel D. Gross made a last-ditch, but futile, attempt to convince his colleagues of the value of bloodletting.[45] "If, now and then, one is bold enough to bleed," Gross complained, "he is sure to be taken to task about it, if he is not actually denounced as a murderer . . . the lancet is an obsolete instrument, the office of the bleeder has departed, venesection has long been unfashionable, and few of the present generation of medical men would, if called upon, be able to open a vein in a scientific and creditable manner. Bloodletting, as I have already declared, is, emphatically, one of the lost arts."[46]

This abandonment of bloodletting as a remedial agent entailed a shift in therapeutic thinking; the early conviction that the disease could be bludgeoned out of the patient gave way to the realization that "building up" and conserving the patient's strength was essential.

In a significant symposium conducted by the Philadelphia County Medical Society in 1860,[47] the reasons for the rapid decline of bloodletting were discussed. Various causes were suggested by speakers to account for the disfavor into which this remedy had fallen. Some insisted that there was a change in the type of diseases encountered and, indeed, even in the constitution of patients themselves.[48] Others pointed to the propaganda activities of sectarian opposition to the practice that had made itself felt upon the medical profession as a whole.[49] Still others singled out empirical grounds for the decline of bloodletting through the realization by observation that the practice was harmful.[50] Also, other means had been found to effect the desired end, namely, the substitution of antiphlogistic agents for the lancet in inflammatory disease.[51] Other factors brought up by symposium speakers were the increase in scientific knowledge[52] (including the influence of Louis's "numerical method")[53] and even the effect of authoritative pronouncements opposed to bleeding, such as those made by the eminent British physician Dr. J. Hughes Bennett.[54]

Surprisingly, one important trend contributing to the overthrow of the old bleeding and purging system was not discussed at the symposium, or if it was, it was not reported in *The Medical and Surgical Reporter.* This trend was the therapeutic skepticism and reliance on the curative powers of nature, as evinced by a number of physicians, beginning in the late 1830s. Jacob Bigelow's essay on "self-limited" diseases, read before the Massachusetts Medical Society in 1835,[55] was influential in this respect, as was the paper by John Forbes published in 1846 in the *British and Foreign Medical Review.*[56] An interesting feature of Forbes' article was that the infinitesimal dosing of homeopathy had unwittingly vindicated the case for therapeutic skepticism, and that the validity of regular therapeutics was thus, by implication, at stake.[57] Dr. Oliver Wendell

Holmes, himself probably the most forceful exponent of this trend, believed that Bigelow's essay had influenced a number of New England physicians.[58] To judge from an address given by Holmes, the trend of "the nature-trusting heresy" had been practiced chiefly in Massachusetts and Boston.[59] He pointed out in the same address that the American pupils of Louis had brought back with them a spirit of skepticism, based on their experiences in Louis's wards, where they had observed that many patients recovered by themselves, with no medication whatsoever.[60] Fifteen years after Bigelow's 1860 address, Gross, in his speech referred to previously, specifically singled out Bigelow's work in Boston, and Forbes' teachings in London, as having had a restraining influence on unbridled medication and bloodletting.[61] Such changes did not occur overnight, however. As Lois N. Magner has pointed out, many American physicians "admired Louis's research, but not his therapeutics. Critics of the numerical system," she adds, "charged Louis's followers with excessive zeal in the art of diagnosis, and negligence in healing the sick. Many doctors believed that Louis's attempt to evaluate the efficacy of bloodletting was a rash, reckless rejection of the wisdom of the ages."[62]

The Medical and Surgical Reporter, commenting editorially on the symposium of the Philadelphia County Medical Society, expressed the view that there had been essentially two ways of interpreting changes in therapy between 1840 and 1860: one group of physicians was convinced that diseases had become asthenic (due to weakness or debility); another, that physicians had simply acquired a fuller understanding of disease and its treatment, and that there had been no change in the type of diseases. The editor then undertook to explain the "revolution" in therapeutics in terms of social change: factory conditions, the rapid growth of urban populations, and the increased tempo of industrial life had a marked effect on the physical constitution of humans and had caused people to become more susceptible to attack by diseases of debility; hence, they could not withstand the former heroic medication.[63]

Dr. Samuel D. Gross accused Robert Bentley Todd (1809-1860), professor of physiology and general and morbid anatomy at King's College, London, of having been the chief proponent of the doctrine of change in disease. According to Gross, Todd had formulated his "absurd" theory as a result of his experience with victims of London factory and slum life, who were unable to tolerate depleting remedies.[64]

Whether "Toddism" is viewed today as an interesting rationalization or as a curious theory, the fact remains that a large number of physicians who held this doctrine modified their therapeutics. This trend must be regarded as having contributed materially to the downfall of heroic therapy.

As for the other reasons advanced at the Philadelphia symposium to account for the volte-face in therapeutic thinking, all appear to possess some validity. The attack on orthodox therapy carried on by the botanics and other medical sects unquestionably aroused public opinion or "public prejudice," as the regulars were inclined to call it. One must also not discount the large number of physicians whom Roberts Bartholow characterized as having "no settled convictions, who are content to drift along, hoping they do good, but whose vaporous therapeutic notions have never crystallized into definite forms."[65] Many of these practitioners gradually abandoned the old methods without being too clear about the reasons. Empirical substitution of various remedies[66] definitely helped to demolish the old practice, and although Louis's numerical method[67] exerted some influence in undermining "active" medication, it is difficult to evaluate other scientific factors, if any, that may have operated in therapeutics prior to 1860.

Despite the general transformation and improvement in therapy by the time of the Civil War, many doctors still showed marked preference for calomel and pushed this remedy to extremes. This situation was dramatically highlighted by Surgeon General Hammond's order in 1863, the infamous Circular no. 6, removing calomel and tartar emetic from the supply table of the army. The surgeon general indicated that reports from his medical inspectors had shown many cases of "profuse salivation" and, not infrequently, "occurrences of mercurial gangrene" brought on by calomel. As for tartar emetic, Hammond justified its removal on the grounds that this remedy had been abused, was not really needed, and its presence on the supply table was "a tacit invitation to its use."[68]

The roar of rage with which Hammond's pronouncement was greeted by the majority of regular physicians drowned out the approbation of his supporters and the gleeful applause of the botanics.[69] A group of irate physicians meeting in Cincinnati drew up a resolution denouncing Hammond and expressed the opinion that "the removal of W. A. Hammond from his position as Surgeon General would meet the approbation of the profession, be of advantage to our soldiers and creditable to the Government."[70] On the heels of this blast came several resolutions from the American Medical Association (AMA), severely censuring Hammond's action; his order was criticized as an insult to the profession and as a "reckless attempt to cut the Gordian knot of intricate pathology by the exercise of official power."[71]

Woodward reported on the basis of evidence he had gathered that prior to the issuance of Hammond's order, "mercurials were abused in certain quarters, but there is by no means so much of it as seems to be implied by the unlucky circular of May 4."[72] Although Woodward claims that Hammond's order was never enforced and that it did not have any appreciable influence on the use of mercurials in the army during the war,[73] the immediate effect of Hammond's circular was threefold. First, it whipped up a furious reaction on the part of organized medicine, with the AMA accusing the surgeon general of having grossly insulted the medical profession and of having maligned two "most invaluable" remedies, mercury and antimony. Second, it bolstered the stand of the botanics who were inveighing against calomel and antimony *and* against the systematic attempt by the regulars to keep them out of the Union medical corps.[74] Finally, Hammond's position, which had been seriously undermined by a feud with Secretary of War Stanton, became even more precarious as the result of his unpopular circular, and it became an important factor leading toward his eventual court martial in the summer of 1864.[75]

In the meantime, evidence gained through animal experimentation in Europe exploded the myth that calomel promoted biliary secretion. The work of H. Nasse (1852), R. A. Kolliker (1853-1854), and F. Mosler (1858) in Germany, and George Scott (1859) in England, showed that calomel actually decreased the secretion of bile.[76] This work, not too well known at first, especially in the United States, was confirmed by the report to the British Medical Association made by the Edinburgh Committee in 1868, under the chairmanship of J. F. Bennett. The findings of this committee, based on experiments with dogs, showed that calomel, blue pill, and podophyllin definitely diminished the flow of bile, while taraxacum had no effect on the liver. This report not only scientifically demolished a cherished fable that the regulars had zealously cultivated, but it also delivered a clear blow to the eclectics who were using podophyllin for the same purpose. Seven years later, William Rutherford of Edinburgh and his associate M. Vignal advanced still more evidence to support the conclusions of the Edinburgh Committee.[77]

This laboratory and clinical evidence notwithstanding, calomel witnessed a painfully slow decline throughout the nineteenth century, and the belief that mercurous chloride affected biliary secretions was tenacious. Prescription ingredient surveys clearly demonstrate that calomel remained a familiar and much-used item in the physician's armamentarium even into the 1920s.[78]

However, the precursors of change were evident. The conflicting views of Alfred Stillé and Roberts Bartholow vied for acceptance in the 1870s, with the victory of Bartholow pointing the direction that modern therapeutics was to take. For Stillé, therapeutics were "continually trespassed upon by pathology, physiology, and chemistry," disciplines that presumed "to dictate what remedies shall be applied, and in what doses and combinations." In the end, Stillé insisted, "they will neither secure the safety of the patient nor afford satisfaction to the physician."[79]

This line of reasoning reflects, of course, the strong influence of the Paris clinical school: the deep faith in empirical observations, the repudiation of theorizing, and, above all, the conviction that therapeutics could not be derived from any of the sciences.[80] Although they helped to demolish the old heroic practice of bloodletting, the brilliant American disciples of Louis also tended to delay the growth of experimental therapeutics and pharmacology in this country and, in some senses, allowed the use of mercurial agents to persist.[81] It was, after all, this same reliance upon empiricism that convinced physicians that the greenish stools produced by their patients dosed with calomel *proved beyond question* its effectiveness as a cholagogue—the experiments be damned! But eyes could deceive. That mercurous chloride's cathartic action did not allow the normal conversion of the bile pigment in the bowel from biliverdin into bilirubin and, hence, produced a green stool that mimicked increased bile secretion was lost upon the well-intentioned bedside observers.[82]

Bartholow's answer to Stillé was to state that "modern physiology has rendered experimental therapeutics possible, and has opened an almost boundless field of research which is being diligently cultivated." Bartholow expressed disappointment at Stillé's "reactionary position" and concluded that "no science of therapeutics can be created out of empirical facts."[83]

Dr. Bartholow buttressed his position by citing Liebig's experiments with chloral (1869), Fraser's work with physostigmine, and Brunton's use of amyl nitrite in angina pectoris as vindicating the physiological method; he also referred to the work of Claude Bernard as demonstrating the validity of animal experimentation to solve problems in therapeutics.

Stillé's views, however, were not entirely erroneous. Today we know that clinical evaluation and experience are still the final test in judging the efficacy of a remedy after it has left the laboratory. Indeed, medicine today is guided by what Richard H. Shryock has called "scientific empiricism"—observations guided by disciplinary theory and theory checked by observation under controlled conditions.[84]

Even in botanic circles changes were in the air. In 1865, a leading physio-medical warned his colleagues "that the old-fashioned methods of Dr. Thomson cannot continue to be popular. . . . Changes are going on; and now the practical question is, shall we cling tenaciously to a course that will drive away our own friends, or shall we turn the changes to our own advantage?"[85]

Yes, the times were demanding new ideas and new approaches. The regular practitioners had, despite the persistent use of calomel and antimony after the Civil War,[86] abandoned the grossest forms of heroic practice, and therapeutics was beginning to be affected by the mounting tempo of scientific progress. The Independent Thomsonians and physio-medicals, caught between the pressure of the regulars, on the one hand, and that of their equally formidable rivals, the eclectics, on the other, fought to retain their shrinking numbers. This pressure was heightened by the competition of other nineteenth-century medical sects such as the homeopaths, hydropaths, and others. Both the physio-medicals and the eclectics sought survival in the acquisition of scientific respectability.[87] To be sure, this had been the policy of the eclectics from the outset, but their inability to rise above scientific mediocrity, their lack of originality, and their espousal of amorphous and ill-defined principles doomed them to extinction. The physiomedicals, never achieving more than a quasiscientific status, contracted into a small, esoteric cult and finally petered out.[88]

The rise and fall of the botanics upon the exigencies of therapeutic change tell only part of the story, however. It is when the social context is examined that the rich and intricate color of the movement emerges, a picture painted in vivid hues of people and personalities.

Chapter 2

The People's Medicine

The end of John Adams' (1735-1826) presidency marked the end of Federalist America. In its stead came the Democratic-Republicans who espoused a more liberal version of the American experiment, certainly one more accommodating to the people than the Federalists' constant fear of the demos. This liberal spirit affected virtually every aspect of American life, including concepts of health and healing. During the antebellum period, many patients and practitioners tried to articulate a brand of medicine that was uniquely suited to the demands of the new republic. In a nation eager to expand and bordered by a vast hinterland, it is not surprising that America's fields and forests took on special importance in developing an indigenous materia medica. How nature's remedies were to be used, however, became issues of serious contention among health care providers, both within and outside mainstream medicine. One unmistakable feature of this period was the development of a people's medicine. Although this egalitarianism was readily accepted and widely adopted by the common folk, the idea that every person could be his or her own physician held serious implications for the medical establishment, not the least of which was the challenge such a brand of healing presented to its professional status and credibility. It is in the nature and extent of this challenge that the American botanics took shape as a discernible movement.

JEFFERSONIAN AND JACKSONIAN INFLUENCES

Thomas Jefferson (1743-1826), one of the most prominent proponents of American republicanism, espoused enough truly democratic rhetoric to make his Federalist counterparts uneasy and some-times downright horrified. Jefferson, however, was no leader of mob rule. His was a democracy built upon an idyllic "natural aris-tocracy," peopled by informed citizens who had achieved their rank and social standing by effort and ingenuity rather than birth and custom. Jefferson pointed to the yeomanry to fulfill this noble charge: "Those who labor in the earth are the chosen people of God," he declared in his *Notes on the State of Virginia* (1785).[1] Years later he told the French economist Jean-Baptiste Say (1767-1832) that it would be better if *every* American were engaged in farming: "Here," he boasted, "the immense extent of uncultivated and fertile lands enables every one who will labor, to marry young, and to raise a family of any size."[2] Democracy, he fervently be-lieved, derived from the countryside, not the city: "The mobs of great cities add just so much to the support of pure government," he wrote in his *Notes on Virginia,* "as sores do to the strength of the human body. It is the manners and spirit of a people which preserve a republic in vigor. A degeneracy in these is a canker which soon eats to the heart of its laws and constitution."[3]

Andrew Jackson (1767-1845), the undisputed symbol of the fron-tier that was gaining political strength and expression in the emerg-ing trans-Appalachian West, took Jefferson's principles to new heights (or as his enemies insisted, *new lows*). Jackson's democracy was born of no fanciful notions of an informed and universally educated yeomanry; his was an egalitarian nation truly of *all* white men. Because of the popularity of his presidency (1829-1837) and his association with an expansionist national project driven by tripartite themes of nature, will, and providence, historians have designated the period as the age of *Jacksonian* democracy.[4] Of course, it was not Jackson himself who created the era that bears his name, but he came to personify it. One of the leading factors in-fluencing the national temper was the frontier itself. Famed Wis-consin professor Frederick Jackson Turner thought he knew the nature of that temper and described it in broad, almost poetic terms. For Turner, the American character emanated from America's for-ests and the influences that the receding wilderness had upon a westward-moving populace constantly challenged by the exigen-cies of pioneer life. It was this, he insisted, that gave Americans their "coarseness and strength combined with acuteness and inquisitiveness."[5]

Nature took on special importance in a nation intimately involved with a vast hinterland. "The forest was not only a surer guide to wisdom because it was pure nature, the word of God without the interlineations of man," writes John William Ward, "but also because it preserved man in the condition of self-reliance since it protected him by geographical distance from the false corruptions of learning."[6]

A cultural and intellectual scene infused with such an egalitarian spirit affected virtually every aspect of the new republic, health care not excepted. Shunning the affectations of European society, Americans became skeptical, perhaps even jaded, in their view of the regular medical profession. Anticipating by nearly thirty years Jacob Bigelow's therapeutic moderation premised upon his concept of self-limited disease, Jefferson wrote to Caspar Wistar, professor of anatomy and surgery at the University of Pennsylvania:

Having been so often a witness to the salutary efforts which nature makes to re-establish the disordered functions, he [the physician] should rather trust in their action, than hazard the interruption of that, and a greater derangement of the system, by conjectural experiments on a machine so complicated and so unknown as the human body, and a subject so sacred as human life. Or, if the appearance of doing something be necessary to keep alive the hope and spirits of the patient, it should be of the most innocent character. One of the most successful physicians I have ever known, has assured me, that he used more bread pills, drops of colored water, and powders of hickory ash, than of all other medicines put together. It was certainly a pious fraud. But the adventurous physician goes on, and substitutes presumption for knowledge. From the scanty field of what is known, he launches into the boundless region of what is unknown. He establishes for his guide some fanciful theory of corpuscular attraction, of chemical agency, of mechanical powers, of stimuli, of irritability accumulated or exhausted, of depletion by the lancet and repletion by mercury, or some other ingenious dream, which lets him into nature's secrets at short hand.[7]

Later, Andrew Jackson would himself suffer from this medical "short hand." Less learned than his presidential predecessor and more stoic about issues of health (especially his own), even America's seventh president knew the cupping and calomel he received at the hands of such eminent regulars as Dr. Philip Syng Physick (1768-1837) were debilitating a body racked by years of respiratory illness and persistent infection; indeed, the latter ultimately led to a fatal nephrotic condition.[8]

Such ineffectual treatments observed and received tended to foster skepticism of, and even disgust with, allopathic practice. More important, if the learned elite could offer the public little more than mysterious disease names accompanied by fees—reasonable or exorbitant was beside the point—then perhaps the answer resided not in the universities but in America's fields and forests, and perhaps, too, answers could be had not in elaborate theories but in common experience accompanied by a judicious observation of nature itself. Everything about the age seemed to suggest it: the rise of egalitarianism, the invigorating and character-building influences of the frontier, the faith in a native intelligence especially suited to democratic republicanism. Consonant with these ideals, self-styled "physicians" were loudly proclaiming a healing art fashioned in the image of the age, and people were listening. A new spirit in the healing arts was afoot.

THE "SPIRIT OF RADICALISM"

Thus, an interplay of social, educational, political, and economic forces associated with Jeffersonian, and particularly Jacksonian, democracy helped shape the character and the direction of the botanico-medical movement. Dr. Worthington Hooker (1806-1867) wrote, in 1849, "As it has been fashionable in the world of business and politics, to denounce moneyed corporations, as being monopolies, so the system of institutions, or corporations (as they may be termed) by which a well educated medical profession is secured in the community, has also been denounced and attacked by this same

spirit of radicalism. Thompsonism [sic] has been one of the principal channels through which this attack has been made. The followers of Thompson [sic] have always spoken of the medical faculty as
a privileged order which must be overthrown."[9]

A number of other nineteenth-century observers also attempted
to formulate a succinct social appraisal of Thomsonianism and botanicism. William Procter Jr. (1817-1874) stated, in the *American
Journal of Pharmacy,* that "the idea that each individual head of a
family should in medicine, as in religion and politics, think and act
for himself, presented so inviting an aspect to the yeomen of the
land, that his [Thomson's] medical system was adopted as a revela-
tion."[10] Oliver Wendell Holmes labeled Thomsonianism as the "common sense scientific radicalism of the barn-yard" and contrasted it
with homeopathy, which he termed "the mystical scientific radicalism of the drawing room."[11] Elisha Bartlett and Worthington Hooker agreed that Thomsonianism appealed largely to the ignorant and
poorer classes, while homeopathy attracted clients from the rich and
educated.[12] This was undoubtedly true in Boston and in some of the
Eastern centers where homeopathy had first taken root. In the Midwest, or on the frontier, however, where homeopathy had not yet
penetrated,[13] the situation was different. From Cincinnati, Daniel
Drake noted, in 1829, that Thomson's *New Guide to Health* was
"not at present limited to the vulgar. Respectable and intelligent
mechaniks, legislative and judicial officers, both state and federal
barristers, ladies, ministers of the gospel, and even some of the
medical profession 'who hold the eel of science by the tail' have
become its converts and puffers."[14]

When it came to fees, the operation of a botanic infirmary, could
boost the proprietor's income to levels comparable with his regular
counterpart. Without it, however, Thomsonian practitioners earned
considerably less than their regular or homeopathic competitors
because of the time spent in administering their therapeutic regimen.[15] An article appearing in a Thomsonian journal ruefully complained of this situation:

> The Thomsonian practice is by far the most laborious, and
> the medicines more expensive. The fashionable calomel gentry
> drive up to the door, are conducted with etiquette to the bed-

side of the patient, and upon the point of a beautiful silver-steel penknife deal out divers little powders, and then mount their "go-cart" and leave, and when they get home mark down $2 or $3. But this will never do for the Thomsonian physician, he must off coat, go to work, and see that the patient's relatives are sometimes violently opposed to having a "steamer" called in, and would about as lief see the poor sufferer die, as cured by means of "roots and herbs." On the score of playing gentleman and making money, the calomel doctor has decidedly the advantage, for while the Thomsonian is giving a course of medicine which requires half a day, and for which he charges $2.50 or $3, the calomizer may visit 20 or 30 patients, and makes ten times as much as the Botanic.[16]

The "extracurricular" activities of the more fanatical and aggressive Thomsonian and botanic practitioners frequently imparted to the movement a quasipolitical, quasireligious orientation. This is typified in the utterance of Elias Smith (1769-1846), the controversial preacher, Thomsonian physician, and ardent supporter of President Jackson, who proclaimed with fervor that "there are three important things in this life to attend to; these are *Medicine, Government,* and *Religion.*"[17] Even more forcefully stated was Wooster Beach's emotional outburst published in the sectarian, religious journal *The Telescope:*[18] "How long, oh! how long, will the people continue to have their pockets picked, their health and lives destroyed by Doctors, under pretense of restoring the health. The world groans under four sore evils, viz. King-craft, Priest-craft, Lawyer-craft, and Doctor-craft, which, sooner or later, God certainly will destroy."[19]

Instances in which devotees of botanicism espoused sectarian and extremist causes crop up persistently. It is startling to discover, for example, that several Thomsonian physicians were implicated, and at least two hanged, in an abortive Mississippi slave insurrection that occurred in 1835.[20] Similarly, if somewhat less dramatically, Thomas Vaughan Morrow (1804-1850), Wooster Beach's missionary apostle, dubbed "the Father of Eclecticism in the West," was an ardent abolitionist and left his native slave state of Kentucky in disgust.[21] Later, and more than two thousand miles away, a number of Thomsonian practitioners were engaged in a mission of a different kind: They were in the vanguard of the Mormon settlement of Utah.[22] Equally surprising is the report given in a Thomsonian journal that a group of missionaries had embarked for Burma, well supplied with Thomsonian remedies "to alleviate the diseases of the heathen." "We rejoice," the article read, "in the introduction of our system among a people who will soon learn to appreciate its value. As there are no prejudices existing against it, we doubt not, but that, by its intrinsic excellence, it will become universal, and prove to be a great blessing."[23]

In 1835, Alva Curtis (1797-1880), then one of Thomson's ablest lieutenants,[24] addressed a number of fiery letters to the *Federal Union* of Georgia under the pseudonym of "Equity." Curtis made it clear that four thousand male adults of the State, all partisans of Samuel Thomson, were prepared to exact political retaliation at the polls, unless legal restrictions against their practice were lifted. There were four thousand votes, he warned, "and the balance of power between our two political parties ascertained to reside in believers in Medical Botany."[25] In another communication to the same newspaper, he announced that Thomsonians were "disgusted with that nominal freedom which leaves them disfranchised and denies them the supervisions of their lives. . . . Woe to the party on whom their vengeance shall alight."[26]

The subsequent successful onslaught against medical regulatory acts made by Thomsonians created a legal vacuum into which the eclectic faction of the botanico-medical movement, as well as other medical sects, rushed in to establish unmolested practice. In 1866, William H. Cook, writing in the *Physio-Medical Recorder,* taunted the eclectics for their pretentiousness in putting "the crown upon their own heads" after the Thomsonians had already "won the victory by forty years of toil."[27] These activities not only added color and piquancy to the movement but are replete with implications of more-than-passing interest to the social historian.

STANDARDS OF MEDICAL EDUCATION

Of all the contemporary strictures leveled at early nineteenth-century medical education in this country, perhaps the most severe were those of Daniel Drake.[28] "I have become acquainted with the literary and professional ignorance of so many students and physicians, in and of, various parts of the Union," he wrote, "that I cannot be mistaken in asserting, that the majority of the profession in America are deficient in common school learning."[29] Drake singled out a number of serious shortcomings in the medical education of his day, such as the shortness of the term of study; the indifference of many preceptors to the needs of their medical faculties; the laxity of the examination for a degree; the incongruity of the two-term *ungraded* course of studies; and the undignified bickering and quarrels among medical educators, to which, unfortunately, Drake himself had contributed a share.

Two terms of formal courses supplementing the three-year apprenticeship was the standard requirement for the Doctor of Medicine (MD) degree up to the time of the Civil War, and even somewhat later. Incredibly, the length of the term in the first years of the nineteenth century declined from fourteen weeks in 1800 to thirteen, and sometimes to twelve weeks; from 1800 to 1830, the term generally consisted of thirteen weeks.[30] Agitation by medical reformers succeeded in having the term increased to fourteen weeks, and a few years later, to sixteen. It was not until 1847 that the American Medical Association recommended as a minimum a six-month term of study.[31] It is even more astounding to discover that the two-term course was really a one-term course because the student took the complete program during the first year and then returned the next year to repeat the identical courses. This precedent was established by the University of Pennsylvania as a result of the shortage of teachers, books, and equipment, so that only by attending two terms could each student thoroughly cover each course at least once. Therefore, what started out to be a functional disorder ended up by becoming the accepted method and duration of study. A two-year graded course for regular medical students did not start until 1859; this was instituted by Lind University, Medical Department, Chicago.[32] Interestingly, the Penn Medical University of Philadelphia, an eclectic institution, offered a four-semester *graded* curriculum six years earlier.[33] American students returning from Paris were surprised by the contrast between the didactic approach of American schools and the clinical approach of the French medical educators.[34]

In the first half of the nineteenth century, clinical teaching and pathological research in American schools were rare.[35]

In contrast to the two terms required at the American schools, Edinburgh University had already required three years of study in 1765, which by 1825 had been raised to four years. During these four years, students took the same subjects as their American confreres.[36]

Deploring the mushroom growth of proprietary medical schools and their inferior standards, a spokesman for organized medicine in Ohio announced in 1847 that "a species of *mania* is prevailing in the profession to *manufacture* doctors."[37] This physician pointed out that most medical students did not even bother to complete the second term of studies for the degree but proceeded to become licensed, "many of them not having read eighteen months under the direction of a respectable preceptor."[38]

By 1870, the number of physicians in the United States had grown to "over 50,000,"[39] but the general level of education remained low. It was authoritatively reported in that year that "ordinary medical students, when commencing their studies, have some acquaintance with the English branches: reading, spelling, writing, arithmetic, geography, and grammar, (though they are frequently so deficient as to make their classmates envy their impudence)."[40] There were exceptions, of course. A few had "some knowledge of natural philosophy, of the rudiments of Latin and Greek, and of algebra and geometry," while still fewer could "claim to have pursued a course of ancient or modern languages, (rarely both), of the higher mathematics, mental and moral philosophy, chemistry, political economy, and logic."[41] By century's end, the glut of physicians had grown to dangerously absurd proportions. Some schools, such as the Medical Department of the University of Louisville, which by one estimate in 1912 was responsible for one-third of all physicians in the United States,[42] were shamelessly flooding the profession with MDs.

The Louisville situation was the natural by-product of medical education conditions that had remained unchecked since they were detailed in the 1870 report. The requirements of regular medical schools were three years of study that included at least two courses of lectures. In practice, however, it was not uncommon for the medical apprenticeship to vary from three months to a year, "during which, if his preceptor is a busy and popular practitioner, he has not been examined on the progress he is making times enough to make it worth mentioning . . ."[43] During this time, the apprentice was expected to read some designated work on anatomy "without any appliances except a deficient set of bones, the relic of his preceptor's dissecting days."[44] The medical apprentice was also expected to acquire at least a superficial acquaintanceship with some works on physiology, materia medica, chemistry, and perhaps theory and practice of medicine, although he was "apt to be bothered by the strange . . . phraseology of these works."[45]

Apparently many students, particularly in the West, took only one course of studies and then went into practice, while those who were financially able or more astute returned for a second and repetitive term of lectures.[46] Anxious for new information and experiences, the returning student was forced to "endure a dreary review of his past instruction."[47] Finally the great day arrived; the student was now ready for the final degree examination. Generally, after less than three years' study, the candidate presented a thesis, paid the fee, and rested comfortably in the conviction that the school wanted the graduation fee as badly as the student wanted the diploma (a conviction grounded in the fact that few ever failed outright).[48]

Somewhat later, Dr. N. S. Davis, reviewing a century of American medical education (1776-1876), reported that one-third of the sixty-four regular medical colleges operating in the United States in 1876 were "so located that they can afford their students no advantages for clinical instruction worthy of mention."[49] Moreover, Davis observed that with the exception of three or four schools, medical colleges were still offering the two-term *ungraded* courses for the MD degree, which in most cases lasted from sixteen to twenty weeks.[50] In the intervening decades, the medical apprenticeship appeared to have undergone a deterioration, with Davis noting that "the relations of the student and preceptor have become merely nominal in practice . . . consisting of little more than the registry of the student's name in the doctor's office, permission to read the books of his library or not, as he chooses, and the giving of a certificate of time of study to the medical college where he expects to graduate."[51]

THE PUBLIC VIEWS THE MEDICAL PROFESSION

When Dr. Joseph N. McDowell took up the cudgels on behalf of his brother-in-law, Daniel Drake, and the Medical Department of Cincinnati College against the rival Medical College of Ohio, he announced publicly, "Give me one year's time and I will blow the d——n Ohio College to hell!"[52] This outburst undoubtedly afforded unending amusement to the good citizens of Cincinnati, although it hardly added prestige to the medical profession. Pickard and Buley have shown that the physicians of the antebellum Midwest were especially prone to medical brawls of this sort,[53] a penchant by no means confined to the West, but prevailing among doctors in other parts of the country as well.

Among the botanic practitioners, the quarreling was even more frequent and acrimonious. Perhaps the most bizarre example of internecine botanic warfare occurred at the Eclectic Medical Institute (Cincinnati) in 1856, when two factions of the faculty fought for the possession of the school building, in the course of which "knives, pistols, chisels, bludgeons, blunderbusses, etc., were freely displayed. . . ."[54] One faction had succeeded in arming itself with a "six-pound cannon," which was subsequently confiscated by the mayor and police, but not before the opposing group of besiegers had "retired in utter disgust."[55]

In the absence of adequate legal support for the procurement of cadavers, many medical schools were forced into clandestine "body snatching" activities during the latter part of the eighteenth and most of the nineteenth century.[56] "Not all who stood around the new grave . . . to witness the farewell ceremony," write Pickard and Buley, "were mourners."[57] An incensed public occasionally gave vent to outraged feelings, resulting in mob attacks on medical schools and physicians.[58]

"One thing is certain," states Shryock. "Such was the popular ferment in the United States by 1840, such was the growing protest against both physicians and their physic, that the regular profession faced a serious crisis involving its entire status in society."[59] Hooker, in a significant contemporary study, attempted to arrive at the reasons for the low social prestige of the medical profession. Bemoaning the fact that medicine lagged far behind the professions of law and theology in public esteem, Hooker complained bitterly about "the whole motley herd of illiterate and reckless quacks"[60] that had infiltrated the healing arts. Hooker was particularly angered by clergymen, whom he considered especially inclined to encourage quackery and nostrums: "Though he [the clergyman] may strain at a gnat in guarding against theological quackery, when he comes to medicine verily he is ready to swallow a camel."[61] "Never," concluded Hooker, "has there been so much of empiricism as there is now. Never has it assumed such a variety of forms to suit all tastes. . . . Never have the opinions of the people been so thoroughly unsettled in regard to different remedies and modes of practice; and the remark is heard every day, even from men of intelligence, 'in medicine I know not what to believe.' " [62]

Both regular and irregular practitioners felt the keen competition from a host of enterprising nostrum manufacturers. A survey of patent medicine advertising in American newspapers reveals that the column inches devoted to nostrum ads during the nineteenth century were exceedingly numerous[63] and, for many newspapers, constituted a crucial source of revenue. Hooker graphically described the situation in 1850 as having become "a monstrous business" with "an enormous machinery of certificates and advertisements."[64]

An interesting feature of the pre–Civil War nostrum trade has been pointed out by Larson in the case of manufacturers who capitalized on the romantic legends associated with the Indians—legends whose appeal was further heightened by the action-packed novels of James Fenimore Cooper. "How the heart of the purchaser—filled, like as not with the heroic exploits of Cooper's Indians—must have warmed as he gazed at the effigy, symbolic of 'Nature's Own Remedy!' "[65]

Low-income families, or individuals living in frontier or other communities not easily accessible to the services of physicians, made frequent use of books on domestic medicine. This genre of nineteenth-century literature was written largely in the tradition of a Culpeper, Salmon, or Buchan; it was decisively shaped by American conditions and constitutes a fascinating source of medical Americana that deserves a comprehensive and systematic study not possible within the scope of this book.[66]

Perhaps no other single work on domestic medicine enjoyed more popularity and sales in this country than John C. Gunn's *Domestic*

Medicine; or, Poor Man's Friend in the Hours of Affliction, Pain and Sickness (Knoxville, 1830, and numerous other editions).[67] With consummate insight and salesmanship, Gunn shrewdly exploited all the insecurity, fear, ignorance, and prejudice that the mass of obscure and ordinary citizens might have had regarding illness. On the front page of his 1838 edition, Gunn announced, "This Book Points Out, In Plain Language Free From Doctor's Terms, The Diseases Of Men, Women And Children And The Latest And Most Approved Means Used In Their Cure . . . Intended Expressly For The Benefit Of Families In The Western And Southern States. It Also Contains Descriptions Of The Medicinal Roots And Herbs Of The Western And Southern Country, And How They Are To Be Used In The Cure Of Diseases. Arranged On A New And Simple Plan, By Which The Practice Of Medicine Is Reduced to Principles Of Common Sense."[68]

As in scores of similar works on popular medicine, Gunn's manual denounced the medical terminology used by physicians as "hostile to the interests of every community"[69] and proceeded to explain the nature and treatment of diseases in language calculated to strip away all mystery from medicine. The science of botany, according to Gunn, consisted of "mere mummery and hard sounding names of plants."[70] Many individuals, stated the author contemptuously, had studied scientific botany and were familiar with plant taxonomy but were nevertheless ignorant of the medical use of the indigenous flora. Gunn wrote derisively of "the refined fripperies and hair-drawn theories of mere science"[71] and revealed his awareness of the yearnings of the "common man" for social and political equality in the Jacksonian era.[72]

When Gunn attacked the alleged mystifications of learned physicians and scientists, he was merely echoing the diatribes of Culpeper and Salmon. It will be observed, however, that Gunn went further, by attempting to identify learning and science with tyranny and antidemocratic forces. This was a calculated attempt to exploit the "spirit of radicalism"; it was the argument ad hominem employed by the old Thomsonians, whose anti-intellectual bias was couched in similar terms.

Unlike the botanic authors of books on domestic medicine, Gunn was not opposed to the prevailing therapeutics of the regular physicians. On the contrary, he was an adherent of the old methods of purging and bleeding, which, he pointed out, could be self-administered without the aid of a physician. All that was necessary was to follow the directions in Gunn's book and thus save the cost of a doctor's services. Aware that large segments of the population were "prejudiced" against calomel, which he considered an excellent remedy, he was nevertheless prepared to offer his readers something just as good, namely, diluted nitric acid.[73]

Books on domestic medicine were as varied in content and emphasis as they were numerous during the nineteenth century. "Indian Doctor" and botanic, layman and regular physician, made their contributions to this literature and vied for readers. These manuals filled a social need as the frontiers of the young nation expanded. "Good or bad, they [the botanic manuals] found their way along all the great highways—on roads, rivers, canals," stated Philip D. Jordan. "They were read when the milk sickness struck on the shores of the Miami and the Wabash, when the scurvy of the trans-Missouri region loosened teeth . . . they were consulted for burns and scalds, for wounds and for inflammations. The housewife learned to make cranberry sauce and apple dumplings from their pages."[74]

THE MEDICAL PROFESSION VIEWS ITSELF

That many regular practitioners in this country were acutely conscious of the shortcomings of their profession and sensitive to the low esteem in which they were held during a greater part of the nineteenth century is evident from the vigorous self-criticism frequently voiced by them in the medical literature of the period.[75] Occasionally, these publications bristle with bitter accusations and self-denunciations. Thus, for example, a letter from a physician to *The Boston Medical and Surgical Journal* in 1854 complained that the profession harbored "a set of Jesuitical practitioners," and that "the medical profession has been sinking in the estimation of the public for a series of years. This is on everybody's tongue. . . ."[76] Similarly, an address before a local medical society, subsequently published and distributed in Ohio, included the following statement: "It is a lamentable truth, that our profession is fast being overstocked—not with men of high mental and moral culture, but with a class assuming the name of DOCTORS, totally unqualified for the solemn duties of the profession."[77]

In 1789, in harmony with Jefferson's agrarianism, Benjamin Rush had advocated a public relations program for country practitioners in which he outlined the advantages to be derived from combining medical practice with agricultural pursuits. He pointed out that country people would respect a physician who was also a successful farmer, "by showing them that you assume no superiority over them from your education."[78] Furthermore, country physicians could augment their income through farming, could study agricultural chemistry, and advantageously accept payment from their patients in produce or labor, in those areas where a money shortage prevailed. "The business of a farm," Rush observed, "will furnish you with employment in healthy seasons of the year, and thereby deliver you from the taedium vitae, or what is worse, from retreating to low or improper company."[79] In addition, the country doctor could thus also avoid sinking into "dram or grog drinking." As a parting piece of advice, Rush warned the prospective country physician to "avoid singular ties of every kind in . . . manners, dress, and general conduct."[80]

Of all the pre–Civil War writings by regular physicians dealing with the public relations of the medical profession, those of Worthington Hooker are certainly the most numerous and, in many ways, the most perceptive. He ascribed the inadequate respect accorded physicians by the public to low standards of education, professional quarrels, the persistence of quakery, a tendency for physicians to ingratiate themselves to their patients, their use and endorsement of secret remedies, the use of unnecessarily complicated terms, and the continued controversy over the use of calomel.[81]

One prominent physician and teacher deplored the fact that by the late 1840s, virtually all legal restrictions on the practice of medicine had been abrogated, thus allowing the errors of sectarian practitioners and quacks to be charged to the medical profession without distinction.[82] But the regular medical profession was powerless—a new wave of medical regulatory acts was not to come until the 1870s.[83] "Empiricism is everywhere rife," stated a report by the Monroe County Medical Society of New York, "and was never more arrogant, and the people love to have it so. That restless agrarian spirit that would always be levelling down, has so long kept up a hue-and-cry against calomel and the lancet that the prejudices of the community are excited against it, and their confidence in the medical profession greatly impaired, and no law could be enforced against the empiric."[84]

SUMMARY

A complex of factors associated with Jacksonian democracy, such as glorification of the common man, intense individualism, laissez-faire sentiment, fear of monopolies, and hatred of moneyed corporations, provided fertile ground for the development of the botanico-medical movement and imparted to it a distinctive American character. The unprofessional conduct and low educational standards of regular physicians resulted in a great loss of social prestige for the medical profession and enabled botanic and other sectarian physicians to practice on an equal footing with the regulars. Under these circumstances, the attack against medical regulatory acts, spearheaded by the Thomsonians, was highly successful by the 1840s, with regular practitioners helpless to stem the tide. When to the foregoing is added the vital factor of popular revulsion against the prevailing therapeutics so adroitly exploited by the botanics, then the background of the botanico-medical movement emerges into clearer focus.

Still, the nineteenth-century botanics must be understood as a group that existed within the context of an extensive materia medica consisting primarily of vegetable products. The herbal character of these substances comprising the dual sciences of botany and medicine animated the discussions of physicians and formed the basis for investigations by the medical community both inside and outside the allopathic pale. Understanding the nature of this lively activity, when added to the larger therapeutic and social dimensions of this period, will complete the historical background for this botanico-medical movement.

Chapter 3

Growth and Utilization
of the Plant Materia Medica

The American medical profession in the nineteenth century became divided by sectarian controversies that centered around a number of issues—education, professional status and organization, statutory regulation, and medical theory. None, however, was as important or as strident as the question of therapeutics. This was an old source of contention, one dating back even to mother England. In the young United States, however, questions surrounding the utilization of indigenous North American plants for medicinal purposes took on special significance and even became emblematic of one's professional affiliation within the medical community.

TOWARD A PLANT MATERIA MEDICA
OF THE UNITED STATES

Almost from the moment that European explorers set foot upon the New World, descriptions of the flora and fauna were cast in idyllic images of paradisaic wonder: *terra incognita* transformed into *terra miraculosa*.[1] Early accounts suggested that much of the North American flora held special medicinal virtues, and physicians such as Nicholas Monardes (1493-1588) tried to promote this Edenic wilderness as nature's apothecary.[2] Although American flora influenced European medicine discernibly with imports of guaiac, sarsaparilla, and sassafras, the long-term economic impact of indigenous North American species upon the overall drug trade in Europe was negligible.[3]

As Great Britain solidified its hold upon the New World, its Old World culture became a more significant feature of colonial life. This was no less true of its medicine. As mentioned earlier, the common folk generally practiced the healing arts with the confidence instilled by some popular medical guide, such as any one of several editions of Nicholas Culpeper's herbal. Armed with their trusty Culpeper, many a colonial household incorporated a few choice herbs commonly used in domestic physic as the first line of defense against illness.[4] Colonial physicians were also tied to the familiar materia medica they had known in England. Mineral agents, such as mercury and antimony, as well as vegetable products common to European practice, such as mandrake, belladonna, asafetida, and henbane, formed prominent articles in every regular physician's armamentarium.

It is tempting to assume that colonial settlers were strongly influenced by the plants they found growing around them in the New World. Native Americans, for example, had an extensive plant-based materia medica of their own, and Robert Turner had stated as early as 1664 that "[f]or what climate so ever is subject to any particular Disease, in the same place there grows a cure." However, the notion that "English herbs were best for English bodies" was also common in early America.[5] The medicinal plants of Native Americans clearly had some influence over domestic medicine, although many of the indigenous plants entering folk practice may have just as readily come from inquisitive and resourceful midwives and other village healers in search of more easily obtainable substitutes for familiar Old World plants. The case for Native American influence over professional practice is even more tenuous. "First it must be noted that the 170 Indian-used drugs that attained official status (not necessarily for the same medical uses) represented but one-third of our basic list. . . . Furthermore," David Cowen has observed, "about half of those that were placed in the 1820 pharmacopoeia were relegated to the secondary list, obviously considered of less importance by the profession."[6]

The general reticence of English colonists to capitalize upon the medicinal potentials of American plants can only be broadly explained by an already preexisting botanical materia medica that tied them to more familiar remedies and a pervasive Eurocentricity that caused them to ignore or discount the ethnobotanical medicines of native tribes. These parochial and narrow-minded tendencies would gradually break down, however, as foreign travelers, colonial civic and religious leaders, and naturalists began to seriously examine the indigenous flora for their therapeutic value. The medicinal plant investigations of Swedish naturalist Peter Kalm (1716-1779), the New England divines Cotton Mather (1663-1728) and Manasseh Cutler (1742-1823), and Pennsylvania botanist John Bartram (1699-1777) became the seminal authorities on an American medical botany that would dominate the healing arts until the opening decades of the twentieth century.[7]

Thus, by the time of American independence, two healing traditions, largely transplanted from Europe, had been established: one composed of home remedies drawn from popular culture, another developed out of professional practice. In this context, the botanico-medical movement presents several paradoxes: First, the botanics sought to attract popular patronage by stressing the superiority of indigenous plant remedies as opposed to the "mineral" and heroic medication of the regulars, at a time when the regulars numbered within their ranks some of the most zealous and productive investigators of indigenous plant drugs; second, the regular medical profession in the United States already possessed an impressive plant materia medica when the botanics appeared on the scene, early in the nineteenth century; third, the regulars had an overwhelming superiority of output in scientific medical botany in comparison with the botanic practitioners.

To the unsuspecting novice, much of the literature of the botanico-medical movement may seem to be concerned predominantly with medical and scientific botany. The casual reader suddenly confronted, for example, with Samuel Robinson's *A Course of Fifteen Lectures on Medical Botany* (1829 and later editions) would expect its contents to correspond to the title. Instead, the reader would discover an impassioned eulogy on the Thomsonian system of medicine, interspersed with frequent references to the Deity, poetical effusions, and quotations from the classics. Many of the journals of the movement, although bearing the term *botanic,* had little to do with that subject; similarly, Thomson and others who styled themselves "botanists" were, in reality, only herb doctors.[8]

As early as 1789, inveterate bleeder and calomel-pusher Benjamin Rush urged his students at the University of Pennsylvania to explore "the untrodden fields and forests" of the United States and to examine the plants found therein for their possible curative properties. "Perhaps," he suggested, "on the Monongahela, or the Potomac, there may grow a root that shall supply, by its tonic powers, the invigorating effects of the savage or military life in the cure of consumptions."[9]

It was certainly worth a try, and even George B. Wood, who, as we have seen, was not backward when it came to wielding a lancet or applying a blister, pointed out to his students that the United States was rich in indigenous drugs and singled out some thirty-six for special mention.[10] Many prominent regular physicians who employed the prevailing heroic methods of treatment were nevertheless keenly interested in scientifically developing an indigenous plant materia medica.

A span of two centuries separated the amateurish botanizing of William Wood (1580-1639) and John Josselyn (fl. 1630-1675) from the two dominating figures in nineteenth-century American botany, John Torrey (1796-1873) and the preeminent Asa Gray (1810-1888). In the intervening period, the development of scientific botany had made possible a systematic study of the medicinal flora based on sound taxonomic principles, much of which was established through the work of Carl Linnaeus (1707-1778).[11]

Botanic exploration and discovery that began on a modest scale in this country with men such as Wood and Josselyn increased in scope throughout the eighteenth century and into the nineteenth.[12] The early exploratory activities of Mark Catesby (1683-1749), John Clayton (1685-1773), John Bartram (1699-1777), Cadwallader Colden (1688-1776), and Peter Kalm (1716-1779) were succeeded by those of Johann David Schoepf (1752-1800), G. H. E. Muehlenberg (1753-1815), André Michaux (1746-1802), François André Michaux (1770-1855), and a host of others. Botanical expeditions were at first made possible through private patronage or personal resources; later, however, a large number of scientifically equipped and well-organized surveys employing naturalists and botanists began to be sponsored by the various states and by the federal government.[13]

According to Andrew D. Rodgers, New York and Philadelphia were early important centers for botanical exploration. Of Philadelphia, he writes, "Early European scientific collectors such as Thomas Nuttall, C. S. Rafinesque, André Michaux and others began their botanical journeys from this city or visited its important scientific circle, which included such men of prominence as John and William Bartram, William Baldwin, B. S. Barton, Zaccheus Collins, and others, to receive knowledge, materials, or provisions."[14]

It has been pointed out that the clergyman G. H. E. Muehlenberg exerted considerable influence on such pioneer investigators as Dr. Schoepf, author of *Materia Medica Americana Potissimum Regni Vegetabilis* (1787), Manasseh Cutler, and Benjamin Smith Barton (1766-1815).[15] Frederick Pursh (1774-1820) paid tribute to Muehlenberg in the preface to his famous *Flora Americae Septentrionalis.* "My first object, after my arrival in America," wrote Pursh, "was to form an acquaintance with all those interested in the study of Botany. Among these I had the pleasure to account one of the earliest, and ever after the most valuable, the Rev. Dr. Muehlenberg of Lancaster, Pennsylvania."[16]

Cutler, also a clergyman, was interested in plant medicinals, and his article "An Account of Some of the Vegetable Productions, Naturally Growing in this Part of America"[17] has been singled out as marking the beginning of systematic botany in New England.[18]

Dr. Benjamin Smith Barton, author of the classic *Collections for an Essay Towards a Materia Medica of the United States* (1798-1804, and later editions),[19] a treatise that has been designated as "the first of its kind written in English but simultaneously a criticism on the work of Schoepf,"[20] occupies an important place in the history of the nineteenth-century plant materia medica. Dedicated to the students of medicine of the University of Pennsylvania, where Barton taught natural history, botany, materia medica, and, after Rush's death, theory and practice of medicine, Barton's treatise was intended "to enlarge the stock of our knowledge concerning the Medicinal Properties of the Indigenous Vegetables of the United States."[21] How influential Barton was may be seen from the relatively large number of theses written by his students. According to George B. Wood, in 1802 alone, "not less than six theses on the subject of our medicinal plants were published by alumni of this school," out of a graduating class of about twenty.[22] It should also be noted that Barton gave financial assistance to Thomas Nuttall (1786-1859), author of the important milestone in American botany *The Genera of North American Plants,* which made it possible for the famous naturalist to embark on significant botanical expeditions.[23] Similarly, Barton's patronage of Frederick Pursh was of mutual benefit to both men. "The collections and observations made in the course of these journeys," wrote Pursh, "all of which I communicated to Dr. Barton, were considerable."[24]

Excluding for the moment the names of sectarian botanic practitioners, one can compile a relatively long list of nineteenth-century authors who had published their observations on indigenous plant medicinals, virtually all of whom were regular physicians: Asahel Clapp, *A Synopsis; or Systematic Catalogue of the Medicinal Plants of the United States* (1852); William Downey, *An Investigation of the Properties of* Sanguinaria Canadensis, *or Puccoon* (1803); Stephen Elliott, *A Sketch of the Botany of South Carolina and Georgia* (1821-1824); R. Egelsfeld Griffith, *Medical Botany* (1847); John S. Mitchell, *On the* Arbutus Uva Ursi *and* Pyrola Umbellata *and* Maculata of Linnaeus (1803); Charles Morris, *An Inaugural Dissertation on the* Prunus virgiana (1802); Francis Peyre Porcher, "Medicinal and Toxicological Properties of the Cryptogamic Plants of the United States," *Transactions of the American Medical Association* 7 (1854), his "Report on the Indigenous Medicinal Plants of South Carolina," *Transactions of the American Medical Association* 2 (1849), and, later, his classic work for the Confederacy, *Resources of the Southern Fields and Forests* (1863); and William Zollickoffer, *Materia Medica of the United States* (1819). In the Midwest, John L. Riddell published his *Synopsis of the Western Plants* (1835), whereas twenty years prior to this Daniel Drake had described sixty genera and about 100 species of plants, many of them medicinal, in his *Natural and Statistical View; or Picture of Cincinnati and the Miami Country* (1815). Active at Transylvania University was the prominent teacher Charles W. Short, who published much valuable material on the indigenous flora in the periodical *Transylvania Journal of Medicine and Associate Sciences,* which he owned jointly with John Esten Cooke.[25] That excellent scientific botanist George Engelmann, of St. Louis, was a very productive investigator despite the distraction of a large medical practice. In the East, Eli Ives and William Tully studied the plants around New Haven and stimulated an interest in botanizing among their medical students at Yale. Regional studies such as Charles A. Lee's *Catalogue of Medicinal Plants . . . in the State of New York* (1848) were fairly common-place. All the men mentioned previously possessed degrees from regular medical schools.[26]

Also of particular interest are Jacob Bigelow's *American Medical Botany* (1817-1820), William P. C. Barton's *Vegetable Materia Medica of the United States* (1817-1819), and the *Medical Flora* (1828-1830) of C. S. Rafinesque. The first work, by the versatile Boston physician, and the second, by the Philadelphia surgeon and professor of botany at the University of Pennsylvania, were extremely influential and popular; the two-volume treatise by the gifted naturalist C. S. Rafinesque, who will be considered in detail later in connection with the botanic movement, was, on the whole, either ignored or unfavorably received by many of his contemporaries.[27] For example, John Torrey and Asa Gray, the doyens of American botany, paid Rafinesque little attention. In the words of James Reveal, "Torrey and Gray were appalled by Rafinesque's proliferation of scientific names and simply ignored most of what he published."[28] Wood, likewise, writing in 1840, failed to mention Rafinesque in discussing contemporary medical botanists, but he was extremely enthusiastic about William P. C. Barton and Jacob Bigelow.

Contributing substantially to the development of the plant materia medica were the botanical herb gardens established during the eighteenth and nineteenth century in this country.[29] A pattern of communication and exchange sprang up early. Pioneer garden owners such as John Bartram of Philadelphia, Dr. A. Garden of South Carolina, John Clayton of Virginia, and Cadwallader Colden of New York wrote and exchanged specimens with Linnaeus, Collinson of London, Gronovius of Leyden, and others. How scientifically stimulating many of these gardens could be may be illustrated in the case of Dr. David Hosack's "Elgin Botanic Garden," cultivated on land purchased by him from the City of New York in 1801. Visited by prominent men of science such as François André Michaux, Thomas Nuttall, Benjamin Smith Barton, Samuel Latham

Mitchill, John LeConte, and many others, the garden curator, for a time, was the famous naturalist Frederick Pursh. Dr. Hosack's plan was ambitious, striving to create a garden similar to the *Jardin des Plantes* of Paris.[30]

According to Martin Wilbert, considerable attention had been directed to the commercial utilization of cultivated medicinal herbs by the early nineteenth century.[31] Spearheading this trend were the Shakers, who had established undisputed leadership in the commercial exploitation of cultivated medicinal plants during the first half of the nineteenth century. Not until the late forties was the Shaker hegemony effectively challenged by Tilden and Company, and subsequently by others.

As mentioned earlier, a domestic medicine had been transplanted among the early settlers of this country that attempted to apply and combine the plant lore of the Old World with indigenous plants. New World plant medicinals were incorporated into the domestic materia medica on the basis of empirical observation, through their imaginary qualities derived from folklore, or through their resemblance to familiar European plants.[32] The literature of English domestic medicine and herbalism was brought to this country by early immigrants as well. It was represented by such works as Gervase Markham's *The English Housewife* (1613) and *The English Husbandman* (1613); the herbals of John Parkinson (1567-1650), John Gerard (1545-1612), and Nicholas Culpeper's astrological herbal, *The English Physician* (1652 and many other editions),[33] to be followed later by such popular works as William Buchan's *Domestic Medicine; or, The Family Physician* (1769 and other editions).

Despite the general reluctance on the part of professional practitioners to adopt Native American herbal remedies, the influence of an indigenous ethnopharmacy upon the general public was considerable. Before long, popular belief began attributing to the Native Americans a certain prowess in the cure of disease, along with the possession of efficacious and secret remedies. Exploitation of this belief, held by many laypeople, resulted in the rise of a class of practitioners known as "Indian Doctors," whose activities will be detailed later.[34]

The leaders of the medical profession were less enthralled. Benjamin Rush wrote contemptuously of Indian medicine: "We are sometimes amused with accounts of Indian remedies for the dropsy, epilepsy, colic, gravel, and gout. If, with all the advantages which modern physicians derive from their knowledge in anatomy, chemistry, botany and philosophy; if, with the benefit of discoveries communicated from abroad, as well as handed down, from our ancestors, . . . we are still ignorant of certain remedies for these diseases; what can we expect from the Indians . . . ."[35] In another passage, Rush categorically proclaimed that "[w]e have no discoveries in the materia medica to hope for from the Indians in North America. It would be a reproach to our schools of physic, if modern physicians were not more successful than the Indians. . . ."[36] One writer had aptly characterized Rush's essay as "a typical product of the Age of Rationalism, reflecting . . . the smug pride of the academician in the unsurpassable achievements within any given field of learning."[37]

The tradition of Culpeper and Buchan, which permeated that large assortment of Americana composed of books on domestic medicine, had become strongly modified and geared to American conditions. These works invariably devoted much space to plant medicinals and recipes and constituted a rich source of empirical plant medicinal lore, frequently intermingled with superstition and charlatanry.

Scientific efforts to promote the growth of a plant materia medica were, in the words of Glenn Sonnedecker, "supplemented by the observations of unscientific empirics. The observations of laymen formed the basis of sectarian movements and later on were subjected to scientific verification."[38]

BOTANIC PRACTITIONERS
AND THE PLANT MATERIA MEDICA

By and large, botanic medical literature was produced on two levels: first, as a literature intended for lay consumption and suited to the needs of uneducated practitioners and, second, as a literature largely designed to attract educated readers, serve as a reference for more ambitious students and practitioners, and in general obtain scientific recognition.

The difficulty of making a clear-cut distinction between botanic and nonbotanic works on domestic medicine has been expressed by

Pickard and Buley, who have attempted to classify the antebellum, nineteenth-century popular medical literature into "Indian medicine and the powwow books"; "household remedy or domestic-medicine books"; and "offerings of the Botanics or Eclectics." Of the third category, these writers state that about the only criterion of difference between them and the general run of domestic medicine books is that the latter include calomel and bloodletting.[39] How difficult some of these works are to classify may be seen in Jordan's analysis of William Mills's *Marrow of Practical Medicine and Family Guide . . . Without Poison or Bloodshed,* St. Clairsville, Ohio, 1848. After perusing this book carefully, Jordan concluded that "it shows the influence of the botanic school . . . the impact of the regulars; and . . . the influence of the frontier itself."[40] The only reliable yardstick that we have found to measure botanicism in works on domestic medicine is their *ideological* content. Certainly, the Thomsonians and their "mongrel" imitators popularized and promoted such medicinals as capsicum, lobelia, myrrh, and bayberry bark, but it was the physio-medicals and eclectics with ambitions toward scientific legitimacy who made a strong, conscious effort to synthesize the works of their less-educated colleagues, to influence the growth of the plant materia medica, and to subject their plant medicinals to "scientific verification."[41] It is at this significant level of botanic output that the contributions of the botanics will be evaluated.

The earliest noteworthy attempt in this direction was the treatise published by Elisha Smith,[42] an independent botanic[43] physician of New York. His book of 624 pages, *The Botanic Physician,* appeared in 1830.[44] In the preface to his work, Smith voiced the aspirations of the few more enlightened botanics of the time. His introductory remarks constituted, in fact, a manifesto that presaged the more ambitious physio-medical and eclectic productions to come. Smith saw "with regret the want of something like a general, systematic treatise upon the different branches appertaining to medicine, on a plan adapted to the peculiar profession of Botanic Physicians."[45]

Smith was one of the most forthright of all botanic writers. He readily admitted that his ideas about causes, symptoms, and description of diseases were lifted from the works of others. "I lay no claim to originality," he wrote and acknowledged his indebtedness particularly to "the estimable Buchan and Thomas."[46] His section on materia medica was strongly influenced by the work of James Thacher, C. S. Rafinesque, and Samuel Henry's *Family Herbal*.[47] Smith was of the opinion that these works had "contributed largely to the development of the medicinal resources of our country."[48] Apparently, Rafinesque's scathing criticism of Henry's *Family Herbal* as an inept piece of work did not lower it in Smith's estimation.[49]

About one-fifth of Smith's book was devoted to plant medicinals. Almost 300 plants were described, their common names followed by scientific binomial nomenclature. Habitat, properties, and uses were given in each case. The section ended with a brief essay on the technique of collecting and preserving plant drugs. The work contained no plant illustrations.

Many of Smith's views undoubtedly shocked the Thomsonians of his day. Although an ardent botanic, he was nevertheless not averse at times to bleeding his patients in moderation,[50] or prescribing "vegetable poisons" and cathartics such as opium, stramonium, digitalis, rhubarb, and similar drugs denounced by Thomsonians. He used "mineral medication" sparingly, and occasionally cantharides plaster and the seton.[51] Mercurial preparations were, of course, strongly denounced by him. A striking feature of his practice was his employment of major surgery, an unusual approach among early botanics.[52] Despite its obvious shortcomings and unoriginality, Smith's *The Botanic Physician* was the first significant attempt to synthesize and systematize the prevailing botanic practice and plant materia medica.

Two years after the appearance of Smith's work, Horton Howard of Columbus, Ohio, published his two-volume treatise *An Improved System of Botanic Medicine* (1832).[53] Howard, a former agent for Samuel Thomson, had become involved in a heated controversy with his employer and had proceeded to set up a botanic faction of his own.[54] The author's section on plant materia medica took up eighty-five pages in the second volume and was titled "New Vegetable Materia Medica." Howard had augmented the seventy plant drugs included in Samuel Thomson's materia medica (see Appendix 1) with forty-two more, making a total of 112 plants. Howard claimed to draw his descriptions "from every available source" yet admittedly credited "but few quotations or authorities which we thought proper to use." Those he did mention included Thomson,

Rafinesque, an unidentified "Rogers," Thacher, Bigelow, Barton, Cullen, and Elisha Smith.[55]

According to Howard, the purpose in writing this treatise was to correct the "imperfections of Dr. Thomson's book, and the circumscribed limits of his materia medica." "I was not satisfied," he announced, "that the knowledge of botanic medicine should remain in so imperfect a state."[56]

Most of the plant medicinals in this work were arranged by scientific binomial names, followed by common names, description, habitat, and medical use. Twenty-two black-and-white illustrations, rather poorly done, were included. By and large, this work was no improvement on Smith's treatise and, in many ways, was actually inferior.

In 1833, the editor of *The Eclectic, and Medical Botanist*,[57] mouthpiece for the Howard faction, denied charges of plagiarism leveled against Howard for lifting material from Henry's *Family Herbal*. "Some of the plates," retorted the editor, "were copies from nature, others from the standard works of Barton, Bigelow and Rafinesque."[58]

Howard's vaunted "Cholera Syrup" proved ineffective when the disease reached Columbus. Both Howard and his chief lieutenant, Harvey D. Little, succumbed in 1833, their demise virtually ending the short-lived "Improved Botanic" faction. Although the faction itself failed to survive, Howard's treatise continued to enjoy posthumous popularity in certain botanic circles, appearing in several editions, and indeed dazzling many a botanic with facile quotations from Wistar's *A System of Anatomy*, Magendie's *Précis élémentaire de physiologie*, and Samuel Robinson's *Fifteen Lectures on Medical Botany*.

In 1833, Wooster Beach published his three-volume work *The American Practice of Medicine*.[59] Its debut was accompanied by a fanfare and publicity campaign unparalleled in the history of botanic literature. Sample copies were distributed to royalty abroad as well as to numerous influential Americans. The resulting deluge of medals and testimonials was subsequently skillfully exploited to promote a large sale of this work.[60] More will be discussed later about this treatise in connection with eclectic pharmacy and medicine, but for the present, attention will be directed to Beach's treatment of the plant materia medica.

The introduction to *The American Practice of Medicine* contained, among other things, a verbatim statement of Smith's manifesto, without, as has been previously indicated, directly crediting Smith. Included also were lengthy quotations from Rafinesque's introductory remarks to his *Medical Flora,* embellished with approving comments by Beach. The section on materia medica included in the third volume was supplemented by superficial essays on botany, chemistry, and natural history. As in Howard's book, illustrations of plants in green ink, rather crudely done, were copied for the most part from Rafinesque, William P. C. Barton, and Jacob Bigelow.[61]

By 1869, *The American Practice Condensed; or the Family Physician,* Fifty-sixth Edition[62] had listed some 134 plant medicinals, 116 of which were stated to have been used frequently in eclectic practice, the remainder being grouped under the heading "Botanical Synopsis of Plants Occasionally Used, and Recommended for Further Investigation."[63] Taxonomy of plants was more elaborately treated by Beach than by Smith and Howard. Not only were genera and species given but class and order as well. Beach's materia medica, although chiefly confined to plant drugs, also listed a number of chemicals. Generally speaking, one is forced to conclude, after reviewing Beach's work on the plant materia medica, that his contribution was noteworthy mainly for its mediocrity and excessive borrowing.

A perceptible stir was created in botanic circles in 1841 with the publication of two pretentious botanic works. The first, by Morris Mattson, titled *The American Vegetable Practice,*[64] was followed immediately by John Thomson's *The Thomsonian Materia Medica; or, Botanic Family Physician.*[65]

Mattson, who for a time had served as editor of the *Boston Thomsonian Manual and Lady's Companion,* had been hired by Samuel Thomson in the late 1830s to help with a revised edition of his *New Guide to Health.* This relationship, as with many previous ones into which Thomson had entered, soon degenerated into a violent feud, and to the consternation of Thomson, Mattson presented to the world his own large tome interspersed with uncomplimentary remarks about the founder of the Thomsonian system.

About 180 pages in *The American Vegetable Practice* devoted to the discussion of plant materia medica were supplemented by twenty-six attractive colored illustrations of plants. In all, some eighty-six plant medicinals were mentioned in monographs that listed common names, botanical names, habitat, history, properties, medical uses, parts used, and time for collecting. Preceding the section on plant materia medica were two very brief essays, one, "Proximate Vegetable Principles," displayed the author's ignorance of chemistry, and the other was "Instructions on Collecting, Drying, and Preserving Plants."

Mattson's work was unquestionably a great advance over Thomson's *New Guide to Health*. It was a far more literate production than any of the preceding works discussed, and there were unmistakable signs that Mattson had made a great effort to read extensively and with discrimination. "In preparing *The American [Vegetable] Practice* for the press," he wrote, "I have availed myself of the usual authorities, where they could be of any service."[66] Of original investigation and scientific acumen, however, there were no indications.

Only the importunate behavior of Samuel Thomson's son, John, and the consuming hatred that the father bore Mattson could have induced the aging Thomson to permit the use of his name on the title page of *The Thomsonian Materia Medica*. The appearance of this book, with its scientific pretensions, evoked hoots of derision and glee from botanic practitioners who were tired of hearing old Thomson's denunciation of education and "mongrel improvements." Thomas Cooke, editor of the independent journal *The Botanic Medical Reformer and Home Physician,* greeted the new book with a scathing editorial:

> John Thomson ("or my son John") of Albany and the "old patriarch," Samuel Thomson of Boston, got up a work in a great hurry, with a view to compete with Dr. Mattson's work, and to help swell out its pages, they copied nearly the whole of a work on Anatomy, (by an English author) a science by the way, that "the old patriarch" has time and again denounced as *humbug,* and forwarded a copy to a "Dutch king" to see whether he liked it. As a mark of common courtesy, the "enlightened Prussian king," Frederick William, sent "my son John" a letter acknowledging the receipt of said "*Anatomical* Vegetable Materia Medica!!" The *king* handed it over to the

faculty to *dissect,* and there is little doubt but that they will give it its deserts [sic]. Did the *American* President receive a copy? . . . Let "my son John" read Dr. B's letters . . . [a reference to Wooster Beach's testimonials]. But we had like to have forgotten, that these are the days of "Improvements."[67]

John Thomson dedicated his 834-page tome to Benjamin Waterhouse, MD, and made a determined bid for scientific recognition. The author announced that he was assisted in his work "upon animal and vegetable life" by consulting such authorities as Hippocrates, Galen, Bacon, Boerhaave, Sylvius, Cullen, Brown, Hunter, Goldsmith, Robinson, Eaton, Tully, Barton, Rush, and, above all, Samuel Thomson. The reader was regaled with essays on the history of botany, plant physiology, plant anatomy, and morphology. An outline of "Linnaeus's System of Vegetables" was succeeded by biographical sketches of Linnaeus, Conrad Gessner, Tournefort, and Mark Catesby. Not content with this show of erudition, John Thomson included an essay on botanical gardens and a fourteen-page glossary of botanical terms. All this, however, was merely a prelude of things to come. Following was a forty-one-page treatise on matter, water, caloric, light, and air, in which the works of Cavendish, Priestley, Lavoisier, Davy, and Dalton were reviewed. Almost 300 pages were next devoted to "Human Anatomy with Plates," followed by eighty-three pages dealing with the "History of the Efforts of Dr. Samuel Thomson to Sustain His System of Vitality In Matter." The author was now ready for his "Description of the Vegetable Substances Used by Samuel Thomson." It should be noted, however, that a number of the substances so described were not used by Samuel Thomson, since the original core of Thomson's seventy plant drugs (see Appendix 1) had been increased by "my son John" to 101. The addition included, among other things, cathartics which the father had vehemently denounced and which John justified on the grounds that they were at least better than taking "the most deadly drugs that are to be found in the [allopathic] shops."[68]

The section on plant medicinals followed the general pattern established by the works of the preceding botanic authors. Monographs on the individual plant drugs gave common and botanical names, properties, and uses in Thomsonian practice. Again, as in Mattson's work, attractive color illustrations of plants were included. *The Thomsonian Materia Medica* was in all respects a worthy competitor for *The American Vegetable Practice.*

All this must have been a severe blow to the "old patriarch," who had steadfastly maintained an honest contempt for education and science, only to see his probity impugned by the ambitious undertaking of his son. The elder Thomson's feelings were perhaps partly mollified by a public statement published at the end of the book, announcing that Dr. Samuel Thomson had disclaimed all responsibility for a number of therapeutic agents recommended by his son:

IMPORTANT NOTICE

The following objections to the different articles and compounds were made by Dr. Samuel Thomson, after the work was printed. And in justice to him, and out of respect to his opinion, we insert them here, that everyone may know that his opinion is not changed in relation to cathartics and that what is said upon that subject is done on our own responsibility, and for which Dr. Thomson is not to be held responsible. The following are the objections, viz.

All cathartic medicine, of every kind; also the compounding of the black salve on page 734 (for which we have inserted a substitute on page 823); borax for sore mouth, page 738; maple charcoal to prevent mortification, page 742; Peruvian bark to clean the teeth, page 740; poke root made into ointment for the piles, page 741; sulphate of zinc compounded in poultices for syphilitic ulcers, page 733; burnt alum for dysentery, page 726; tobacco ointment for salt rheum, page 713; gin to quiet nervous irritability, page 711; emetic pills, page 700; asafetida for hysteria, page 634; blood root for emetic, page 684; black cohosh to cure rheumatism, and to regulate the monthly turns with females, page 643; and, page 695, the injection should be given before steaming.

It is to be understood, that he objects to the use of those articles, in every form or shape whatever, except the enemas.

John Thomson[69]

PROCTER'S CRITIQUE OF KOST AND KING

Historians are indebted to William Procter Jr. (1817-1874) for a penetrating and objective appraisal of the work of John Kost, a leading physio-medical practitioner, and of John King, one of the most prominent exponents of eclecticism. Procter's reviews of Kost's *Elements of Materia Medica and Therapeutics* (1858)[70] and King's *American Eclectic Dispensatory* (1854 and 1859 "editions")[71] consti-tute, not only a valuable critique of botanicism and eclecticism as seen through the eyes of one of the most distinguished pharmacists of the time, but are also among the very few dispassionate critical analyses of botanicism to appear in nineteenth-century literature.[72] Not being a physician, Procter carefully refrained from passing judgment on the medical and clinical pretensions of eclecticism, confining his critical analysis to fields in which he was eminently competent to speak, namely, pharmacy, chemistry, and materia medica. There will be occasion to refer again to Procter's critique during the course of an extended appraisal of neo-Thomsonian and, especially, eclectic pharmacy; for the present, however, the discus-sion will center on Procter's cogent observations concerning the treatment of the plant materia medica in the works of Kost and King.

In 1849, John Kost published the first edition of his *Elements of Materia Medica and Therapeutics.* This treatise was intended to be used in the "new physiological system of practice," an elegant and euphemistic phrase coined by neo-Thomsonian practitioners to de-scribe the new Thomsonian methods and to forestall such uncouth epithets as "steamers" and "puke doctors," which were constantly being hurled at them by their enemies. The author, who announced himself on the title page as an honorary member of the Thomsonian Medical Society of New York, had taught materia medica, botany, and therapeutics at a number of physio-medical schools. A new and revised edition of Kost's work appeared in 1858, and it was this edition that was reviewed by William Procter in the *American Jour-nal of Pharmacy.*

The new and enlarged volume of 829 pages was still called *Ele-ments of Materia Medica and Therapeutics,* but the descriptive phrase "Adapted to the New Physiological System of Practice," which appeared on the title page of the first edition, had been significantly changed to "Adapted to the American Reformed and Eclectic Practice." Reluctant to lose his followers among the new Thomsonians but at the same time eager for a large sale of his book to the eclectics, Kost, for many years, managed to maintain a delicate balance, poised between the two hostile camps and maneuvering with singular adroitness. This would account for Procter's impression that Kost's treatise was a product of the eclectic school,[73] despite strong evidences to the contrary, some of which Procter himself recognized in his review.[74]

Some of Procter's conclusions were forcefully stated: "We look in vain," he wrote, "for evidences of that laborious research which has ransacked the primary depositions of scientific knowledge."[75] He pointed out that Kost had "been careful to keep beyond the reach of the law of copyright in making copious quotations from Royle and Pereira, which are interspersed through his pages, like patches of silk on garments of cotton."[76] As a pharmacist, Procter was free from the emotional block that characterized the attitude of regular physicians when confronted with botanic literature. "There are many things in the volume of Dr. Kost which merit the attention of the regular physician,"[77] Procter observed. "Practice and experience have materially modified the standing and quality of the body called Eclectics; much they have gained by observation, much from hearsay from inferior sources, of the use and qualities of many indigenous plants, unknown or slightly understood by regular practitioners. These they are verifying by trial, and undoubtedly are developing many valuable facts."[78] In contrast, Procter observed that "[t]he contracted therapeutics of Thompsonianism [sic], and its limited materia medica, are disappearing in the voluminous admixture of regular medicine, and new discoveries in the literature of Eclecticism, and in a few years it will be difficult to detect the stern features of the doctrine of its founder."[79]

Finally, Procter pointed out certain plant drugs that the eclectics were using as meriting attention, namely podophyllum, leptandra, sanguinaria, caulophyllum, cypripedium, "and some other plants, which to some extent have been tried by physicians, and in some instances highly approved."[80]

John King (1813-1893) was unquestionably one of the most important spokesmen for eclecticism. His 1854 edition of the *American Eclectic Dispensatory* (1,391 pages) and the 1859 version, the *American Dispensatory* (1,475 pages), were reviewed at length by William Procter in the pages of the *American Journal of Pharmacy.* Procter prefaced his critical analysis of King's 1854 edition by remarking that the rise of eclecticism in this country, with its medical schools, societies, and "a materia medica, to a large extent botanical and indigenous, . . . is certainly a phenomenon in medical history of the United States of no ordinary interest."[81] Briefly sketching the rise of Thomsonian and eclectic medicine, Procter concluded that this development "may be esteemed a remarkable episode in the history of American medicine and pharmacy."[82] Procter's review of King's work as it related to the plant materia medica is an important window into the attitude of mainstream pharmacy for the eclectic materia medica. He believed that improper and insufficient attention to medicinal chemistry represented "a stigma on the science of the Eclectics" and cited the work of the graduates of the Philadelphia College of Pharmacy as having done more work on popular eclectic plants, such as lobelia, hydrastis, podophyllum, and rhus, "than any other class of investigators."[83] Procter went on to praise the eclectics for their work on an indigenous plant materia medica but added "we may look for their greater progress when more real science becomes commingled with their recorded observations," and although he believed King's efforts were of "very considerable value," he also suggested that King's lack of scientific training made him less than "a master workman."[84] Procter's review went on to note that King's descriptions of plants were based upon Gray or Wood and that, although his book was quite readable, "its inaccuracies are so numerous, and its patchwork character so unmistakable, that it will have no scientific authority except so far as each individual quotation is concerned."[85] Procter concluded with a list of eclectic medicinal plants:

Among the plants which have attracted most attention we may name the following, attaching an asterisk to each of those which are particularly relied on in their practice, viz.:

Aletris farinosa
Ambrosia trifida
* Apocynum cannabinum
Asclepias incarnata
* Asclepias tuberosa
* Baptisia tinctoria
* Caulophyllum thalictroides
Chelone glabra
* Cimicifuga racemosa
Coralorhiza odontorhiza
Corydalis formosa
* Cypripedium pubescens
* Dioscorea villosa
* Epigea repens
Erechthites hieracifolius
* Euonymus atropurpureus
* Eupatorium purpureum

* Geranium maculatum
Helianthemum canadense
* Hydrastis canadensis
* Iris versicolor
Kalmia latifolia
* Leptandra virginica
* Lobelia inflata
Myrica cerifera
* Phytolacca decandra
* Podophyllum peltatum
Ptelea trifoliata
* Sanguinaria canadense
* Scutellaria lateriflora
* Senecio aureus
* Stillingia sylvatica
* Viburnum opulus
* Xanthoxylum fraxineum[86]

A number of observations are made in these passages that apply not only to King's work but to that of other botanics and eclectics as well. The laudable objective of investigating indigenous plants for curative purposes could not be realized as long as botanic practitioners were not scientifically trained in this direction. Moreover, mere appropriation and compilation of facts established through investigation by nonbotanics could not be substituted for original research on the plant materia medica. Finally, the botanic practitioners as a group evinced a marked disinclination and lack of ability to conduct phytochemical work. This last point is particularly important in connection with the subsequent evolution of eclectic pharmacy, and as Procter so forcefully indicated.

The eclectics had long evaded the responsibility for the chemical examination of their plant medicinals, many of which had been subjected to proximate analyses at the Philadelphia College of Pharmacy. Instead, the eclectics were instrumental in promoting a large-scale manufacture of "eclectic medicines" derived from plants, consisting of heterogeneous and ill-defined substances, without bothering to ascertain their chemical nature. By the 1850s, many firms had entered the field. "All of these firms," wrote John Uri Lloyd, "listed their products under various titles, such as Alkaloids, Resinoids, Resins, and Concentrated Medicines, some even attempting to group or classify the various substances. But, as a rule, no attempt was made to distinguish between useful agents and those questionable, or between the unworthy and those entitled to a systematic position, by legitimate scientific nomenclature."[87]

WILLIAM H. COOK'S DISPENSATORY

Of considerable historical interest is the now forgotten and exceedingly rare treatise by William H. Cook, titled the *Physio-Medical Dispensatory,* Cincinnati, 1869. Written by a prominent physio-medical leader, teacher, and editor, this volume of 832 pages represents perhaps the most ambitious attempt to synthesize the therapeutics, materia medica, and pharmacy in vogue among the neo-Thomsonians of the post–Civil War period. The initial printing of this book was very meager[88] and probably accounts for the virtual absence of references to Cook's work in the literature, although Lloyd commented briefly on it in a paper devoted to American pharmacopoeias and dispensatories.[89]

As would be expected, the preface to the *Physio-Medical Dispensatory* contained a savage attack on regular medicine. The author made the observation that mercurials, antimony, bloodletting, and arsenic, "which had been the pride of allopathy for one and two hundred years were now being pushed aside to make room for opium, aconite, veratrum, bromine, bismuth, woorara [curare?], prussic acid, and strychnine."[90] Dr. Cook believed that the allopaths had "established nothing reliable in therapeutics" and "with a list of poisons for sheet-anchors" were "in no position to lay claim to public confidence."[91] Then, in a display of divisiveness that the botanics could ill afford, Cook brought the homeopaths in for their share of castigation. The bitterest denunciation of all, however, was directed against the eclectics, "a sect without a tenet in science, and claiming a merit for the number and boldness of its conflicting plagiarisms. The little good it contains," concluded Cook, "lies in the few remedies it has surreptitiously taken from Physio-Medicalism."[92]

Dr. Cook devoted a major portion of his book to a discussion of physio-medical materia medica (557 pages). Some 350 items were arranged alphabetically, the vast majority being plant drugs, with only a sprinkling of "minerals." The monographs consisted of the Latin binomial nomenclature of plants, their common names, their botanical descriptions (including order, genus, habitat, etc.), their properties and uses (including parts of plant used and therapeutic indications), posology, and pharmaceutical preparations and dosages.

By this time, the longstanding Thomsonian outcry against "minerals" had been modified to an attack against "poisons," whether of mineral or plant origin. This made for a more consistent policy, permitting the inclusion of such chemicals as Creta Preparata, magnesium carbonate, etc., in Cook's "sanative materia medica." Physio-medical practitioners would have been quick to deny that their rejection of a substance as a poison or their acceptance of some remedy as "sanative" was dictated by subjective and arbitrary factors. Acceptance or rejection, they would have stoutly maintained, was determined by bedside experience and observation. Thus, for example, according to Cook, bitter root *(Apocynum androsaemifolium)* "has by some been called poisonous, but we are abundantly able to certify the contrary."[93] Similarly, cinchona and quinine, which had been violently spurned by the Thomsonians, were accepted by Cook after reassuring his disciples that "[i]t is a common suspicion that this article quinine is poisonous, and I was at one time inclined to share in this belief, but careful observation has satisfied me that such is not the case."[94]

It is safe to say that Cook's treatise was little known beyond the circle of his followers, who were then mainly concentrated in the Midwest. Nevertheless, the *Physio-Medical Dispensatory* is an invaluable source of information for the historian, and it shall be referred to again in discussing the neo-Thomsonian trend.

A notable exception to the general run of eclectic compilations was the quarterly publication *Drugs and Medicines of North America,* written by the eminent pharmacist John Uri Lloyd, preeminent among the eclectics, in collaboration with his brother, Curtis G. Lloyd. This valuable and original study of the indigenous plant materia medica was published at irregular intervals from 1884 to 1887. Volume one, completed in 1886, but unfortunately terminating publication with the fifth number in 1887, considered in detail medicinal plants occurring in several other orders. John Uri Lloyd assumed responsibility for those sections of the work dealing with phytochemistry, pharmacy, and commercial history, while his brother, a prominent botanist and mycologist, undertook to elucidate the purely botanical aspects of the study.[95]

RAFINESQUE:
UNIQUE AND CONTROVERSIAL MEDICAL BOTANIST

Earlier studies on Rafinesque expressed the opinion that the distinguished naturalist deserves consideration by historians of pharmacy and medicine as a challenging figure in the context of the nineteenth-century botanico-medical movement and, moreover, that Rafinesque's major contribution to medical botany (his *Medical Flora*, 1828-1830) was the first such work to delineate an authoritative and enduring vegetable materia medica of the trans-Appalachian West.[96] Although further investigation has confirmed this view, the task of clearly defining Rafinesque's position in the current of botanico-medical activity is not an easy one. This is principally due to two factors: Rafinesque's intensely individualistic and unconventional attitude, which prevented his formal affiliation with any particular group, and the necessity to demolish many unsupported statements about Rafinesque, zealously propagated, for the most part, by later eclectic writers. Nevertheless, Rafinesque's position in the mainstream of the botanico-medical movement can be established by botanic practitioners' widespread use of his *Medical Flora*, in contrast to the hostility or indifference evinced by regular physicians toward this work; the relationship of Rafinesque to the eclectics; Rafinesque's critical attitude toward regular medicine; and his own brief venture into medical practice as a lung specialist or "pulmist."

Francis R. Packard's reference to the *Medical Flora* as a book that became the vade mecum of the botanic physicians is generally correct,[97] but it should be kept in mind that this was true only of the more educated botanics, and that the botanic writers previously mentioned borrowed from many other authorities besides Rafinesque. Not only did botanic authors such as Elisha Smith, Horton Howard, Wooster Beach, Morris Mattson, and others make use of

Rafinesque's *Medical Flora,* but copious references and abstracts appear in such periodicals as Alva Curtis's *The Botanico-Medical Recorder*[98] and in the independent *Botanico-Medical Reformer,* under the editorship of Thomas Cooke, who later became an eclectic. Cooke had purchased the plates of the plant illustrations of the *Medical Flora* soon after Rafinesque's death and began publishing them in 1841 in his journal.[99] Subsequently, these plates came into the possession of Wooster Beach, who used them to illustrate later editions of his *The American Practice of Medicine.*[100] Whereas the *Medical Flora* met with a favorable reception among botanics and was used as a reference book, Rafinesque's treatise received a cold reception by the regular physicians and was ignored (e.g., by George B. Wood) or severely criticized by such authors as R. Egelsfeld Griffith[101] and Asahel Clapp.[102] The reasons for this were his unorthodox views, his eccentricity, and his reputation for being unreliable. Moreover, he had also antagonized the regular medical profession at this time by setting himself up in practice as a "pulmist," or a specialist in the treatment of consumption, without benefit of a license or an MD degree.

The favorable acceptance of Rafinesque's treatise by the botanics and its hostile treatment at the hands of the regulars has led to some startling statements in the literature, the most fantastic being Otto Juettner's assertion that "C. S. Rafinesque, author of a book on 'the Medical Flora of North America' (Philadelphia, 1828), is really the originator of the botanical movement."[103] Curiously, slight variations on this notion have been carried forward into modern scholarship, most notably with a rather topsy-turvy perspective that has Rafinesque naming the eclectics (rather than the eclectics borrowing the term from Rafinesque) and has the naturalist-turned-medical botanist "belonging to the Reformed Practice [i.e., eclectics]" (rather than the eclectics attaching themselves to Rafinesque).[104] On more careful investigation, the Rafinesque connection rests more upon persistent promotion than historical fact.

In the 1890s, Wilder, Felter, and other eclectic writers began to build up Rafinesque as one of the early founders of eclecticism. Editorial comment and articles in the *Eclectic Medical Journal,* for example, referred to the *Medical Flora* as "the first work in science that complimented the eclectic profession,"[105] and to Rafinesque as one who had "divined the advent of the new [eclectic] school of medicine."[106] An excerpt from a letter that Rafinesque had written to Beach in 1840, which had been buried for years among the dozens of testimonials printed in various editions of *The American Practice,* was dusted off and submitted as prima facie evidence. "I must now state again that I think highly of your Medical work," reads one excerpt. "I belong, like yourself, to the Reformed School of Medicine, and agree with you much better than with Thomsonian, Homeopathic, and Botanical Empirics. Your system is a good one, if not perfect."[107]

Just as it appeared that a good case had been made for claiming Rafinesque as an early eclectic, and that much-needed luster had been gained by eclecticism, a very disconcerting episode occurred. Professor Herbert T. Webster, a prominent Western eclectic and editor of the *California Medical Journal,* shocked his colleagues by publishing an editorial in 1898 in which he declared, among other things, that Rafinesque "never claimed to be an eclectic." Out of the clear blue, Webster had presumed to challenge the cherished Rafinesque-eclectic relationship, had impugned the originality of his colleagues, and had accused John Milton Scudder (1829-1894), a name revered in eclectic circles for his long tenure at the Eclectic Medical Institute and his doctrine of "specific diagnosis" and "specific medication," of borrowing the majority of his remedies from Rafinesque. This challenge could not go unanswered. John King Scudder (1865-1930) sought to vindicate his deceased father's reputation through the pages of the *Eclectic Medical Journal,* the most influential publication of the movement, and trained the sights of his editorial guns on Webster, while another journal, the *Eclectic Medical Gleaner,* launched a series of ad hominem attacks on the California professor. In a spirited rebuttal vindicated by objective historical investigation, Webster steadfastly maintained that no evidence supported that Rafinesque had ever been an eclectic, and that most eclectic remedies "have been used by others prior to their adoption by our school."[108]

The net effect of Webster's action, and the ensuing dispute, was not only to cripple the attempt to portray Rafinesque as a champion of early eclecticism but also gave ammunition to the enemies of the movement, who had always maintained that the eclectic slogan

borrowed from Rafinesque[109] was a convenient excuse to appropriate and plagiarize from others.

In November 1827, under the pseudonym "Medicus," Rafinesque
began a series of advertisements in *The Saturday Evening Post* of
Philadelphia, in which he announced to the public his discovery of
"Pulmel" as a "cure" for consumption. Two years later, in 1829, Rafinesque published a brochure under his own name, titled "The Pulmist,
or the Art to Cure and Prevent Consumption." This work was subsequently translated into French and published in Paris in 1833.[110]

In his introduction, Rafinesque stated that when he was ill with
consumption, he had treated himself with his own methods and had
recovered. "My previous skill in practical and medical botany," he
wrote, "enabled me to discover . . . the probable effect of some
active plants; and by their mixture . . . I restored myself to perfect
health." He also informed his readers that he was "prepared to con-
tend with a host of prejudices and the established routine of the
faculty," and he justified the secret composition of remedies on the
grounds that "anyone has a right to withhold for a time the results of
his experience, until he is remunerated." As far as can be learned,
the precise nature of his medication, which he called Pulmel, was
never divulged. Pulmel was described by Rafinesque as follows: "It
is a peculiar compound substance, formed by the chemical combination of several powerful vegetable principles, acting on the
lungs and whole system. It contains no pernicious nor poisonous
substance. The taste and smell are fragrant, and balsamic."[111]

An original manuscript of a medical consultation by Rafinesque
is in the possession of the New York Public Library. This "medical
consultation" has been edited and annotated by Mabel Clare Weaks.
It is the opinion of Weaks that "the 'consultation' shows that the
treatment recommended by Rafinesque was in advance of his period."[112] While his allopathic contemporaries were treating phthisis,
or consumption, with a depletive regimen of venesection, blistering,
and application of leeches, Rafinesque discouraged bloodletting
and advised a restorative therapy designed to build up the general
health of the patient through a balanced diet, including milk, fruit,
and green vegetables.

As might be expected, the regular practitioners reacted very
strongly against Rafinesque's intrusion into their field. Dr. Daniel

Drake, writing in the *Western Journal of Medical and Physical Sciences,* in 1829, denounced Rafinesque as a quack and classed him with Samuel Thomson, William Salmon, William Swaim, and Samuel Robinson.[113] Curiously enough, there does not appear to be a single reference in any botanic work to Rafinesque's venture into medical practice as a pulmist.

Regardless of the attacks made upon Rafinesque by the regulars, the quality of the eccentric naturalist's *Medical Flora* appears to be exonerated by the test of time, both from *botanical* as well as *medicinal* perspectives. Many contemporaries sneered at the genera-splitting pursuits of the peripatetic naturalist and suggested that, even from a botanical standpoint, Rafinesque's work was unworthy of consideration. Modern botanists, reexamining these efforts, have greatly revised this view, however.[114] Echoing Mabel Clare Weaks, Ronald Stuckey concluded, "In many respects, Rafinesque's pioneering efforts were not ready for acceptance, nor were his readers prepared to grasp or see the relevance of the new information being provided. Actually, in many respects he was distinctly ahead of the botanical writers of his time."[115] Medically speaking, detailed analysis of each of the 100 monographed species in the *Medical Flora* shows that the vast majority of the plants listed did have, or would attain, pharmacopoeial and/or dispensatory status, and, perhaps even more interestingly, a majority are still in use today, primarily in Europe, where herbal medicine has remained a viable part of medical practice.[116]

Given the demonstrable merit of Rafinesque's contribution to American medical botany, plus his obvious influence over the botanico-medical movement, one is left to assess the mutual—perhaps even symbiotic—relationship between both. Although Webster generated some vitriolic copy in the journals, no doubt a good many eclectic readers smiled at the Californian's accusation that John Milton Scudder had borrowed from so honored a figure as Rafinesque, since to borrow that which worked in practice was a hallmark of eclecticism. Regardless of who borrowed what from whom, there can be little doubt that the materia medica described and elucidated in Rafinesque's *Medical Flora* exerted a tremendous influence over *all* the botanics. While eclectics sang the praises of the *Medical Flora,* physio-medicals such as Alva Curtis and independent botanics such as Elisha Smith readily admitted their intellectual debt to Rafinesque as well.[117] Since 91 out of 100 hundred plants described in Rafinesque's *Medical Flora* were eventually incorporated into major mainstream medical compendia past and present, the adoption of Rafinesque's medicinal plants by the botanics can hardly be called an embarrassment. Indeed, the affinity of the botanics for Rafinesque inclines one to view their materia medica with a greater degree of generosity than might otherwise be the case.

The affinity for Rafinesque's medical progressivism would be a boon to the botanics in other ways. When that great American eclectic John Uri Lloyd issued a call to systematically investigate North American medicinal plants in the 1870s,[118] he was echoing the plea made years before by this radical naturalist. "Rafinesque . . . ," writes historian Glenn Sonnedecker, "laid down rules for the pharmaceutical manipulation of plants in order to get efficient medicaments. Moreover, he believed that 'The active principles of medical plants may be obtained in a concentrated form by chemical operations' and he urged American research in plant chemistry, particularly praising the work of the Society of Pharmacists of Paris."[119]

Rafinesque held a high position in the botanico-medical movement, and his *Medical Flora* was used extensively by all botanic factions. He thought highly of Beach's system of medicine but never became affiliated with any botanic sect, although eclectics later attempted to use his name for propaganda purposes. Rafinesque was critical of the regular medical profession, as can be seen from reading the introduction to his *Medical Flora.* He preferred to use plant medicinals rather than mineral ones and, for a brief period, competed with the regular physicians by setting himself up as a pulmist. His role as an unlicensed physician was strictly on a free-lance basis. Nonetheless, Rafinesque's careful selection of medicinal plants and the thorough analysis of his materia medica redounds to the credit of the botanics who acknowledged their debt to this unique and controversial naturalist.

VOX POPULI!

"It has been a cause of profound regret and humiliation," wrote Alexander Wilder, "that so few practitioners, even among those who profess to belong to a school of botanic medicine, have been disposed to acquire any thorough or even any considerable knowledge of scientific botany."[120] This observation would have been appropriate to the vast majority of nineteenth-century regular physicians as well as to the botanics. To the man in the street, however, it meant nothing that among the regulars were found a number of excellent medical botanists, vastly superior to the best that the botanics could offer. The botanics could point out that the regulars were killing their patients with heroic medication and were trying to create a medical monopoly. This was a very effective argument in an era of Jacksonian democracy.

Though Dr. Daniel Drake might sneer at the "People's Doctors," the champion of Thomsonianism and botanicism, Samuel Robinson, addressed his fellow citizens in ringing tones and identified this grassroots herbalism as the epitome of *vox populi vox Dei*.[121]

PART II:
THE BOTANICO-MEDICAL
REVOLT, DECLINE, AND REVIVAL

With *Latin prescriptions,* and *letting of blood,*
They do all the people, with poverty flood;
Some bear it in silence, while others complain,
And speak of all doctors, with perfect disdain.

Elias Smith
*The American Physician
and Family Assistant*
Fourth Edition
Boston, 1837, p. 252

Chapter 4

The Thomsonians

With the exception of a few small groups of independent botanic practitioners, whose antecedents and activities are difficult to reconstruct,[1] the organizational and factional history of the botanico-medical movement prior to 1840 can be traced with relative ease to the followers of Samuel Thomson. After 1840, the situation becomes increasingly complex. Affiliations and names change rapidly; ephemeral botanic medical schools and journals appear and vanish; local and national societies succeed each other with kaleidoscopic speed; and uneasy alliances spring up between warring botanic factions. Investigating the data bearing on the movement in the Midwest during the 1840s and 1850s, Pickard and Buley conclude that the prevailing confusion was such as to defy analysis.[2] Similar conditions existed in the East and South.

A ROSTER OF BOTANIC GROUPS

The Disorganized Fringe Groups

For a good part of the nineteenth century, a number of freelance botanic practitioners operated on the periphery of the movement. Known as "root" or "herb" doctors, "Indian" doctors,[3] and occasionally by other names, these individuals developed either itinerant or local practices based on the use of remedies prepared from indigenous plants. We know that some of these irregular physicians were active in this country as early as the eighteenth century, for Samuel Thomson described his contacts with them in 1785 and 1791.[4] Wooster Beach stated that his knowledge of the botanic practice was largely derived from herb, root, and botanic physicians, and from a period of tutelage with botanic doctor Jacob Tidd.[5] Although the activities and literary productions of these empirics are of considerable interest to students of American medical folklore and early American plant materia medica, their disorganized status and individualistic behavior prevented them from playing any significant role in the botanico-medical movement.

The Thomsonians

In 1805, Samuel Thomson (1769-1843), a New Hampshire farmer, made the momentous decision to pit his botanical medical system against the pretensions and therapeutics of the regular medical profession.[6] Thomson's teachings were quickly accepted by large segments of the population. In 1813, 1823, and 1836, the founder and first organizer of the botanico-medical movement received patents for his system. Purchasers of "Thomson's Patent," which was bought by thousands of people, were organized into Friendly Botanic Societies. Delegates from these societies held seven annual United States Botanic Conventions, from 1832 to 1838. During the 1838 meeting, the Convention split into two irreconcilable factions, an event of singular importance to the nineteenth-century botanico-medical movement that will be examined in the subsequent pages. This latter society ceased to exist after a few annual meetings. By midcentury, the old-fashioned, fanatical Thomsonian patent holders had shrunk in numbers, were disorganized, and lacked leadership. By this time, too, virtually all botanic groups and journals had dropped the name "Thomsonian."

The Neo-Thomsonians

Conflict with Thomson over policies involving education, therapeutics, as well as sale of "rights" and remedies had caused serious defections in the movement. In 1832, Horton Howard formed a faction in the Midwest, called the Improved Botanics, whose purpose was to streamline and improve Thomson's system. This was the first of the neo-Thomsonian groups to arise, but its progress was cut short by the death of Howard in 1833. The advent of Curtis's

Independent Thomsonian Botanic Society in 1838 marked the beginning of neo-Thomsonian activity that was to extend into the twentieth century. In the course of succeeding decades, various names were adopted by new Thomsonian practitioners, such as botanico-medical, physo-medical, physio-medical, physiopathist, and reform medical physicians. The neo-Thomsonian physicians sponsored such organizations as the Reformed Medical Association of the United States (1852), which initiated the Baltimore Platform;[7] the Middle States Reformed Medical Society (1852), whose membership came from New Jersey, Delaware, Virginia, Maryland, and Pennsylvania; and the Southern Reform Medical Association, organized about the same time, composed of members residing in Virginia, Alabama, Mississippi, Arkansas, Tennessee, and Kentucky. These organizations were infiltrated by the followers of Beach, and their memberships in the East and South succumbed in droves to the blandishments of the eclectics. Thanks to the vigilance of Alva Curtis, the organizational activity of the neo-Thomsonians in the Midwest remained fairly intact, and they preserved their identity under the name of physio-medical. In 1883, they formed the American Association of Physio-Medical Physicians and Surgeons, which continued to function as late as 1907.[8]

Besides the physio-medicals, other botanics laid claim to the Thomsonian healing arts and therefore deserve consideration under the broad umbrella of neo-Thomsonianism. These include Albert Isaiah Coffin (1790-1866), a New York Thomsonian who carried botanicism to England, and R. Swinburne Clymer (1878-1966), who promoted Thomsonianism from his residence in Allentown, Pennsylvania, well into the twentieth century.[9]

The Eclectics

It has been stated in the literature that the eclectic group was an offshoot from Thomsonianism, a dissident faction that gravitated toward the leadership of Wooster Beach (1794-1868),[10] but this statement has to be modified in light of the available evidence. Beach organized his sect independently in 1829, applying the generic designation "Reform" to his practice (reformed system of medicine or reformed practice of medicine), and simultaneously organized the Reformed Medical Society of the United States (1829) in New York.[11]

From the outset, Beach's group differed markedly in many of its practices and therapeutic measures from the Thomsonians.[12] In the words of historian John S. Haller Jr., "Although allopaths claimed that Wooster Beach and Samuel Thomson were spun from the same heretical cloth, reformed medical practice was as unlike Thomsonianism as was allopathy."[13] This did not prevent the "Beachites" from adopting some of the features of Thomsonianism and independent botanicism, as well as borrowing extensively from the regulars. Indeed, "borrowing" was developed into a fine art by the eclectics under the high-sounding slogan appropriated from Rafinesque; they were proud to be known as "those who select and adopt in practice, whatever is found most beneficial, and who change their prescriptions according to emergencies, circumstances and acquired knowledge."[14] In 1848, the American Eclectic Association was formed; its name was changed to National Eclectic Medical Association during the succeeding year. This organization, moribund after 1857, was revived again in 1870. The last of the eclectic medical schools, the Eclectic Medical Institute of Cincinnati, closed in 1939.[15]

The Organized, Independent Botanic Groups (Unaffiliated with the Thomsonians or Eclectics)

As indicated earlier, there is a baffling paucity of data concerning the activities, programs, strength, etc., of the organizations calling themselves New York Association of Botanic Physicians and Pennsylvania Associate Medical Society of Botanic Physicians. The New York group came into existence primarily as a defensive measure against restrictive medical legislation passed by the state legislature in 1827.[16] Credit for organizing this group belongs to Elisha Smith (d. ca. 1830), who became its president and, as we have seen in the previous chapter, produced the first treatise to attempt a scientific synthesis of the botanic practice.

After the death of Smith, the association became inactive but was revived by his son, Isaac S. Smith, who also founded an uncharted botanic medical school in the state, which ceased operation in 1846.[17] The Pennsylvania group was organized about 1833 by a Dr. John B. Howell (d. 1839), "earliest practitioner of Botanic medicine in Philadelphia," who emigrated to this country from England in 1793, subsequently becoming the society's first president.[18] The most important figure, however, to be associated with the Pennsylvania group was Thomas Cooke (d. 1855), of Philadelphia, student of Howell and editor of the influential journal *The Botanic Medical Reformer and Home Physician,* which was published in Philadelphia for three years—from 1840 to 1842.

From the very outset, Cooke made it clear that his group took "an *independent stand.*"[19] He announced his intention of working for a union of all botanic factions[20] and singled out for special praise Nicholas Culpeper, Samuel Thomson, Elisha Smith, Wooster Beach, and Horton Howard, as having contributed most to the development of botanicism.[21] A few years later, Cooke went over—lock, stock, and barrel—to the "Beachites," and in 1850, he helped found the Eclectic Medical College of Pennsylvania.[22]

SAMUEL THOMSON AND HIS FOLLOWERS

The nineteenth century witnessed the growth of numerous medical sects in the United States.[23] Of these, Thomsonianism, perhaps the most vociferous and belligerent, is of interest not only to the historian of pharmacy and medicine but also to the student of Americana. Thomsonianism was not confined to advocating a medical system of plant and steam therapy allegedly superior to the regular practice, nor did it base its appeal entirely on censuring chemical (especially calomel) medication and bleeding. The sincere Thomsonians also regarded their cause as a crusade to protect the people against the monopolistic designs of the "Mineral Faculty."

Thomsonianism gained adherents rapidly and was the first of the botanico-medical groups in the United States that rose up in revolt against orthodox medicine during the nineteenth century. The movement spread so rapidly that John Thomson, writing in 1841 about the success of his father's system, exclaimed enthusiastically, "who can look upon the prosperity of the Thomsonian practice of the present day without admiration—spread as it has from Mexico to Canada, and from the sea shore back to the Pacific, also in Europe and South America, originating with the illiterate New Hampshire farmer, less than fifty years since."[24]

This estimate of the popularity of Samuel Thomson's theories was undoubtedly exaggerated, but Thomsonianism did gain a foothold abroad, especially in England, where it was vigorously promoted by A. I. Coffin.[25] Coffin came to botanical healing through his own bout with what was undoubtedly a serious upper respiratory infection. Unable to get satisfactory treatment from the medical establishment, Coffin accepted the ministrations of a Seneca Indian woman who restored him to health with "an apronful of herbs."[26] Coffin's loss of faith in the regular medical profession was replaced by a belief in the healing power of herbs. "Indulgent nature," he declared, "provides a fitting remedy for every ill that flesh is heir to."[27] Moreover, he disdained the pretensions of the learned physicians and insisted that "the children of nature in their wild unlettered state, have knowledge sufficient to enable them to overcome the power of disease, and protract life to a very advanced age."[28] Much to his delight and surprise he found that he was not the first to express these ideas. Samuel Thomson had been doing so for some time, and Coffin was determined to meet this medical savant. Coffin became a Thomsonian agent in Troy, New York, but soon decided that Europe would be a more suitable arena for his system of health and healing than the provincial towns of a fledgling republic. In 1837, he moved to France but had most of his unlicensed medicines confiscated by the post-Napoleonic customs authorities at Le Havre.[29] Coffin found a more receptive audience in England, where, after a few false starts, he began lecturing to appreciative working-class throngs in the urban slums of the northern districts. Similar to his mentor in America, Coffin appointed agents who then established "Friendly Botanico-Medical Societies." "The movement spread like a prairie fire," writes historian Barbara Griggs. "By 1850 there were branches in every major city in the industrial North—the Coffin heartland—as well as London, where he now had a handsome house at 24 Montague Place . . ."[30] As popular as he was, however, he modeled himself too closely on his beloved Thomson. A general contentiousness and bitter rivalry with John Skelton, an herbalist from Devon who had done for eclecticism what Coffin had done for Thomsonianism, caused Coffin's botanical movement to disintegrate. By the time of Coffin's death in 1866, he was all but forgotten. When he was remembered, it was usually with a sardonic comment that failed to appreciate his pioneer efforts in bringing a truly American brand of herbalism to the mother country, proving only that fame and reputation in popular medicine can be as ephemeral as any other endeavor that rests upon the whim of the crowd.

Biographical Note on Samuel Thomson

At at an early age, Samuel Thomson had shown a keen interest in the therapeutic possibilities of the plants growing in profusion throughout the countryside. In his autobiography, bound with his *New Guide to Health,* he related that, while working in the fields, "My mind was bent on learning the medical properties of such vegetables as I met with, and was constantly in the habit of tasting everything of the kind I saw."[31]

Repelled by the curative measures of the regular physicians, Thomson began to treat his family and neighbors with his herbs, and soon, becoming convinced that he had a gift for treating the sick, he decided to abandon farming. In his own words, "I finally concluded to make use of the gift which I thought nature or the God of nature had implanted in me; and if I possessed such a gift, I had no need of learning, for no one can learn that gift."[32]

In due time, he formulated a highly speculative theory of disease that, despite all its pretensions to originality, was merely a modified version of Galen's humoral pathology. "I found, after maturely considering the subject," wrote Thomson, "that all animal bodies are formed of the four elements, earth, air, fire, and water. Earth and water constitute the solids, and air and fire, or heat, are the cause of life and motion. That cold, or lessening the power of heat, is the cause of all disease . . . that a state of perfect health arises from a due balance or temperature of the four elements."[33]

At first Thomson attempted to use lobelia as a universal remedy, by which he meant a medication that would "increase the internal heat, remove all obstruction to the system, restore the digestive powers of the stomach, and produce a natural perspiration," and so be applicable in all cases of disease.[34] Finding that lobelia alone did not meet the requirements of a single cure-all, he decided to supplement this drug with other medication, such as capsicum and bayberry. Eventually, he employed some sixty-five or more plant drugs, a list of which was published in the *Lobelia Advocate* in 1838.[35]

Subsequently, the Thomsonian armamentarium consisted not only of plant drugs but also of steam baths, medicated enemas, and emetics, especially lobelia. Regular physicians were quick to refer to Thomsonian practitioners as "steam doctors" or "puke doctors." Chemical medication and any substance that Thomson considered poisonous were strictly proscribed.

A large part of Thomson's *Narrative of the Life and Medical Discoveries of Samuel Thomson* is devoted to a recital of diseases cured by him with monotonous regularity. Other parts of his autobiography describe such vicissitudes as his struggle with regular physicians, the duplicity of his agents, and his many sacrifices for the common good. A high point in the *Narrative* is his account of his imprisonment and trial in 1809 on a charge of having killed a patient with lobelia. In a taxonomic faux pas of major proportions, Manasseh Cutler (1742-1823), the famous botanist, testified in court that what the prosecution considered lobelia was in reality marsh rosemary, a relatively harmless herb. The prisoner was thereupon acquitted for lack of evidence, after his trial had become a cause célèbre of the time.

Thomson was consistent to the end. According to Lloyd, "Fanatically zealous in his cause, an advocate of the Thomsonian course of medication in all that the course implied, he passed from life heroically partaking of lobelia, enemas, and the recognized Thomsonian syrups, teas, etc."[36]

PATENTS, AGENCIES, AND SALE OF RIGHTS

The Thomsonian patents were unique because they covered not only Thomson's medications but his system of medical practice as well. Thomson was granted his first patent in 1813 and applied for and received a second one in 1823 to eliminate existing loopholes. At the request and advice of the National Thomsonian Convention, Thomson had this patent renewed in 1836.

According to Kebler,[37] "The word 'patent' means open, not secret. A patent cannot be granted for a medicine of secret composition. The term 'Patent Medicine' applied to a medicine of secret composition is a misnomer." Kebler hastens to add, however, that "patenting a product does not preclude fairy tales about it. In fact, therapeutic claims contained in the description of some of the patents for medicines are grossly false and fraudulent. . . ."[38] This was particularly true in the early days of the Patent Office.[39]

It is interesting to note that while literally hundreds of nostrums and secret remedies flooded the American market during Thomson's lifetime,[40] only about seventy-five patents were granted for medicines from 1790 to 1836, an average of less than two per year. The first medical patent was issued in 1796 to Dr. Perkins for his "metallic tractors." Thomson's 1813 patent was the twenty-sixth granted in the United States for medical purposes and is listed as *Fever Medicine.* The one he obtained in 1823 is simply referred to as *Medicine* in the Index of *Unnumbered* patents.[41]

Thomson's 1836 patent reads "Thomson's Improved System of Botanic Practice of Medicine." Kebler states that "[t]he Patent as written up in the 'Restored Patents' volumes covers nearly four pages of foolscap paper in excellent longhand. It is the last of the unnumbered patents granted for medicines by the United States Patents office."[42]

Samuel Thomson's purpose in obtaining his patents was twofold. First, to use his own words:

> In obtaining a patent it was my principal object to get protection of the government against the machinations of my enemies more than to take advantage of a monopoly; for in selling family rights, I convey to the purchaser the information gained by thirty years practice, and for which I am paid a sum of money as an equivalent.[43]

In the second place, Thomson sought this type of legal protection to circumvent, in some degree, the medical legislation aimed at restricting his movement. As he expressed it:

> [I wanted to] put myself and medicine under the protection of the laws of my country which would not only secure to me the exclusive right to my system and medicine, but would put me above the reach of the laws of any state.[44]

Family rights were sold by his agents, subagents, and by Thomson himself. The following family right issued to one Joseph Chapman will illustrate the modus operandi:[45]

No. 1398   *Seventh Edition*[46]

This may certify that we have received of Joseph Chapman, Twenty Dollars, in full for the right of preparing and using, for himself and family, the medicine and System of Practice secured to Samuel Thomson by Letters Patent from the President of the United States, and that he is thereby constituted a member of the Friendly Botanic Society, and is entitled to an enjoyment of all the privileges attached to membership therein.

Dated at Alton this 19th day . . . 1839.

R. P. Maxey
Agt. for Pike, Platt and Co.
Agents for Samuel Thomson

All Purchasers of Rights can have intercourse with each other for advice, by showing their Receipt. All those who partake, or have no right to sell, can show no receipt, either from me or any of my agents, and are not to be patronized by you or any honest man, as they are liable to sixty dollars fine for each and every trespass. Hold no counsel or advice with them or with any who shall pretend to have made any improvement on my System of Practice, as I cannot be responsible for the effect of any such improvement. "Resist the devil and he will flee from you." (James 4:7)

Samuel Thomson

The number of agents that Thomson had in the field is difficult to specifically ascertain. During his lifetime, Thomson frequently had cause to revoke agencies and often entered into litigation against them. Despite the internal strife of these sectarians, however, their impact was appreciable. John Haller has indicated that "regulars and botanics alike acknowledged that at least a million people were practicing Thomsonian medicine."[47]

THE DECLINE OF THOMSONIANISM

The tremendous grassroots appeal of Thomson's populist medicine could not be maintained, however. Thomson's inability to control his own agents, legal wrangling over patent rights, and Thomson's intransigent refusal to establish a formal educational structure for the movement would spell its demise.

Annual national conventions—marked by contention and acrimony—were held from 1832 until 1838. At the second gathering (Pittsburgh, 1833), a resolution was passed to establish a national Thomsonian Infirmary in Baltimore. The following year, in Boston, the convention voted to boycott apothecary shops. Finally, at the 1838 meetings in Philadelphia, Thomson requested that the convention be permanently dissolved, since the irreconcilable divisions in the ranks, which he had foreseen, had indeed materialized.[48]

It was at this 1838 convention that Alva Curtis, the editor of *The Thomsonian Recorder,* who had replaced Thomas Hersey, split with Thomson and formed the "Independent Thomsonian Botanic Society," while those Thomsonians loyal to the founder formed the "United States Thomsonian Society."[49] Thereafter, according to Wilder, "Only the State Society of Delaware signified its adherence to the old ways. The evidences of disintegration were manifest."[50]

Alva Curtis (1797-1880) was the foremost advocate of medical school education among the Thomsonians. In 1834, Curtis had arrived at Columbus, Ohio, from Richmond, Virginia, where he had been teaching languages at a girls' school.[51] While residing in Richmond, he had purchased Thomsonian rights and had become a practitioner. Waite states that Curtis's advocacy of abolitionist principles made him persona non grata in Richmond.[52] Soon after his arrival in Columbus, Curtis replaced Hersey as editor of *The Thomsonian Recorder,* then in its third volume. For a while, he professed complete loyalty to the principles of Samuel Thomson, but it soon became apparent to the founder that Curtis had plans and ambitions of his own.

At the fourth national convention that had been held in Richmond, in 1835, a resolution was passed in connection with the proposed National Infirmary at Baltimore. It established professorships in the theory and practice of medicine, physiology and midwifery, surgery and surgical anatomy, and chemistry and medical botany. It also proclaimed that "this school shall be in strict accordance with the principles and practice of Dr. Thomson, as laid down in his Guide" and provided for the dismissal of any professor whose "departure from the principles (medical) of Dr. Thomson shall be detected."[53]

This was obviously a move by the Curtis faction to pull the wool over the founder's eyes. Not content with this subterfuge, Curtis also published a garbled version of Thomson's address at the fourth national convention, making it appear that Thomson supported wholeheartedly the proposed scheme for a medical school.[54] Moreover, Alva Curtis also expressed his grandiose plans in an editorial, calling for the establishment of botanic schools in Maryland, Georgia, Mississippi, Tennessee, Ohio, New York, and "several among the Yankees."[55]

Thomson's response was immediate and unequivocal. "I . . . hereby give notice," he fumed, "that I never will subscribe to any Literary College, or any other institution wherein and whereby books are to take the lead. . . . The object of the Hospital, or Infirmary, which I proposed to the Convention at the beginning, and which I continued to urge the necessity of, was to be mechanical, like a carpenter's shop. . . . But the moment you blend the simplicity of my discoveries with the abstruse sciences, such as chemistry and other discoveries that have nothing to do with medicine, that moment the benefit of my discoveries will be taken from the people generally, and, like all other crafts, monopolized by a few learned individuals."[56]

Despite all his efforts, Samuel Thomson could not deter the increasingly numerous advocates of formal medical education, and in April 1836, he withdrew his support from *The Thomsonian Recorder.*[57] Curtis expressed pained surprise and bewilderment at this move, but he was probably secretly glad that such a break had occurred—a break that was to become final in 1838.

In the meantime, Curtis had founded a Botanico-Medical School and Infirmary in Columbus and had begun to petition the Ohio legislature for a charter. Soon Curtis was able to report to his readers that the "infant school" was prospering (twelve students at the first session).[58] Five months later, Alva Curtis proclaimed in *The Thomsonian Recorder* that a comprehensive course of instruction, lasting from six to eighteen months, was available to those who wished a thorough knowledge of the botanic practice. Furthermore, he was prepared to offer to ambitious students all the instruction available in regular proprietary medical schools. He cautioned, however, that "[a] minute acquaintance with Anatomy, Surgery and other branches of the old theories and practices, demand a longer period."[59]

The followers of Wooster Beach, at the Worthington Medical School, Ohio, wrote scathingly of Curtis's school and of his attempt to obtain a charter: "For a single individual at this enlightened day of investigation, to spring up in the midst of an intelligent community and proclaim himself a flourishing Medical Institution . . . is what in our opinion, would justly stagger human belief," they scoffed. Calling Curtis's efforts the product of "overgrown pretensions" and a remarkable example of "modern arrogance and impudence," they doubted its equal in "the annals of human folly."[60]

Nonetheless, in 1839, Curtis's efforts were crowned with success. The Legislature of the State of Ohio granted a charter to the Literary and Botanico-Medical Institute of Ohio, which then became the second chartered sectarian medical school in the country.

Thomsonianism is credited by most historians of medicine as having produced several chartered botanico-medical schools. Although these schools were a far departure from the principles laid down by Samuel Thomson, it seems clear that the Thomsonian impulse sparked more than a few schools. "Several dozen colleges opened between 1829 and 1860," writes Haller, "nine by the Independent Thomsonians, including one begun initially as a combination of Thomsonian and eclectic; the remaining schools were based on the teachings of Wooster Beach and his American school of reform. . . . Most reform schools began as botanically-based institutions and transformed over time into more liberal eclectic schools."[61]

Perhaps more enduring than these botanic schools was the impact of Thomsonianism on pharmacy and materia medica. By the 1840s and 1850s, even mainstream pharmacy was influenced by the repurcussions of the movement. "Thomsonism had clearly entered the public domain," concludes Haller, "as apothecaries and retail houses that earlier refused to use the name now accepted it as part of the lexicon of American botanic practice."[62]

ATTITUDE TOWARD REGULAR PHARMACY

Thomsonian and early botanic physicians regarded regular apothecaries and pharmacists of the period with undisguised hostility. These practitioners considered the druggist or apothecary a purveyor of poisons, in league with the "mineral doctors" and not above adulterating drugs.

It is not surprising, then, that the Thomsonians, aided by the total absence of legislative regulation, developed a pharmaceutical practice peculiar to their needs and system. They operated infirmaries, depots, and stores where medication was compounded and sold *in direct competition* with regular apothecaries and druggists.

As has been pointed out earlier, the third national Thomsonian convention at Baltimore, in 1834, passed a resolution boycotting regular drug and apothecary stores. Thomson's followers and some of the early botanic practitioners held emphatic views on patronizing regular pharmacies, to judge from the editorial commentary in their journals.

In 1841, the letter of a perplexed reader was printed in *The Botanic Medical Reformer:* "I should like to hear your opinion on the druggists of these United States selling medicines of the Botanic order. I think no Botanic should buy of a druggist. I should like to see something relative to that matter in the Recorder." To which the editor replied, "We have always been of the opinion that the Botanic as well as the Thomsonian medicines should be kept separate, and under no considerations ought we to encourage apothecaries in vending our medicines."[63]

Alva Curtis, commenting on this policy, wrote:

> We do believe that, as a general rule, it is not safe to buy Botanic medicines of the regular apothecaries. They are liable to be poisoned by the accidental dropping of a portion of the scientific Samsons. Whether by accident or not, cayenne bought of apothecaries has been found adulterated with red lead, and ginger with corn meal. But we have not much confidence in the moral honesty of men, who for filthy lucre, will sell in this enlightened age, poisons for medicines, to anyone that will buy them. Besides, if anything can be honestly made by dealing in genuine medicines, it should be conscientiously

given to those who have suffered for their adoption of truth and adherence to its dictates.[64]

In 1842, this same journal warned its subscribers, "We have frequently cautioned our readers as well as the friends of Botanic and Thomsonian medicines generally, to beware of purchasing the articles we make use of from what is generally termed, regular apothecary shops."[65]

The generally low standards of training and education of pharmacists, the absence of licensing, the widespread adulteration of imported drugs, led the Thomsonians and botanics of that period to make wild accusations. Benjamin Colby, a follower of Thomson, wrote in the preface of his book *A Guide to Health*, "The imposition practiced by medical men in writing their prescriptions in Latin, and the evils resulting from it by the ignorance or carelessness of apothecaries or their clerks, who may know nothing about the language in which the prescription is written—the mistakes of whom have destroyed thousands of lives, are too obvious to be misunderstood."[66]

Despite all exhortations by leaders of Thomsonian and early botanic factions, some of the trade trickled into regular drug channels, as illustrated by an advertisement that appeared in the *Richmond Enquirer* of November 13, 1846. Peyton Johnson, druggist, was offering for sale "Thomsonian Medicines . . . Nerve Powder, Lobelia, Golden Seal, Bayberry No. 6, Cholera Syrup and all other herbs and medicines used in the practice."[67] Evidence indicates that certain regular druggists were imitating and selling Thomsonian remedies, since occasional warnings appear in the Thomsonian journals informing the public to beware of buying imitation Thomsonian medicine from regular pharmacists.[68]

In the main, the views expressed by Elias Smith (1769-1846),[69] regarding pharmacy, typify the thinking of many Thomsonian practitioners. This self-styled "Minister of the New Testament and Botanic Physician" was opposed to the separation of pharmacy and medicine: "There must be some craft in all this," he hinted darkly.[70] "A *physician* is the only man suitable for an *apothecary,* and an *apothecary,* the only man capable of being a *physician,*" Smith announced.[71] Smith boasted that he had opened up an establishment in Boston despite his modest resources and the hostility of the regular druggists.[72] Characteristic also of the Thomsonian and early botanic attitude toward pharmacy was Smith's condemnation of the traditional Latin prescription, which he regarded as an insidious stratagem to fool the people.[73]

MANUFACTURE, SALE, AND DISTRIBUTION OF REMEDIES

A large-scale distribution and sale of Thomsonian remedies existed in the United States during the height of the movement. John Uri Lloyd, writing in 1909, observed that stocks of medications carried by some Thomsonian agents would have appeared extensive enough to astonish drug dealers in the first decade of the twentieth century.[74] A careful examination of the available data has been made by the authors of this study in an attempt to evaluate the pharmaceutical activity of the Thomsonian movement.

Advertisements in Thomsonian and lay publications offer some indication of the scope of pharmaceutical practice carried on by infirmaries, depots, and itinerant agents. For this reason, it is appropriate to cite some typical advertisements, not only for their pharmaceutical significance, but also to illustrate their distinctive phraseology. Thus, for example, the Thomsonian firm of Godfrey Meyer and Company of Columbus, Ohio, proclaimed in 1835 that it had secured a steam mill with an eight-horsepower engine for the exclusive purpose of manufacturing and selling Thomsonian botanic medicines.

John Thomson frequently advertised his wholesale and retail establishment at 343 Broome Street, in New York City, where he offered the "sale of his valuable medicines, which will be administered by competent hands to all who may desire them and to such as can get no relief from the physicians. Also constantly on hand, wholesale and retail, his celebrated Anti-Dyspeptic Wine Bitters, an anti-scorbutic syrup for Scrofula and all impurities of the Blood." As an added attraction, Thomson offered to show his customers letters from the Kings of France and Prussia, as well as a gold medal from Louis Phillippe.[75] John Thomson had received these letters and the gold medal by the simple expedient of sending to these royal personages his 1841 edition of the *Thomsonian Materia Medica,* which bore his father's name on the front page. He was thus belatedly borrowing the advertising technique of Wooster Beach, who had been deluged with medals and testimonials from foreign potentates, including the Pope, for his book *The American Practice of Medicine.*

D. L. Hale advertised the "New England Thomsonian Depot" of Boston, in Samuel Emmons's book, *The Vegetable Family Physician.* Among the items listed were dental instruments, trusses, nursing bottles, "Anti-Dyspeptic Bread," "Injection Powder," Shaker herbs, syringes, etc. Hale boasted that his establishment was the largest and conducted a more extensive trade than any other Thomsonian depot in America, stating that his medicines were sent to all the states, to Mexico, the British provinces, Europe, Asia, and Africa[76] (see Appendix 8).

Referring to numerous people who had set themselves up surreptitiously as Thomsonian dealers in medicine, Thomson bitterly complained that

> many persons are practising by my system, who are in the habit of pretending that they have made great improvements and in some instances it is well-known that poisonous drugs have been made use of under the name of my medicine, which has counteracted its operation and thereby tended to destroy the confidence of the public in my system of practice; this has never been authorized by me.

Alluding to the misuse of his system and his materia medica, he stated,

> The avarice of designing and dishonest men stepped in to do what the whole learned Faculty of mineral doctors could not do, viz., put it down by making the people lose confidence in it. These men pretended to be my agents, stole my name, and under it put forth spurious medicines, to speculate upon the public health. Some that were regular agents at first, violated their contracts, and set up for themselves under my name and manufactured inferior medicines or compounded new ones which they called Thomsonian.[77]

In vain did Samuel Thomson resort to lawsuits, exhortations, and public announcements in an attempt to control the manufacture, sale, and distribution of Thomsonian medications. Unauthorized dealers, attracted by lucrative possibilities, continued to crop up as quickly as Thomson could put them down. With the disintegration of the movement mentioned earlier, the sale of Thomsonian remedies ceased, by and large, to be a profitable venture.

In 1839, Thomson was prosecuted for a libel against Paine D. Badger, a self-styled Thomsonian doctor who had set himself up in general practice without authorization from the founder *(Commonwealth of Massachusetts v. Samuel Thomson)*. Although the defense was able to show that Badger had been operating surreptitiously, it could not prove the accusation made by Thomson that Badger had opened a letter addressed to Thomson, with the intention to defraud. As a result, Thomson was fined fifty dollars.

Badger's prosecution of Thomson was prompted by a notice appearing in the *Boston Traveller* of January 25, 1839, illustrating a frequent technique that the founder used to discredit troublesome competitors:

BEWARE OF IMPOSTERS

Mr. Editor: Seeing in your paper a notice that P. D. Badger, Botanic Physician, has returned to this city and resumed his professional duties (not impositions;) said Badger has strove hard to sail under my flag for several years, both in this city and Nashua, where he has been met with deserved contempt and put down. He finding himself not able to sail under Thomsonian, has substituted Botanic Physician, (not impostor.) I would ask said Dr. Badger a few questions. Did you or did you not open a letter of mine, at 554 Washington-street, and agree to answer for medicine of fifty dollars, and have it ready for Wm. Kinsley by tomorrow noon, which I discovered and answered myself? Did you not sell and clear out to escape an indictment? Depend on it Sir, you are not yet out of danger. You had better clear again and hire some more Lectures written for you to read to your imposed audience; when questioned you could not answer a word nor show a particle of my medicine or authority from me. When you were advertised in Nashua, did you not clear out with the loss of several hundred dollars, as your patients would not pay for your deceptions, as neither law or justice demands it? I say beware of the man; also Clark and Wilder, who sail under a Thomsonian flag in Pleasant-street. Also H. Winchester and William Johnson, Hanover-place, Dealers in spurious Medicines.

Boston, Jan. 25, 1839
Samuel Thomson[78]

On the witness stand, Badger made several significant statements and admissions under questioning: "My patients refused to pay me several hundred dollars," Badger testified, "because they said Thomson called me an imposter, which I was not. . . . Most all Dr. Thomson's agents are charged with being impostors. Most all the Infirmaries of Boston have run down on that account. Dr. Thomson wants to monopolize it all to himself."[79] Badger admitted under examination that he had no authorization from Thomson to sell or compound medications or to operate an infirmary.

Several important points regarding Thomsonian pharmacy were brought out during the course of the trial. First of all, to prevent spurious medicines from being compounded, Thomson required a bond of $5,000 from his agents. How many agents were thus bonded is not clear. This measure seems to have been adopted in the 1930s to ensure that the agents sold *only* bonafide Thomsonian medicines, a lesson learned after many painful experiences with some of his agents. Second, this bond was accompanied by a schedule of prices above which the agent was not permitted to sell his medicines. The schedule was intended by Thomson to protect the public and maintain standard prices. Last, the agent was not permitted to compound his own medicines but had to purchase them from Thomson or his designated principal agents.

David L. Cowen has unearthed an interesting legal statement concerning the licensing of botanic or Thomsonian "apothecaries" in the state of Georgia.[80] In 1847, the Georgia Legislature had enacted a law establishing a Botanico-Medical Board of Physicians, whose purpose was to regulate the botanic or Thomsonian practice of medicine. The law provided, among other things, that

. . . no Botanic or Thomsonian apothecary within this State unless he be a graduate [of the local Thomsonian medical school] . . . or a licensed Botanic or Thomsonian physician, shall be permitted to vend or expose to sale Botanic or Thomsonian medicines, without previously obtaining a license from the Board created by this act. . . . Provided that nothing herein be so construed as to prevent merchants or shop-keepers from vending or exposing to sale Botanic or Thomsonian medicines already prepared.

. . . The Board of Physicians created by this act shall have the power to examine any apothecary who may apply to it for a license, touching their knowledge of drugs and pharmacy, and on finding such persons qualified shall grant such license.[81]

Virtually all the early Thomsonian and botanic physicians compounded and dispensed their own medications. However, as we have already seen, some persons were devoted full time to the manufacture and sale of Thomsonian remedies, for example, Ward Sears and Company; Godfrey Meyer and Company; as well as others. We have been unable to discover any evidence to indicate whether the 1847 Georgia act relating to Thomsonian apothecaries was ever enforced.[82]

THOMSON'S "SIX NUMBERS" AND OTHER REMEDIES

A large portion of the Thomsonian materia medica (see Appendix 1) was divided by the founder into six classes based on the properties and uses of the respective drug or drugs. These plant drugs were administered as powders, tinctures, syrups, infusions, in enemas, etc.

"No. 1" consisted of only *Lobelia inflata,* Thomson's most vaunted and cherished medicine, which was employed in tincture form for asthma. In addition, the powdered leaves and pods were steeped in warm water to make infusions. Lobelia was also mixed in prescribed amounts with other plant ingredients or added to medicated enemas. The emetic property of No. 1 was guaranteed by Thomson "[t]o cleanse the stomach, overpower the cold, and promote a free perspiration."[83]

Capsicum was the drug of choice in the second class of medications, referred to as "No. 2." Other drugs in this group were ginger
(Zingiber officinale) and black pepper *(Piper nigrum).* This group
of preparations was calculated "to retain the internal vital heat of
the system and cause a free perspiration."[84]

"No. 3," or the third group, included bayberry *(Myrica cerifera);*
white pond lily root *(Nymphaea odorata);* the inner bark of hemlock spruce *(Tsuga canadensis);* marsh rosemary root *(Limonium
carolinianum);* sumac bark, leaves, and berries *(Rhus glabra);*
witch hazel leaves *(Hamamelis virginiana);* wild red raspberry
leaves *(Rubus idaeus);* and squaw weed (Thomson called this *Erigeron purpureum,* although most *Erigeron* spp. are known commonly as fleabane; squaw weed is generally considered *Senecio aureus,*
so Thomson's usage here is open to speculation). According to
Thomson, these drugs, alone or in combination, were able to "scour
the stomach and Bowels, and remove the Canker." Thomson
thought highly of this class of remedy. For example, he described
the medical virtues of bayberry as follows: "an excellent medicine,
either taken by itself or compounded with other articles; and is the
best thing for canker of any article I have ever found."[85]

The fourth group, or "No. 4," consisted of "Bitters to correct the
Bile, and restore Digestion." Barberry *(Berberis vulgaris),* balmony
(Chelone glabra), poplar bark *(Populus* spp.), bitter root *(Apocynum androsaemifolium),* and Ohio kercuma *(Frasera verticillata)*
made up this class of drugs.[86]

Thomson referred to his "No. 5" as "Syrup for the Dysentery, to
strengthen the Stomach and Bowels, and restore weak patients . . .
the articles used in this preparation are the bark of poplar and
bayberry, which have been described, peach-meats, or meats of
cherry-stones, sugar and brandy."[87]

"No. 6" was his famous "Rheumatic Drops," made with "high
wines, or fourth proof brandy, gum myrrh and cayenne; for external
application spirits of turpentine is added, and sometimes gum camphor."[88]

In addition, orthodox Thomsonian preparations included other
popular remedies, such as his "Nerve Powder," made up of cypripedium root used in half-teaspoon doses, and his "Composition or

Vegetable Powder," a preparation primarily of bayberry and ginger with a small amount of cayenne and clove. The drugs were pounded and triturated to a fine powder and sifted through a fine sieve. The dose was a teaspoonful of the powder and a teaspoonful of sugar mixed in a teacup of warm water. This remedy was reputed to be effective in cases of "relax, dysentery, pain in the stomach and bowels, etc." Other popular remedies were a "Strengthening Plaster," made with the extract of burdock and mullen leaves, rosin, and turpentine, and a "Nerve Ointment," made with bittersweet root, wormwood, chamomile, and animal fat.

The remainder of crude plants given in the list in Appendix 1 were widely used, alone or in combination with other drugs. In due time, Thomson's agents began to compound numerous remedies, using all sorts of combinations from the materia medica and, then, to the consternation of the founder, introduced new drugs and "improvements."

Thomson's reaction was to issue one of his typical proclamations to his followers:

> Those who have family rights are hereby cautioned against being imposed upon by spurious or adulterated articles, under the name of *Thomsonian Medicine,* as *Wine Bitters, Cholera Syrup, Cholera Preventive,* etc., etc., which, although they may have some value, yet, still, they are rather an imposition on the public than otherwise.[89]

This type of pronouncement obviously did not gladden his agents—it was bad for business. Nor was his recommendation for a "stock of medicine for a family" consisting of 1 ounce of emetic herb, 2 ounces of cayenne, ½ pound of bayberry root (in powder), 1 pound of poplar bark, 1 pound of ginger, and 1 pint of Rheumatic Drops conducive to large-scale enterprise.[90]

Despite the founder's exhortations, mentioned earlier, the agents went blithely on their way, some impelled to improve on Thomson, others feeling that doctrine should not interfere with business. The formulas of some typical preparations sold in Thomsonian establishments are given in Appendix 10.

Thomson and his agents bought crude plant drugs in enormous quantities. For example, Thomson wrote the following in his *Narrative:*

> I have collected about three hundredweight of the goldenseal the year past, and a large quantity of cayenne from the Island of Madagascar; nearly three tons. I have sent to the southern states nearly twenty barrels, floured, which is a great help in the agues of that country."[91]

It is worthy of more than passing notice that a careful analysis of Thomson's materia medica leaves one distinctly unimpressed. Thomson's botanical nomenclature—all-important in the proper identification of the plants to be used—was flawed; in some cases, it is unclear exactly what plant he was really recommending. The confusion of squaw weed with fleabane has already been noted parenthetically. However, Thomson also apparently identified goldenseal (generally known as *Hydrastis canadensis*) as *Frasera verticillata* (today known as *F. carolinensis* or American columbo). These confusions are all the more surprising given the fact that even a nodding acquaintance with the botanical and medical authorities of the period would readily have avoided these errors.[92]

CONCLUSION

A number of Thomsonian plant medicinals that were widely used by botanic practitioners eventually attracted the interest of pharmacists connected with the Philadelphia College of Pharmacy. It is interesting to note that William Procter's inaugural essay, published in 1837, was on *Lobelia inflata*.[93] This work has been described by John Uri Lloyd as being "the first credible chemical investigation of the plant."[94] Procter's interest in the pharmaceutical aspects of lobelia continued, for in 1842 he published an important paper in which he stated, "It has been generally admitted by Thomsonians and others that heat exercises an injurious influence on the activity of this plant, and hence preparations in which heat is requisite have been necessarily dispensed with."[95] Drawing on the experience of the Thomsonians, Procter then suggested four preparations of lobelia made without the use of heat, which would supplement the official tincture, namely, an acetous extract, a vinegar, a syrup, and an infusion.[96] Lloyd not only credited the old Thomsonians with realizing that heat destroyed the stability of their lobelia preparations but pointed out that Thomson's followers soon discovered that they could stabilize their lobelia recipes with acetic acid. "Empiricism demonstrated what chemistry supports."[97]

Edward Parrish, in his inaugural essay of 1842, published a pioneer chemical analysis of the root of *Statice caroliniana* (marsh rosemary, today known as *Limonium carolinianum*), a plant frequently used by the Thomsonians. Parrish wrote:

> Statice occupies an important place in the Materia Medica of the Thomsonian or Botanical system of medicine, and it is extensively used by Thomsonians as a tonic and emollient, as well as an astringent. A compound decoction, infusion and plaster, are recommended by them in the treatment of putrid sore throat, and they frequently employ it in other diseases.[98]

Similarly, Lawrence Turnbull published that same year a thesis on *Populus tremuloides,* in which he discussed its use in Thomsonian pharmacy and medicine, and presented a proximate analysis of the plant.[99]

The confusion resulting from the transformation and contraction of the old Thomsonian medical and pharmaceutical movement, the emergence of a neo-Thomsonian cult, and the rise of a strong eclectic movement are reflected in a significant statement read at a meeting of the American Pharmaceutical Association in 1853:

Committee Report

> We are not able to report satisfactorily to the amount of Botanic medicines sold. As this branch of the trade has undergone considerable change within a few years; what was then confined to a few herbs and simples, now embraces a wide range of vegetable medicines. Indeed, the present *"Eclectic System"* bids fair to annihilate the old Thompsonian [sic] practice. The practitioners of this school place but comparatively

few of our officinal articles under their ban,—and these mostly corrosive poisons,—while they are introducing new vegetable preparations, (Alkaloids, so called). If we understand the term "Eclectic" in the sense they use it, we may soon see them educated in the regular practice.[100]

More than any other botanico-medical group, the eclectics were destined to play an important role in nineteenth-century American pharmacy, but not before Thomson's followers had made a concerted bid for scientific respectability.

Chapter 5

The Neo-Thomsonians

Stated in broad terms, neo-Thomsonianism represented the transformation of a movement that had for its base a mass of unevenly educated, fanatical patent right holders into a botanic movement seeking survival in scientific respectability. It most prominently manifested itself among the physio-medicals, who broadened the Thomsonian perspective to include educational institutions and a vitalistic doctrine that rested upon pseudoscientific concepts that bordered on the mystical. Also within the neo-Thomsonian fold, however, were botanics who continued to carry the Thomsonian banner long after the founder had departed, most notably A. I. Coffin, already discussed, and R. Swinburne Clymer, whose "Natura System" brought Thomson's healing arts into the twentieth century.[1]

This neo-Thomsonian trend was very marked by mid-nineteenth century and was most obvious in the emergence of the physio-medicals, a development that did not escape the attention of the discerning Worthington Hooker, who acutely appreciated the irony of the situation. Here was a group of botanic practitioners, sheepishly dropping the name "Thomsonian," forming medical schools, state medical societies, and boards of censors, and issuing diplomas in imitation of the regulars. Indeed, "they had thus the effrontery," wrote Hooker indignantly, "to ask that they might possess, in common with us, that which they have always branded an unjust and odious monopoly. This is a *morceau* in the history of Thomsonism [sic], too precious to be lost."[2] Besides appropriating some of the organizational and educational trappings of the regulars, Hooker also noted that the physios were expanding their materia medica, were using steam and emetics less frequently and with more caution, and were beginning to vaccinate for smallpox and employ cathartics, in contrast to the practice of the Thomsonians.[3] The implications of these changes, along with the pharmaceutical efforts of the physio-medicals, are worth noting.

THE NEW THERAPEUTICS

Despite all exhortations and opposition by Thomson, a considerable expansion in the Thomsonian materia medica had already taken place during the founder's lifetime. Ironically enough, while denouncing Howard and Mattson for their "mongrel improvements," Thomson himself had reluctantly, and with reservations, permitted his name to be used in connection with the pretentious 1841 edition of the *Thomsonian Materia Medica,* thus materially contributing to this neo-Thomsonian trend. As stated earlier, the original core of seventy plant drugs employed by the Thomsonians had been augmented fivefold and included, moreover, a number of minerals as well by the time Cook's *Physio-Medical Dispensatory* was published in 1869.

This was not all. Samuel Thomson's crude pronouncements about the nature of disease were elaborately restated by the physio-medical practitioners in quasiscientific and metaphysical terms. A vitalistic pathology was formulated in which disease was regarded as a unit, and fever proclaimed as a beneficent manifestation of the "life principle." The most authoritative expression of these views occurred in the Baltimore Platform of 1852 (see Appendix 2) and continued to be promulgated, with certain refinements, by this sect until the time of its virtual extinction in 1911.[4]

Great emphasis was laid by physio-medicals on the use of "sanative" or "nonpoisonous" medication. The regular practitioners, as well as physicians of other schools, were accused by William H. Cook of using poisonous and disease-producing remedies. Of the "allopathic" practitioners, Cook wrote as follows:

> The Allopathic rule in treatment seeks the removal of one disease by making another disease in its place . . . and this doctrine permeates everything that comes from Allopathy. Out of this springs its other proposition, *Ubi virus, ibi virtus—* where there is poison, there is virtue. If disease is to be made,

poisons must be used for the purpose; and it is only on this ground that calomel, antimony, arsenic, blisters, iodine, opium, veratrum, gelsemium, strychnine and other destructive agents were introduced as remedies. . . . Hence while that school has made much progress in Anatomy, Physiology, Symptomology, Diagnosis and kindred topics, it has steadily conformed its Materia Medica to the rule of using poisons; and its entire numbers and influence have ever been used to oppose every suggestion in practice that did not accord with its primeval pathology.[5]

In a savage attack against the eclectics, Cook denounced them for using "deleterious agents" and compiled a list of "poisons" that he claimed the eclectics were administering.[6]

A pertinent question to ask at this point is, How did the neo-Thomsonians define or determine what was "poisonous"? All their definitions were obscure and subjective, apparently being influenced by either grossly speculative or empirical factors. Definitions such as the following are given for a "poison": "Any article to which human experience attaches the term *poison* is dangerous to the human frame and at war with vitality,"[7] or "every means and process, which, in its nature and tendency, in authorized medicinal quantities, degrees or modes of application, has been known to have directly destroyed human life, or permanently injured the tissue or deranged the physiological action" (Baltimore Platform, see Appendix 2), or "every article, means or process of cure which . . . is directly antagonistic to the laws of vitality" (Union Platform of Principles, see Appendix 3). For example, during the meeting of the Illinois Physio-Medical Association in 1865, gelsemium and veratrum were considered deleterious within the meaning of these definitions and officially proscribed.[8] Taunted by his enemies for not having effective drugs to alleviate pain in the physio-medical materia medica, Cook retorted:

It is often charged against Physio-Medicalism, that it cannot relieve pain as effectively as can be done by the narcotics of Allopathy and Eclecticism. This is a mistake. Our agents can secure more effective relief . . . the [Physio-Medical] list already known is far greater than is generally supposed. Among them may be mentioned blue cohosh, mullen, bugle weed, cockle burr, Greek valerian, twin leaf, yellow poplar, and at least a dozen others. They are positive and reliable in giving relief to pain . . .[9]

Necessity sometimes forced the physios to accept medicinal agents or adopt curative measures that had been authoritatively pronounced deleterious by their leaders. An early, interesting example occurred in 1837, when the respectable editor of *The Southern Botanic Journal,* Dr. D. K. Nardin, scandalized his Thomsonian colleagues by advocating the use of quinine sulfate in "chills."[10] Nardin was severely scolded by William H. Fonerden, a prominent Thomsonian, who argued that "if Dr. Nardin may add one article to the [Thomsonian] materia medica I may add another, and so may others ad infinitum, until we have a volume as ponderous as Wood and Bache's American Dispensatory."[11] Furthermore, maintained Fonerden, Nardin was violating a basic principle of Thomsonian therapeutics, which always called for the use of general remedies: "A local specific is a general poison," Fonerden reminded Nardin. "This is a favorite axiom with Thomsonian physicians. To those I may add, 'a limited remedy is a general bane.' Is the sulphate of quinine, doctor, a limited or general remedy? Would you prescribe it in every case of disease? I know you would not."[12] Other arguments advanced by Fonerden against the use of quinine were that Dr. Thomson proscribed minerals, and since quinine sulfate was a combination of "a tonic extract of Peruvian bark and sulphuric acid," it could not be safely administered; also, it was "equivocal" in action, causing many side effects.

To these arguments, Nardin retorted that he could not see why quinine was more "equivocal" than many remedies in Dr. Thomson's materia medica; that although common table salt was composed of two deadly mineral poisons, and eggs contained sulfur, they were nevertheless consumed by everyone; and, finally, that Fonerden's remarks about general remedies were "overstrained."[13] As late as 1865, no agreement could be reached at a meeting of physio-medical practitioners as to whether to sanction the use of quinine,[14] and it was not until 1869 that all taint was removed from the drug, through its inclusion in Cook's *Physio-Medical Dispensatory* as a "sanative" remedy.[15]

There is reason to believe that the influence of independent botanic leaders such as Elisha Smith and Thomas Cooke served to accelerate the neo-Thomsonian trend. It will be recalled that Smith's *The Botanic Physician* (1830) was the first significant attempt at a scientific synthesis of the botanic practice. This work strongly emphasized the need for an expanded plant materia medica, and a judicious inclusion of some mineral remedies. It was noteworthy for its stress on the need to study all branches of medicine, including surgery. This approach was also taken by Thomas Cooke in the pages of his journal, *The Botanic Medical Reformer and Home Physician.* In a significant editorial, Cooke pointed to the contrast between the therapeutic practice of the independent botanic and the old-fashioned Thomsonian physician:

> The Thomsonian practitioners, it is pretty generally known, adhere strictly to the manner of practice recommended by Dr. Samuel Thomson, which consists principally of giving *courses* of medicine, such as stimulating, puking, steaming, and the shower bath, with such other directions as Dr. Thomson gives in his "New Guide," discarding in toto Cathartics, Laxatives, and other means recommended by well experienced Botanic authors. And we will here state that Botanic physicians, make use of all the articles recommended by Dr. Samuel Thomson, when they deem them necessary: hence, a Botanic practitioner has all the Thomsonian remedies, while the Thomsonian has no other except those which are laid down in the "New Guide." And we believe there is not a person living but would rather take any of our mild remedies, than resort to the *coursing* practice.[16]

By the 1840s, many physio-medicals had begun to practice what the independent botanic physicians had been preaching for considerably more than a decade. In 1865, William H. Cook announced heatedly that "very many people still think our system can do little else than give emetics and baths; and only a limited number of persons understand that we have an extended system of scientific principles."[17] Try as they might, however, the physios could never achieve more than a pseudoscientific therapeutics. As the century wore on, it became apparent that the dogma-ridden leaders of this ever-shrinking sect were unable to grasp the implications in the dramatic emergence of bacteriology, immunology, and synthetic organic medicinals. In 1907, a professor at the Physio-Medical College of Indiana warned his students that "if you ever hope to become expert in diagnosis and treatment of the sick, you must throw aside the pernicious doctrine of *disease-entity,* a *bacterial* pathology or a microbe disease maker, and *chemical therapeutics* or the doctrine that the living body is simply a chemical laboratory to be ruled only by the chemist. I do declare to you that the so-called 'disease germ' is a monumental medical bugbear, it is the greatest romanticism of the age."[18] Even as late as the 1920s, R. Swinburne Clymer talked about "[t]he coming enlightened practice" that would "gradually replace all forms of serums and toxins now used in the field of therapeutics."[19] Clymer went on to bemoan the end of Thomsonianism because, as he believed, "these natural remedies are coming into favor once again and may replace the great number of complicated chemical compounds many of which have been highly dangerous in practice."[20] Alas, Clymer's optimism was un-founded.

It seems appropriate to end this discussion of neo-Thomsonian therapeutics on a somewhat bizarre note. In 1906, a woman gradu-ate of the Physio-Medical College of Indiana received permission to matriculate for a course in obstetrics and gynecology in the medical school of the University of Strassburg on the strength of her diplo-ma and her Indiana State license. She addressed a letter to the editor of the *Physio-Medical Recorder* in which she praised the remarkable technical facilities of the University but contemptuously dismissed the prevailing therapeutics. "Of course," she wrote, "I would not for all the world give up my knowledge of Physio-Medical treatment for their superior technic."[21] She then proceeded to tell of her successful treatment of patients with "leptandra virg. and zingiber," and "as I had nothing else on hand I made a strong solution of No. 6 and bathed a burned hand. . . . The patient said 'it was a little hot,' but she thought it healed very fast."[22] For a fleeting instant, the ghost of Samuel Thomson, vindicated, hovered over the Medical Faculty of the University of Strassburg!

ORGANIZATIONAL PHASES
OF NEO-THOMSONIANISM

Not only did the Thomsonian materia medica and therapeutics begin to undergo transformations during the founder's lifetime, but serious organizational changes had also occurred. Toward the end of his life, the vision that Thomson had so hopefully nurtured over the years of a gigantic Friendly Botanic Society composed of citizens happily treating one another with Thomson's patented system, and avidly reading his *New Guide to Health,* was fast fading away. The first serious blow to this dream had been Howard's abortive defection in 1832, and the formation of the dissident "Improved Botanics." Thomson had surmounted this obstacle, however, only to be confronted six years later with the Curtis split.

One of Curtis's first acts in 1838 as the spearhead of this formidable rival group, the Independent Thomsonian Society, was to issue a policy statement:

> This result is to be regretted, as it has the appearance of a split in the Thomsonian ranks, and affords the regulars a plausible pretext for saying that the opposition to their abominable quackery is already divided, and will soon be conquered. . . . They [the regulars] need expect no sympathy from the "Independents" in their battles with Thomsonism [sic], nor any conniving with their quackery and murder. Thomsonians are divided, to be sure, into right and left wings, but the regulars will find the columns in both divisions sufficiently deep, active, and persevering, for all their purposes. The steam and lobelia practice, in its most essential features (which for Dr. Thomson's abuse of many of its purest friends and warmest advocates might forever have been called Thomsonian) under whatever name it may hereafter pass, is destined to out-live all others; and will yet be the fashionable practice of this nation and the world.[23]

Curtis's confident prediction that the two factions would present a solid front to the regulars never materialized; the gap between the left-wing Independent Thomsonians and the right-wing orthodox followers of Thomson widened rapidly. For a few years, the "old patriarch" was able to retain a modicum of organization among his dwindling followers through his United States Thomsonian Society. With the death of the founder in 1843, however, disorganization set in quickly among his remaining loyal supporters.

In little more than a decade after the 1838 schism, a remarkable transformation was discernible. The old Thomsonian crusading zeal, with all its color and fanaticism, was gone. With the abrogation of virtually all restrictive medical regulatory acts, a sense of security permeated the ranks of the neo-Thomsonian practitioners. To be sure, there were still the "poisons of Allopathy" to inveigh against, but the old cry against the monopolizing schemes of the "Mineral Faculty" was no longer tenable, since by this time the physios had erected a monopolistic apparatus of their own in the form of state societies, medical schools, boards of censors, diplomas, etc. The mass base of patent right-holding citizenry, which had formed the strength of the old Thomsonian movement and had given it an impressive grassroots flavor, had by this time almost melted away. In short, what had been a remarkable sociomedical movement was to become, as the century progressed, merely a small, ineffectual, pseudoscientific cult.

A series of important events occurred in 1852. That year a national meeting took place in Baltimore. After debating the adoption of various names, the convention decided to organize itself into the Reformed Medical Association of the United States, and Alva Curtis was elected as its first president.[24] Significantly, a resolution was passed to the effect that "those members of the Reformed Medical Profession who choose to assume the cognomen of *Thomsonian* or *Physio-Medical,* be considered as advocates of true sentiments, and be eligible to membership with us by signing our platform of principles." Curtis tried to pressure the convention to adopt physio-medical as the official name of the organization, but the majority voted to continue the name Medical Reform. In the end, however, Curtis had his way, since the term was soon adopted in practice after the Baltimore Convention.[25] In addition, practitioners from the five eastern states of Pennsylvania, Delaware, New Jersey, Maryland, and Virginia held their first annual meeting of the newly founded Middle States Reformed Medical Society.[26] Shortly thereafter, the Southern wing formed the Southern Reform Medical Association.[27]

Probably the most important result of the 1852 meeting of the Reformed Medical Association of the United States was the formulation of the Baltimore Platform. In the words of one of the speakers at this meeting, its object was to present to the world "a code of medical principles that the community may know what we propose . . . as substitutes for the various systems of medicine popular in our day, and to guard them against the injustice and injury to themselves and us, of attributing to us doctrines which we do not sanction."[28] What made this document significant was that it served as a test or standard as to who was or was not a genuine physio-medical. It also spelled out the basic tenets of their pathology and therapeutics.

In addition, a number of important resolutions were adopted by the Reformed Medical Association of the United States.[29] The members present pledged support of the three principal physio-medical schools then in existence.[30] It was also decided that three specified medical journals should be supported as reflecting the views of the assembled delegates.[31] One resolution stessed "the importance of encouraging the preparation of genuine sanative agents, and that our new school druggists, *in all cases,* should be patronized in preference to those of other schools,"[32] and another fixed a uniform scale of fees. Finally, it was decided to publish a "United States Reformed Medical Dispensatory," with the responsibility for the task assigned to the faculty of the Metropolitan Medical College in New York City.[33] It is interesting to note that the Reformed Medical Association of the United States ceased to exist after its first meeting in 1852,[34] and it was not until 1883 that a small group of physio-medical physicians were to organize another national body, called the American Association of Physio-Medical Physicians and Surgeons.

For several years, the Middle States Reformed Medical Society held annual meetings, but despite its pretentious claims, its membership remained very small. In 1854, the society's journal, *The Middle States Medical Reformer,* stated that the organization had only fifty members[35] but hastened to assure its readers that "[t]hese however, constitute, by no means, the whole number of New-School Practitioners in the five states composing our organization. The precise numbers we do not know, but so far as our information extends, there are over 500."[36] Requirements for membership in the

society were graduation from "any respectable and regularly organized medical college" or an apprenticeship of two years with satisfactory evidence of competence, as judged by the society's board of
censors.[37] Of course, adherence to the code and principles of physio-
medicalism was a sine qua non.

Of particular interest are the relations between the Middle States
Reformed Medical Society and the eclectics. In 1854, the society
made an alliance with the Eclectic Medical College of Pennsylvania, in which a Union Platform of Principles was signed by representatives of both organizations (see Appendix 3). This move was
greeted by Alva Curtis in the Midwest with a suspicious outburst:
"We are glad to learn that the Eclectic College has adopted this
resolution," he wrote, "but we must watch them . . . we have been
told that one of the doctrines of Eclecticism is, that every man is
responsible only for himself—that they reject all authority, and
make no pledges."[38]

At first it appeared as if the physios had swallowed up the eclectics. The editors of *The Middle States Medical Reformer* could not
contain their excitement and enthusiasm and proclaimed, "A new
era in medicine has commenced. The great brilliant science of medicine is now rising majestically above the horizon."[39]

The following year, the Middle States Reformed Medical Society
appointed five delegates to represent it in negotiations with the
National Eclectic Medical Association.[40] As it turned out, Curtis's
warning should have been heeded, for in the course of a few years,
the eastern eclectics gobbled up the society and its followers. A
similar fate overtook the Southern Reform Medical Association.[41]

All staunch and incorruptible physios rallied around Curtis and
Cook in the Midwest, where, henceforth, the sect demonstrated its
greatest strength. Wounded by the encroachments of the eclectics in
the East and South, Cook could only rage ineffectually: "It [eclecti-
cism] is today a more dangerous enemy to medical reform, than the
bitterest Allopathy is."[42]

For years after the "great schism" of 1838, the neo-Thomsonians
faced a dilemma in naming their organization. It will be recalled
that immediately after the split of 1838, the followers of Curtis
called themselves Independent Thomsonians, but this designation
was quickly changed to Botanico-Medicals. In 1851, Curtis, dis-

gruntled, announced, "We never liked the name 'Botanico-Medical' because botany includes all vegetables, bad as well as good. Still it answered our purpose well for thirteen years, and we resume it for the sake of uniformity."[43] The following year, just before the Baltimore convention, Curtis issued an ex cathedra statement:

> Let the *name*, then, be not Eclectic which signifies merely choosing and refusing (as all doctors do); nor Botanic, which signifies vegetable *poisoning* as well as *curing;* nor Thomsonian, which directs the mind as much to Thomson as his principles; nor Physopathic which signifies windy disease—But Physio-Medical, which signifies natural-medical, or curing according to nature. . . . This is the most appropriate name yet proposed.[44]

As mentioned earlier, Curtis's attempt to pressure the convention to adopt the name physio-medical failed to move the majority, but in the course of a few years, physio-medical became the recognized designation for those who identified with the organization.

No further organizational activity on a national level occurred among the physios until 1883, when a call was sent out "to every *true and genuine* Physio-Medicalist on the American Continent, to meet in a grand convention in the City of Indianapolis, Indiana, on the first Wednesday in May 1883, for the purpose of organizing a National Association."[45] The circular letter announcing this call was initiated by three state physio-medical societies (Indiana, Ohio, and Illinois)[46] and was signed by ninety-three names from "twenty-three States and Provinces."[47] Meeting at the designated time and place, the convention created the American Association of Physio-Medical Physicians and Surgeons. Forty-eight persons were designated charter members, and a Platform of Principles, Constitution, and By-Laws, along with a public statement, titled "An Address to the Public," were drawn up (see Appendix 4).

There is a record of the American Association of Physio-Medical Physicians and Surgeons meeting for a three-day annual convention in Dallas, Texas, as late as May 1907.[48] After this date, the fate of this organization, if it still existed, is completely obscured through lack of data.

THE PHYSIO-MEDICAL MEDICAL SCHOOLS

The establishment of the first chartered medical school by Alva Curtis in 1839 in Columbus, Ohio, was not only greeted with derision by the regulars and the "Beachites," but it also became the target of savage and sarcastic criticism by the orthodox Thomsonians. "It appears that the Curtico-Botanico-Medical College has been chartered by the Ohio Legislature," sneered the editor of *The Boston Thomsonian Manual.* "We had heard a great deal about Dr. Curtis and his school, and the wicked Legislature of Ohio, who would not grant him a charter, but we never dreamed that it was his intention to make the healing art an odious monopoly and imitate the regular medical profession by conferring a sheep-skin diploma. But so it is; and the Thomsonians must endeavor to rub along as well as they can without the aid of diplomas and colleges."[49]

To make matters worse, all staunch followers of Samuel Thomson were thrown into deep consternation when Dr. Lanier Bankston, the "Curtis of the South," secured a charter from the Georgia Legislature for the Southern Botanico-Medical College at Forsyth, Georgia, that same year.[50] Thus, with two schools opening in 1839, the new trend in education among the left-wing Thomsonian faction was off to a good start. Six more schools were to be chartered before 1861.

The following eight schools were chartered before the Civil War:[51]

1. *Literary and Botanico-Medical Institute of Ohio* (1839), Columbus, Ohio. This institution moved to Cincinnati in 1841. After many vicissitudes and changes of name, it finally became the Physio-Medical College of Ohio, closing in 1880.
2. *Southern Botanico-Medical College,* chartered 1839 at Forsyth, Georgia. Two grants of $5,000 each were voted to this school by the state legislature. The name of the college was changed to Reformed Medical College of Georgia in 1854. It was suspended in 1861. Revived in 1867, it again underwent a change in name, becoming the American College of Medicine in 1874. Finally, it merged with the Georgia Eclectic College in 1881.

3. *Alabama Medical Institute,* Wetumpka, Alabama. Received a charter in 1844, but closed the next year in 1845, after only one session. The faculty had been composed of seceding professors from the Southern Botanico-Medical College. Nonetheless, in an ironic twist, for a movement that had spent so much of its time opposed to formal medical training, the short-lived institute at Wetumpka holds the distinction of being Alabama's first medical school, preceding the Graefenburg Medical Institute by eight years and the medical school at Mobile by fifteen.[52]

4. *Botanico-Medical College of Memphis,* Memphis, Tennessee. Chartered in 1846, the faculty had come largely from the defunct Alabama Medical Institute. In 1859, the institution became eclectic, changing its name to Eclectic Medical Institute of Memphis. The college closed in 1861.

5. *Scientific and Eclectic Medical Institute of Virginia,* Petersburg, Virginia. Chartered in 1847, this school was eclectic in name only.[53] Torn asunder by faculty squabbles, the college lasted only a few years.

6. *Worcester Medical School,* Worcester, Massachusetts. This school was established in 1846 but was unsuccessful in obtaining a charter from the Massachusetts legislature. To circumvent this situation, the Worcester school made an ingenious arrangement to become a branch of the Southern Botanico-Medical College, located approximately 700 miles away. In this capacity, and using the name Worcester Botanico-Medical College, it was able to grant degrees in 1846 and 1847 under the charter of the Georgia institution. Terminating its connection with the Georgia school in 1848, it entered into a similar arrangement that same year with the Scientific and Eclectic Medical Institute of Virginia. Under the terms of this agreement, the Worcester school again changed its name to New England Botanico-Medical College. Finally, in 1851, it obtained a Massachusetts charter and operated independently until its demise in 1859.[54] It is interesting to note that probably the most erudite neo-Thomsonian, Dr. Calvin Newton, was the founder of this school and, until 1853, its chief attraction.[55] In 1852, Newton joined the eclectics and became, that year, the president of the National Eclectic Medical Association.

7. *Metropolitan Medical College* in New York City.[56] A charter for this school was secured in 1850. During its last few years of existence, it was captured by the eclectics. Dissension among the faculty as well as insufficient students caused the school to close in 1862.

8. *Physio-Medical Institute,* Cincinnati, Ohio. Established in 1859 as a rival of the Physio-Medical College, this school closed in 1885. This institution had only fifteen graduates prior to 1861. After the Civil War, the number of graduates continued to be very small.

Three of the previous schools continued to operate after the Civil War, with the last one, the Physio-Medical Institute, closing in 1885. In the meantime, the following three physio-medical schools came into existence in the postwar period and were still functioning in the first decade of the twentieth century:

1. *The Physio-Medical College of Indiana,* Indianapolis, organized in 1873

2. *College of Medicine and Surgery,* Chicago, Illinois, organized in 1885 as the Chicago Physio-Medical Institute

3. *Physio-Medical College of Texas,* Dallas, organized in 1902

By 1910, only the Illinois school was still in existence; after this date, it, too, became defunct.

It is difficult to evaluate the quality of these schools, but as William G. Rothstein has pointed out, *all* nineteenth-century medical schools—sectarian or regular—were characterized by large amounts of didactic instruction, very infrequent (if any) real opportunities for clinical experience, and a general tendency to view formal medical school training as a complement for, rather than a replacement of, the time-honored apprenticeship.[57] The distinctive therapeutics and peculiar pathologies of the neo-Thomsonians blurred into a larger curricular regimen indistinguishable from the allopathic schools of the day. As the new century heralded a modern research-based curriculum largely transplanted from Germany, sectarian schools found it more and more difficult to keep pace with essential changes. By 1907, the American Medical Association's Council on Medical Education issued its first report based upon site inspections of degree-granting institutions. Not surprisingly, the physio-medical schools were found wanting in clinical instruction. "In an age when both the laboratory and the hospital had become significant sources of therapeutic knowledge," concludes John Haller, "the limited use of this important agency had weakened the physios' professional legitimacy."[58]

By the opening decade of the twentieth century, the end of the neo-Thomsonian movement was all but complete, as the last remaining schools sputtered to their demise. The ridiculously small number of students graduating from the three combined neo-Thomsonian medical colleges from 1901 through 1908 can be seen from the following statistics published in the *Journal of the American Medical Association:*[59]

1901 = 18	1905 = 22
1902 = 16	1906 = 22
1903 = 24	1907 = 11
1904 = 20	1908 = 12

PHARMACEUTICAL RESOURCES OF NEO-THOMSONIANISM

The neo-Thomsonian trend was accompanied by not only its own unique therapeutics, organizational structure, and education but also a different kind of pharmaceutical activity. The large-scale manufacture, distribution, and sale of Thomsonian remedies involving numerous agents and many unauthorized persons, which had been such a remarkable feature of the old movement, had disappeared by mid-nineteenth century. By this time, there were no longer thousands of patent right-holding followers of Thomson to support such activity.

Indeed, as one scrutinizes this trend closely, it becomes increasingly difficult to speak of neo-Thomsonian pharmacy per se. The old Thomsonians had been able to build up an extensive pharmaceutical apparatus to serve the needs of their adherents, but the physio-medical practitioners, the only organized group of neo-Thomsonians in America, were relatively too weak and few in number to muster pharmaceutical resources comparable to those of their crusading forebears. Moreover, the rapid rise of an impressive eclectic pharmaceutical industry in the 1850s completely submerged and overshadowed the few ineffectual attempts of physio-medical physicians to create a distinctive pharmacy of their own. For a good part of the century, neo-Thomsonian pharmacy may properly be regarded as an appendage of eclectic pharmacy, as subsequent discussion will show.

Intense excitement prevailed among the eclectics in the late 1840s when William S. Merrell of Cincinnati began marketing "concentrated" eclectic remedies. Numerous competing manufacturers immediately followed suit, and before long, a lucrative industry had evolved. The physios were quick to endorse the new concentrated remedies. An editorial appearing in the *Physo-Medical Recorder*, organ of the Physo-Medical College of Cincinnati,[60] praised the advent of these medications as "a glorious work of Medical Reform,"[61] without bothering to give the eclectics credit for this development. "No one is a greater lover of the different baths [vapor] than ourself, or has a higher appreciation of emetics and enemas," the editor reassured his readers.[62] But if the new concentrated preparations worked as well and were easier for the patient to take and for the physician to administer, he argued, then why not adopt them? Attacking the regular physicians for their employment of poisonous alkaloids, the writer conceded that these plant derivatives had done much to make the allopathic practice "acceptable and popular." Then, contrasting the regular alkaloidal pharmacy with the "New School" pharmacy, the editor wrote:

> . . . but how different their articles are from ours. They extract proximate principles, many of which are most deadly in their character . . . from the poppy they extract their morphine; from the strychnos (nux vomica), they extract their strychnine, two grains of which will kill; from cinchona they extract their quinine, etc., etc.

> Now our agents are reduced to a concentrated form without breaking up the relations existing between the proximate principles. For example, we reduce lobelia to so concentrated a form, that from three to five or ten drops upon loaf sugar, or dropped

into water, are sufficient to produce emesis; still this article is not lobelina, one of the proximate principles of lobelia . . .[63]

Finally, the writer, in a burst of enthusiasm, concluded that because of this "great improvement . . . we feel more than ever inclined to the belief that the Physo-Medical Practice will soon, very soon, become the most popular and successful practice of medicine."[64]

As mentioned earlier, a resolution had been passed at the Baltimore Convention urging patronage of "New School Druggists . . . in preference to those of other schools." Who these New School Druggists were can be seen by examining the advertisements in the physio-medical journals of the period. The Physio-Medical practitioners in the Cincinnati area apparently favored the concentrated remedies of F. D. Hill and Company of Cincinnati, who advertised "the Most Improved Method of preparing the concentrated Medicines . . . all articles belonging to the list of Drugs and Medicines used by Thomsonian and Botanic Physicians."[65] From the available data, it would seem that the eclectic establishments were well patronized. For example, the concentrated preparations of the American Chemical Institute, an eclectic firm controlled by B. Keith and Company, for whom the wholesale botanic house of Coolidge, Adams, and Bond acted as agents, were advertised in the *Journal of Medical Reform*. Similarly, the wholesale botanic druggists, Law and Boyd, offered for sale their concentrated preparations in the same journal, without, however, divulging the manufacturer.

The Middle States Medical Reformer was an ardent champion of concentrated preparations. In 1856, the Middle States Reformed Medical Society unreservedly endorsed the use of concentrated medicines at its fifth annual meeting in Philadelphia.[66] By this time, the physio-medical practitioners were patronizing eclectic establishments, wholesale botanic druggists who stocked eclectic remedies, and even regular drugstores. The new concentrated eclectic remedies were being sold through regular retail drug channels soon after their appearance on the market. Advertisements for these products are to be found in the very first volume of the *American Druggists' Circular and Chemical Gazette* (1857).[67]

This does not mean that the physio-medical practitioners used only eclectic concentrated remedies. In a report delivered at the convention of the Middle States Reformed Medical Society referred to earlier, it was authoritatively recommended that infusions, decoctions, and syrups should be retained as "adjunctive aids," and that extracts and tinctures should not be completely abandoned in favor of concentrates.[68]

In the succeeding years, the physio-medical physicians occasionally expressed their dissatisfaction at their inability to establish physio-medical pharmacies, as well as with the shortcomings of the botanic wholesale houses and regular drugstores. For example, in 1858, a disgruntled physio-medical practitioner wrote to the editor of the *Physio-Medical Recorder* to complain about drug adulteration:

> I am satisfied that our Reform physicians are not careful enough in selecting their medicinal agents. The manufacture of botanic medicines has become a lucrative business; and unprincipled men, disregarding the direful consequences, are adulterating our most sanative preparations. It is not uncommon to find, in our wholesale drug stores lobelia seed adulterated with tobacco, pulverized capsicum with logwood, ginger with corn meal, cream of tartar with alum, jalap with sawdust, etc. . . . Brothers in medical reform, if we can not get pure articles prepared for our immediate use, let us go into the laboratory prepared by the God of nature, and find for ourselves, in this crude state the healing remedies of a beneficent Creator.[69]

It was, of course, commonplace for many of the old "steam and puke doctors" to go out into the country and gather medicinal plants. These new practitioners, however, were a different breed of men. Many of them were now the proud possessors of diplomas and MD degrees, and the threat to "go into the laboratory prepared by the God of nature" was purely rhetorical.

At an annual meeting of the Indiana Physio-Medical Association, which met in 1895, a prominent spokesman of the cult complained bitterly that "[w]e are depending too much on the pharmacists of the old school . . . we should have a Physio-Medical Pharmacy."[70]

Another speaker joined in to approve the sentiments of his colleague: "We need efficient, conscientious Physio-Medical pharmacists to manufacture and prepare Physio-Medical remedies for Physio-Medical physicians."[71] The physios, however, were unable to attain this goal.

Procter's review of Kost's *Elements of Materia Medica and Therapeutics* (1858 edition) has already been discussed, but the strong links between Kost's book and the botanics serve to heighten the importance of Procter's critique. This book, used as a text in a number of physio-medical and eclectic medical schools, attempted, among other things, to display the author's pharmaceutical erudition. In his review, Procter quickly demolished Kost's pretensions by stating bluntly that "if the volume of Dr. Kost should get to another edition he will do well to submit his pages to the revision of a practical pharmaceutist, who will correct the numerous chemical and pharmaceutical defects which occur in the pharmaceutical portion."[72] The *Physio-Medical Dispensatory* of Cook, which contained a short section on pharmacy (42 out of 800 pages were devoted to this subject), was completely ignored in the pharmaceutical press and was virtually unknown outside the small circle of physios.

From the foregoing discussion, it must be concluded that the physio-medicals exerted little tangible influence on American pharmacy. Unlike their belligerent predecessors and their eclectic rivals whose pharmaceutical activities are of considerable interest and importance, these new Thomsonian practitioners caused hardly a ripple or stir on the pharmaceutical scene.

PHOTO 1. Title Page from *The English Physician*

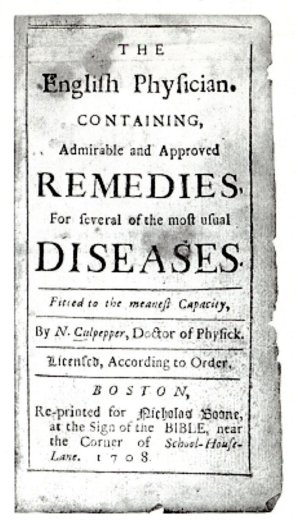

THE

English Physician.

CONTAINING,

Admirable and Approved

REMEDIES,

For several of the most usual

DISEASES.

Fitted to the meanest Capacity,

By *N. Culpepper*, Doctor of Physick.

Licensed, According to Order.

BOSTON,

Re-printed for Nicholas Boone,
at the Sign of the BIBLE, near
the Corner of School-House-
Lane. 1708.

The English Physician was the first medical book published in America. Although attributed to Nicholas Culpeper (1616-1654), it is likely the work of Nicholas Boone (1679-1738), known for his compilations of pocketbooks and assorted guides. Today, this small twelve-mo. herbal is quite rare. The example shown here, one of only four known copies in existence, is owned by the Reynolds Historical Library, University of Alabama at Birmingham, and is reprinted with permission.

PHOTO 2. Valentine's *The Triumphal Chariot of Antimony*

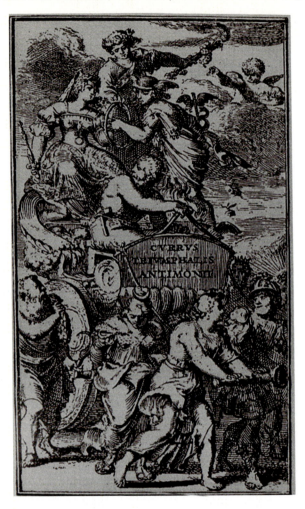

Through the ages, no two substances attained higher status among Western physicians than calomel and antimony. As the American botanics railed against their use, the medical profession persisted in giving them high priority in their therapeutics. Nothing epitomizes this more than the glorious frontispiece to Basil Valentine's *The Triumphal Chariot of Antimony,* first published in Amsterdam in 1685. The image here is from Arthur Edward Waite's reprinting of that venerated work in 1893. The illustration is the property of the Lloyd Library and Museum, Cincinnati, Ohio, and is reprinted with permission.

PHOTO 3. Samuel Thomson

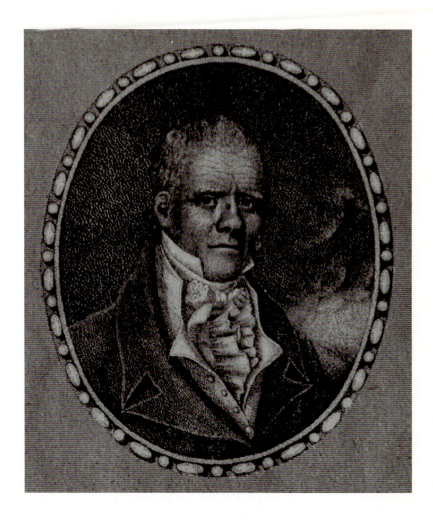

Samuel Thomson (1769-1843) began practicing his homely brand of botanic medicine in 1790, but it was the publication of his *New Guide to Health* in 1825 that sparked the American botanico-medical movement. The illustration is the property of the Lloyd Library and Museum, Cincinnati, Ohio, and is reprinted with permission.

PHOTO 4. *Lobelia inflata*

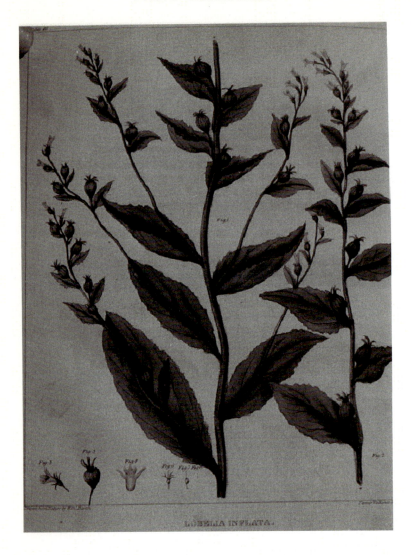

Samuel Thomson's favorite remedy, *Lobelia inflata,* sometimes referred to as Indian tobacco or "puke weed" because of its emetic properties. The illustration is from William P. C. Barton's *Vegetable Materia Medica of the United States,* 1817. The illustration is the property of the Lloyd Library and Museum, Cincinnati, Ohio, and is reprinted with permission.

PHOTO 5. Thomson's Patent Rights Certificate

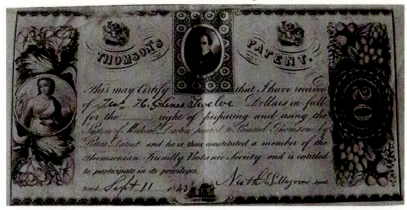

Samuel Thomson sustained his botanic system of medicine through the sale of patent rights distributed through designated agents such as the one shown here. The illustration is the property of the Lloyd Library and Museum, Cincinnati, Ohio, and is reprinted with permission.

PHOTO 6. Russell's Patent Rights Certificate

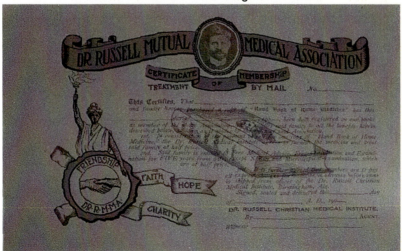

Thomson's sale of patent rights persisted in some curious forms, such as R. M. Russell's "Mutual Medical Association," a regional system of domestic health care, whereby agents designated by Russell sold not only his *Handbook of Home Medicine* but association membership as well. The example shown here is from the 1911 edition of Russell's work. The illustration is courtesy of the Reynolds Library, University of Alabama at Birmingham, and is reprinted with permission.

PHOTO 7. Russell's Botanical Remedies

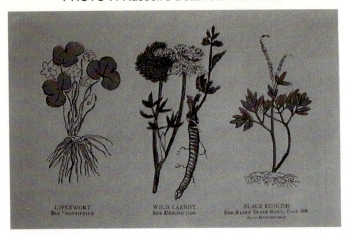

Russell was a Birmingham, Alabama, resident who, similar to Thomson, promoted botanical remedies indigenous to the people he served, such as these plants common to the South. The illustration is from his *Handbook of Home Medicine*, courtesy of the Reynolds Library, University of Alabama at Birmingham, and is reprinted with permission.

PHOTO 8. Thomsonian Advertisement

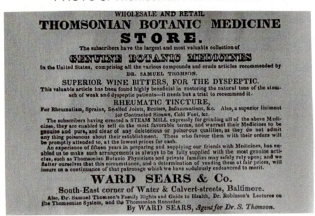

Thomsonian medicines were sold in a variety of forms by numerous agents. This one, featuring "Superior Wine Bitters" and "Rheumatic Tincture," was run in *The Thomsonian Recorder*, 1835-1836, by Ward Sears, Agent for Dr. S. Thomson. The illustration is the property of the Lloyd Library and Museum, Cincinnati, Ohio, and is reprinted with permission.

PHOTO 9. Typical Botanic Ad

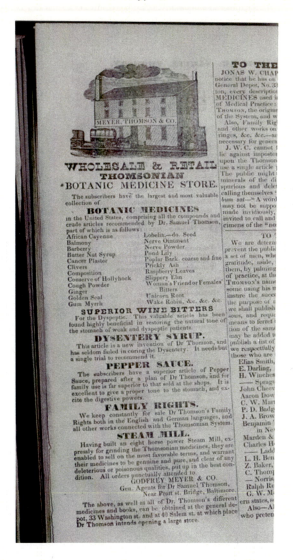

Advertisement from *The Thomsonian Manual,* 1835. The illustration is the property of the Lloyd Library and Museum, Cincinnati, Ohio, and is reprinted with permission.

PHOTO 10. *The Botanic Medical Reformer*

THE

BOTANIC MEDICAL REFORMER,

AND

HOME PHYSICIAN.

A CONDENSED RECORD OF REFORM VEGETABLE MEDICINE, AND USEFUL
INFORMATION FOR FAMILIES.

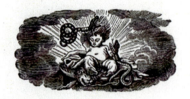

VOLUME I.

EDITED BY DR. THOMAS COOKE.

PUBLISHED BY HENRY HOLLEMBAEK & Co.

PHILADELPHIA:
C. B. BARRETT, PRINTER.
1841.

Thomas Cooke (d. 1855) became the most important Pennsylvania botanic with his *Botanic Medical Reformer,* which ran from 1841 to 1842. Cooke took great pains to explain his interesting emblem: "The 'frightful child' is young Hercules (an emblem of the Botanic System of Medicine), and the 'writhing serpents,' which he is strangling, are the branches of the old or Mineral Faculty—merculializing and blood-letting—the 'dead or sleeping lion,' is the great or many headed Hydra (the Faculty), which it will be observed, the infant Hercules has got pretty well subdued." Cooke pointed out, of course, that the rays of light were shining from the brilliant emanations of the Thomsonians. The illustration is the property of the Lloyd Library and Museum, Cincinnati, Ohio, and is reprinted with permission.

PHOTO 11. Alva Curtis

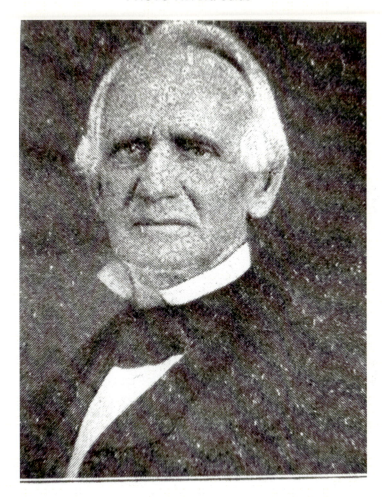

ALVA CURTIS

Alva Curtis (1797-1881) was a protégé of Samuel Thomson. The chartering of his Botanico-Medical School of Columbus, Ohio, in 1839 marked a break with his contentious mentor and would spawn the neo-Thomsonian movement. The illustration is the property of the Lloyd Library and Museum, Cincinnati, Ohio, and is reprinted with permission.

PHOTO 12. William H. Cook

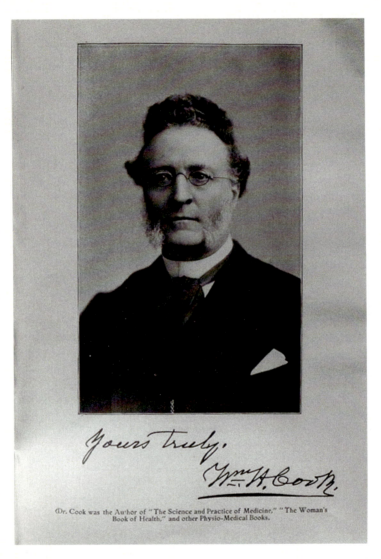

Dr. Cook was the Author of "The Science and Practice of Medicine," "The Woman's Book of Health," and other Physio-Medical Books.

William H. Cook (1832-1899), former eclectic and zealous physio-medical convert, became an intellectual leader of neo-Thomsonianism with his *Physio-Medical Dispensatory* (1869). The illustration is the property of the Lloyd Library and Museum, Cincinnati, Ohio, and is reprinted with permission.

PHOTO 13. A. I. Coffin

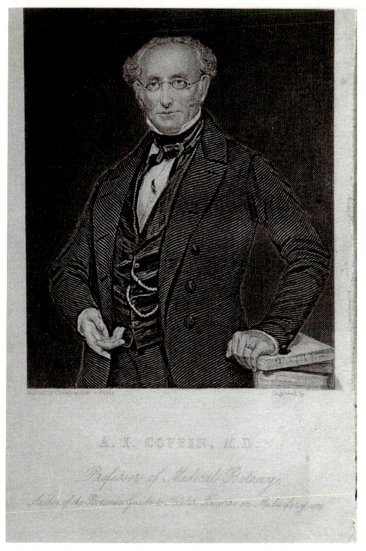

A. I. Coffin (1790-1866) carried Thomsonian medicine to England where the American brand of botanicism took hold and spread among the working classes through his "Friendly Botanico-Medical Societies." The illustration is the property of the Lloyd Library and Museum, Cincinnati, Ohio, and is reprinted with permission.

PHOTO 14. *The Thomsonian System of Medicine*

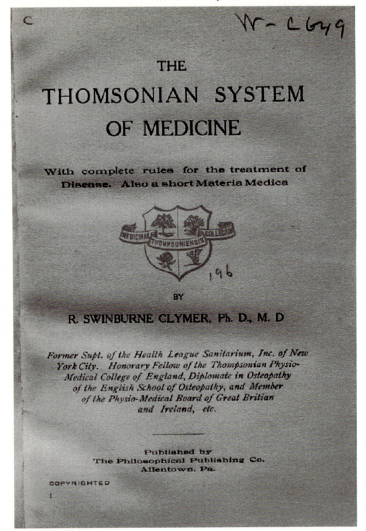

This curious work, published in 1905, shows the persistence of Thomsonian medicine years after the death of its controversial founder. While most of Samuel Thomson's followers had long since allied themselves under the physio-medical banner, some, such as R. Swinburne Clymer of Allentown, Pennsylvania, adhered to the founder in both principle *and* name. The illustration is the property of the Lloyd Library and Museum, Cincinnati, Ohio, and is reprinted with permission.

PHOTO 15. Rafinesque's *Medical Flora*

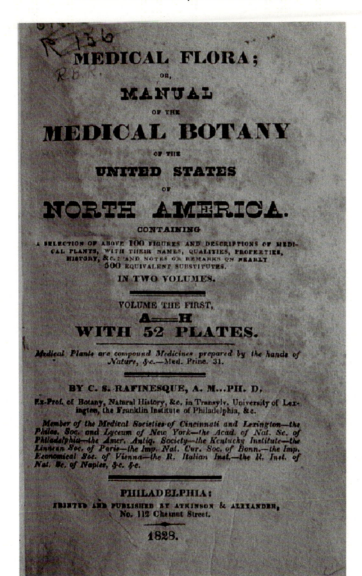

Rafinesque's *Medical Flora* (1828-1829) exerted a profound influence over the American botanico-medical movement. The illustration is the property of the Lloyd Library and Museum, Cincinnati, Ohio, and is reprinted with permission.

PHOTO 16. Constantine Rafinesque

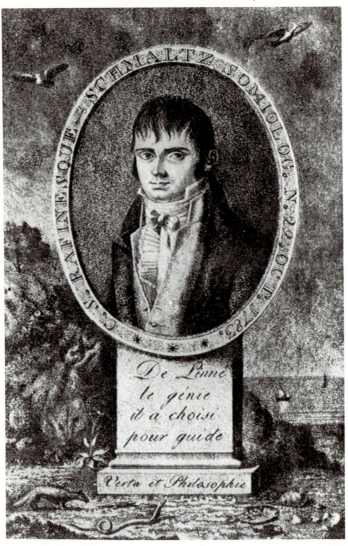

Although not directly associated with the botanical movement, Constantine Rafinesque (1783-1840) was highly regarded by physio-medicals and eclectics alike. The illustration is from Richard Ellsworth Call's *The Life and Writings of Rafinesque,* Filson Club Publications, no. 10, 1895, courtesy of the Reynolds Library, University of Alabama at Birmingham, and is reprinted with permission.

PHOTO 17. Wooster Beach

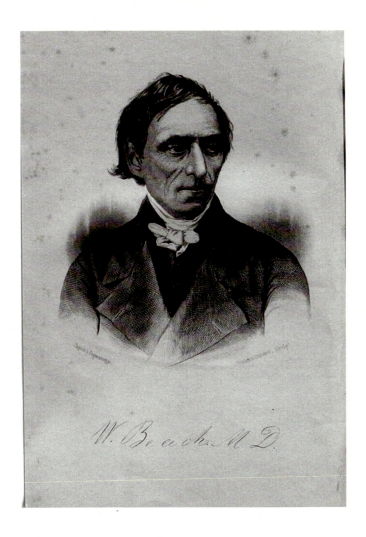

Wooster Beach (1794-1868) founded the American eclectic medical movement with his United States Infirmary (1827), later renamed the Reformed Medical Academy (1829), of New York City. The illustration is the property of the Lloyd Library and Museum, Cincinnati, Ohio, and is reprinted with permission.

PHOTO 18. William S. Merrell

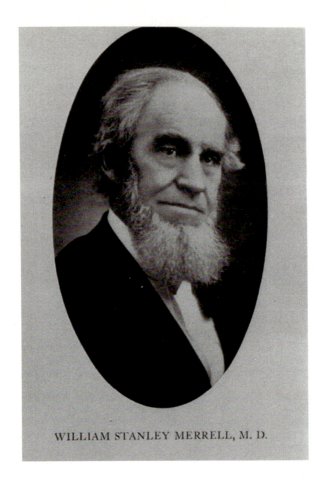

WILLIAM STANLEY MERRELL, M. D.

William S. Merrell (1798-1880) was widely regarded as the "Father of Eclectic Medicine." Merrell started in the drug business with the establishment of his Western Market Drug Store in Cincinnati in 1828. Soon, Merrell developed a strong and devoted following among eclectic practitioners. The illustration is the property of the Lloyd Library and Museum, Cincinnati, Ohio, and is reprinted with permission.

PHOTO 19. Concentrated Medicines

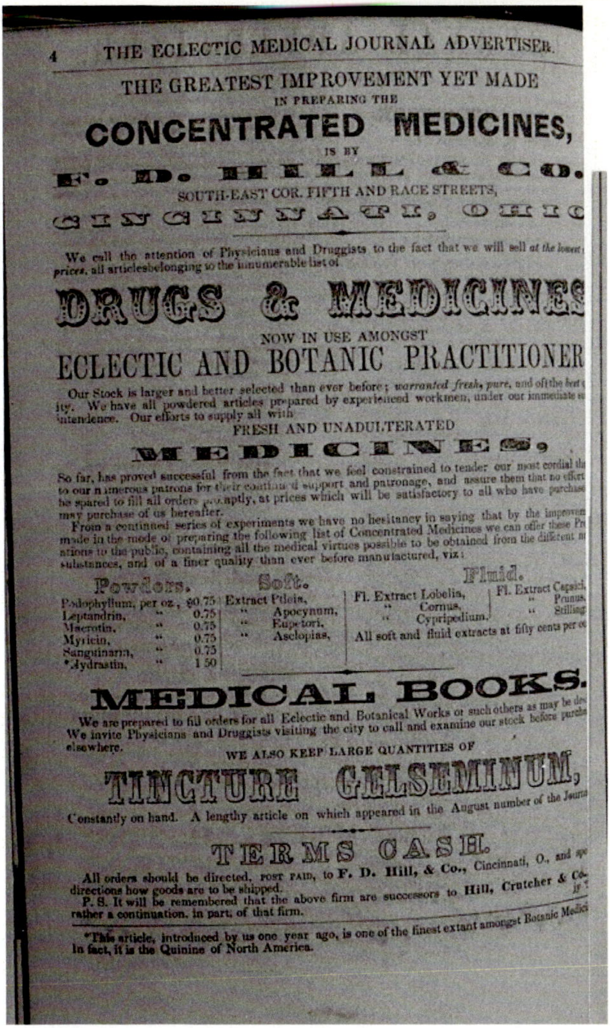

4 THE ECLECTIC MEDICAL JOURNAL ADVERTISER.

THE GREATEST IMPROVEMENT YET MADE
IN PREPARING THE
CONCENTRATED MEDICINES,
IS BY
F. D. HILL & CO.
SOUTH-EAST COR. FIFTH AND RACE STREETS,
CINCINNATI, OHIO

We call the attention of Physicians and Druggists to the fact that we will sell *at the lowest prices*, all articles belonging to the innumerable list of

DRUGS & MEDICINES
NOW IN USE AMONGST
ECLECTIC AND BOTANIC PRACTITIONER

Our Stock is larger and better selected than ever before; *warranted fresh, pure,* and of the best ity. We have all powdered articles prepared by experienced workmen, under our immediate intendence. Our efforts to supply all with

FRESH AND UNADULTERATED
MEDICINES,

So far, has proved successful from the fact that we feel constrained to tender our most cordial to our numerous patrons for their continued support and patronage, and assure them that no effort be spared to fill all orders promptly, at prices which will be satisfactory to all who have purchase may purchase of us hereafter.

From a continued series of experiments we have no hesitancy in saying that by the improvem made in the mode of preparing the following list of Concentrated Medicines we can offer these Pr ations to the public, containing all the medical virtues possible to be obtained from the different substances, and of a finer quality than ever before manufactured, viz:

Powders.			Soft.	Fluid.	
Podophyllum, per oz.,		$0.75	Extract Ptleis,	Fl. Extract Lobelia,	Fl. Extract Capsici,
Leptandrin,	"	0.75	" Apocynum,	" Cornus,	" Prunus,
Macrotin,	"	0.75	" Eupetori,	" Cypripedium,	" Stilling
Myricin,	"	0.75	" Asclepias,	All soft and fluid extracts at fifty cents per o	
Sanguinarin,	"	0.75			
*Hydrastin,	"	1 50			

MEDICAL BOOKS.

We are prepared to fill orders for all Eclectic and Botanical Works or such others as may be de We invite Physicians and Druggists visiting the city to call and examine our stock before purch elsewhere.

WE ALSO KEEP LARGE QUANTITIES OF
TINCTURE GELSEMINUM,

Constantly on hand. A lengthy article on which appeared in the August number of the Journ

TERMS CASH.

All orders should be directed, POST PAID, to **F. D. Hill, & Co.,** Cincinnati, O., and sp directions how goods are to be shipped.

P. S. It will be remembered that the above firm are successors to **Hill, Crutcher & Co.** rather a continuation, in part, of that firm.

*This article, introduced by us one year ago, is one of the finest extant amongst Botanic Medici In fact, it is the Quinine of North America.

The so-called "concentrations craze" captured the attentions of many eclectics. Subsequent analysis soon quashed those high expectations. From the *Eclectic Medical Journal,* 1853. The illustration is the property of the Lloyd Library and Museum, Cincinnati, Ohio, and is reprinted with permission.

PHOTO 20. John King and John Milton Scudder

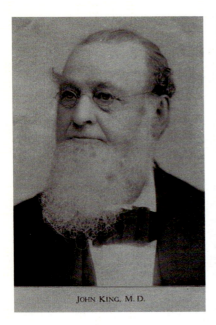
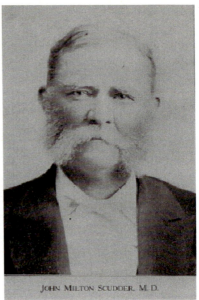

JOHN KING, M. D.

JOHN MILTON SCUDDER, M. D.

John King (1813-1893) and John Milton Scudder (1829-1894) became leaders of the Eclectic Medical Institute of Cincinnati. Their influence defined eclectic therapeutics in its last and perhaps greatest phase, specific diagnosis and specific medication. The illustration is the property of the Lloyd Library and Museum, Cincinnati, Ohio, and is reprinted with permission.

PHOTO 21. William Procter Jr.

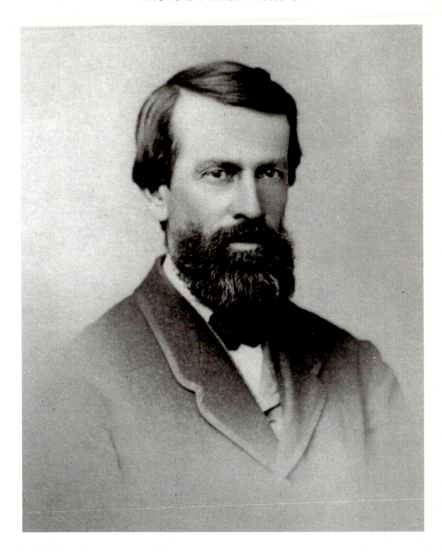

William Procter Jr. (1817-1874), leader of American pharmacy in 1867, gave a frank but fair assessment of King's *Dispensatory* and of the American botanical movement in 1854 and 1859. The illustration is courtesy of the American Institute of the History of Pharmacy, Madison, Wisconsin, and is reprinted with permission.

PHOTO 22. King's *Dispensatory*

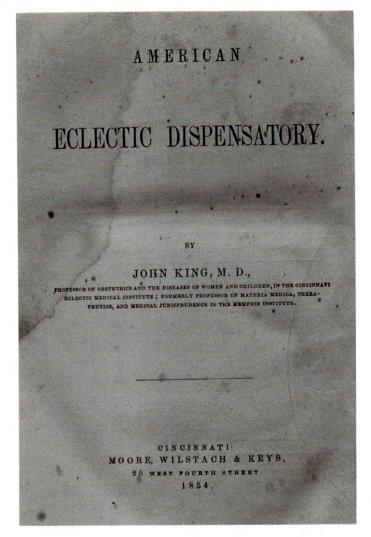

King's *Dispensatory,* despite Procter's mixed review, soon attained high status among eclectic practitioners. First published in 1852, it went through numerous editions, with the final revision appearing in 1909 under the editorial guidance of John Uri Lloyd and Harvey Wickes Felter. The illustration is the property of the Lloyd Library and Museum, Cincinnati, Ohio, and is reprinted with permission.

PHOTO 23. Scudder's *Specific Medication*

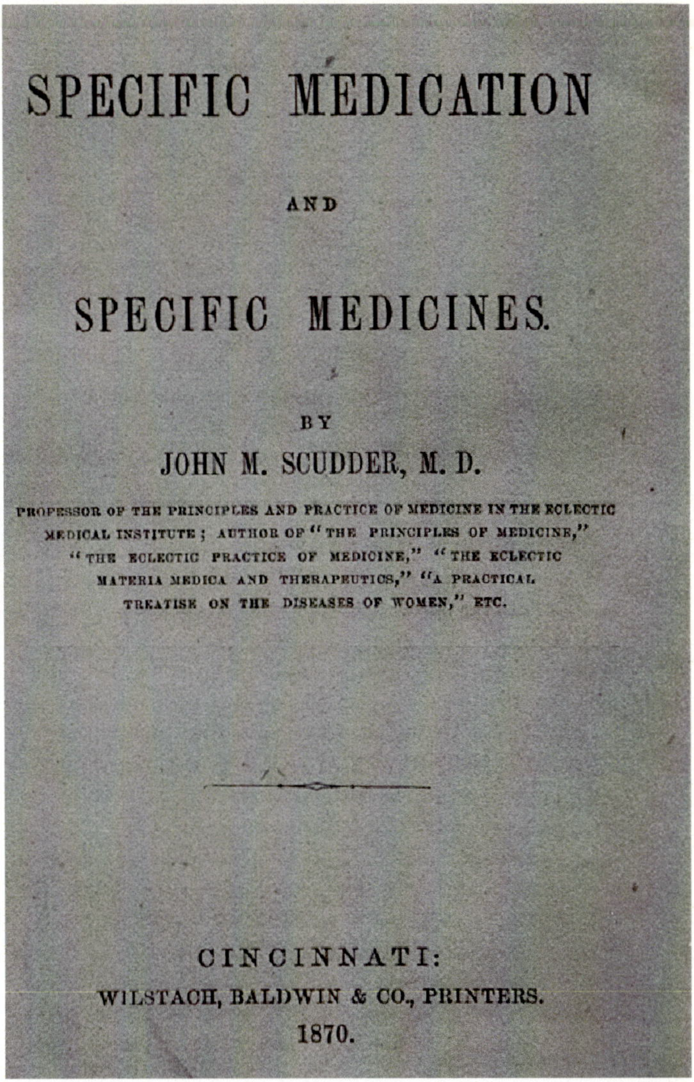

SPECIFIC MEDICATION

AND

SPECIFIC MEDICINES.

BY

JOHN M. SCUDDER, M. D.

PROFESSOR OF THE PRINCIPLES AND PRACTICE OF MEDICINE IN THE ECLECTIC
MEDICAL INSTITUTE; AUTHOR OF "THE PRINCIPLES OF MEDICINE,"
"THE ECLECTIC PRACTICE OF MEDICINE," "THE ECLECTIC
MATERIA MEDICA AND THERAPEUTICS," "A PRACTICAL
TREATISE ON THE DISEASES OF WOMEN," ETC.

CINCINNATI:

WILSTACH, BALDWIN & CO., PRINTERS.

1870.

Next to King's *Dispensatory,* the most important guide to eclectic therapeutics
during the last quarter of the nineteenth century was John Milton Scudder's
Specific Medication and Specific Medicines, which appeared in several editions after its first issue in 1870. The illustration is the property of the Lloyd
Library and Museum, Cincinnati, Ohio, and is reprinted with permission.

PHOTO 24. Typical Eclectic Ad

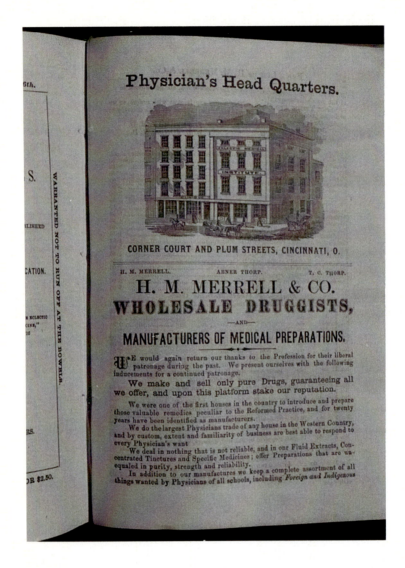

From the *Eclectic Medical Journal,* 1874. The illustration is the property of the Lloyd Library and Museum, Cincinnati, Ohio, and is reprinted with permission.

PHOTO 25. John Uri Lloyd

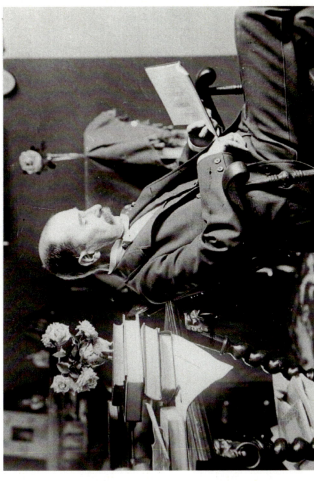

John Uri Lloyd (1849-1936) in one of his more relaxed moments. President of the American Pharmaceutical Association, 1887; winner of three Ebert Prizes for original research in pharmacy; and recipient of pharmacy's highest honor, the Remington Medal, Lloyd is arguably the American botanico-medical movement's greatest figure. The illustration is the property of the Lloyd Library and Museum, Cincinnati, Ohio, and is reprinted with permission.

PHOTO 26. Lloyd Brothers Specific Medicines

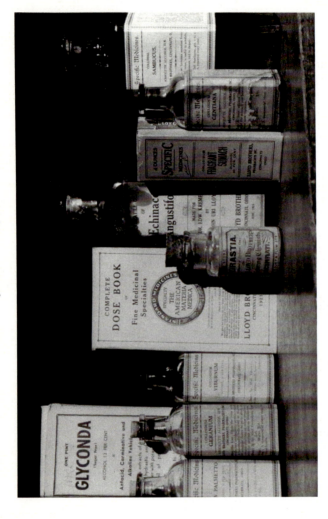

The Specific Medicines of the Lloyd Brothers became some of the most widely sold botanics in America. The illustration is the property of the Lloyd Library and Museum, Cincinnati, Ohio, and is reprinted with permission.

PHOTO 27. Bennett Medical College

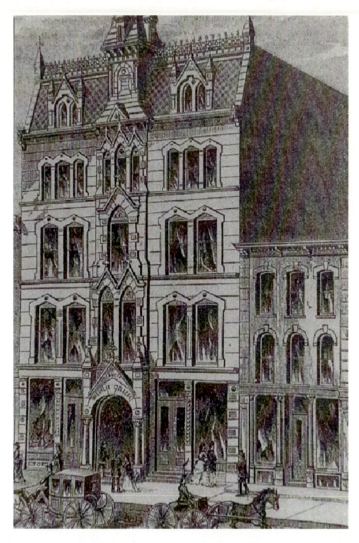

Incorporated in 1868, this school was described by historian John S. Haller Jr. as Chicago's "pillar of reform medicine." It was named after John Hughes Bennett (1812-1875) of Edinburgh, a physician who had apparently captured the attentions and hearts of American eclectics. The illustration is the property of the Lloyd Library and Museum, Cincinnati, Ohio, and is reprinted with permission.

PHOTO 28. The Eclectic Medical Institute

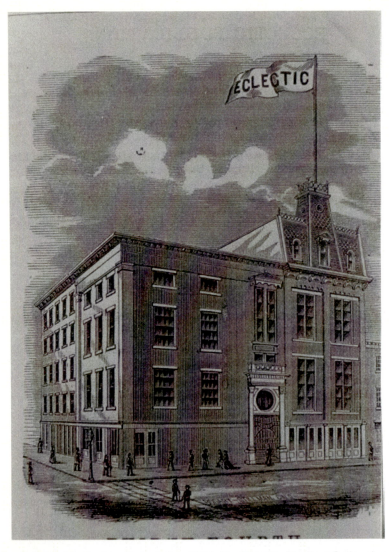

The Eclectic Medical Institute (after 1910, the Eclectic Medical College) was the center of American eclecticism from its first charter in Cincinnati in 1845 to its last graduating class nearly a century later in 1939. The illustration is the property of the Lloyd Library and Museum, Cincinnati, Ohio, and is reprinted with permission.

PHOTO 29. Milestones in Pharmaceutical Botany (A Symposium of the American Institute of the History of Pharmacy, Orlando, Florida, March 20, 1995)

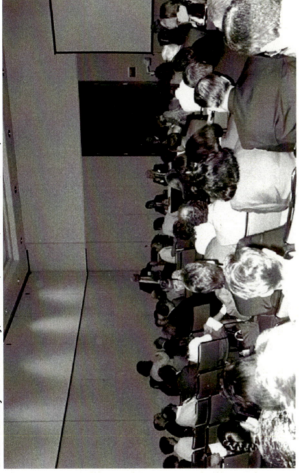

The 1990s were witness to a tremendous revitalization of interest in medical botany, past and present. Typical was the well-attended symposium sponsored by the American Institute of the History of Pharmacy as part of the American Pharmaceutical Association's annual conference. Featured presenters were Ara Der Marderosian, Varro Tyler, and Mark Blumenthal. The illustration is courtesy of the American Institute of the History of Pharmacy, Madison, Wisconsin, and is reprinted with permission.

Chapter 6

The Eclectics

If the botanico-medical movement had included only the Thomsonians, physio-medicals, and an assorted array of neo-Thomsonians, the impact upon American pharmacy and medicine would have been negligible. The eclectics, however, brought a new dimension to therapeutics and to medicinal plant inquiry. Not only did the eclectics gain a stronghold in the Midwest, but they also developed in several distinct therapeutic phases, the sum total of which appreciably influenced pharmaceutical research, the mainstream pharmaceutical profession, the drug manufacturing industry, and, ultimately, practicing physicians, both irregular and regular. Emerging concomitant with Thomsonianism, the eclectics were able to attract faculty and students more effectively and for longer periods than their physio-medical counterparts. The story of the botanico-medicals may begin with Thomson, but its influence and lasting importance for the historian reside with the eclectics.

WOOSTER BEACH (1794-1868)

It is in the development of a distinctive pharmacy of indigenous plant remedies that the eclectics made their strongest bid for scientific recognition.[1] But before the eclectic impact on American pharmacy can be understood properly, a brief historical sketch and appraisal of the botanic sect created by Wooster Beach is necessary.[2] In some ways, Wooster Beach, the acknowledged founder of eclecticism, forcibly reminds one of Elias Smith. Both were engaged in religious and medical controversy, warring against the regular theological and medical beliefs of the day; both had Messianic complexes; and both were acutely conscious of the value of publicity. Beach's personality and outlook are best revealed in his crusading articles against the "craft of Doctors and Priests," published in his religious newspaper, *The Telescope,* during the late 1820s. The laudatory statements about him that later appeared in the eclectic press do not give the same picture.

Beach was born in Trumbull, Connecticut, in 1794. As a young man, he became obsessed with the idea of reforming current religious and medical practices. Learning of the alleged medical prowess of Jacob Tidd, an herb doctor who lived in a secluded section of New Jersey, Beach lost no time in visiting this gentleman to request that he be accepted as Tidd's student. Though at first reluctant, Tidd finally consented. After a period of tutelage, Beach, in his own words, "attended a course of lectures in the University of the State of New York during the time of Drs. Post, Hosack, Mott, and others were professors. I concluded this was best, were it only to detect the errors of the modern practice; and subsequently I obtained a *diploma,* according to the law of the State, which should any wish to pursue, they will find it recorded in the County Clerk's Office, in the City Hall, New York."[3]

About 1825, we find Beach a member of the New York County Medical Society, pursuing a busy medical practice in New York City and instructing students. In 1827, he announced the opening of a clinical institution that he designated by the grandiose title of United States Infirmary. Two years later, Beach founded a medical school, first called the Reformed Medical Academy (1829), later changed in 1830 to the Reformed Medical College of the City of New York. This medical school was never chartered by the State of New York and finally closed in 1838.

Under the leadership of Beach, there was organized in New York City during 1829 a national organization called the Reformed Medical Society of the United States. One of the first acts of the society was to establish a chartered medical school at Worthington, Ohio, in 1830, whose purpose was to make available to the people of the West "a scientific knowledge of Botanic Medicine." Along with Beach, several of the charter members of this society, such as John King, Thomas Vaughan Morrow, and I. G. Jones, were destined to play major roles in the history of eclecticism.

In subsequent years, Beach became involved in religious polemical writing, publishing at least two other periodicals, *The Battle-Axe* and *The Ishmaelite*. Despite this activity, he found time to engage in extensive medical writing, producing in 1833 his very popular three-volume work *The American Practice of Medicine*, discussed earlier in this study (see p. 48). Two other works by Beach were well received in Botanic circles: his *Medical and Botanic Dictionary* (1847) and his *An Improved System of Midwifery* (1847).

Beach lectured briefly at the Eclectic Medical Institute (EMI) in 1845 as a professor of clinical surgery and medicine. In 1848, he visited England and made a number of converts to his cause. During 1855, he was elected president of the National Eclectic Medical Association. After this date, Wilder and Felter mention that his relations with other teachers of "reformed" and eclectic medicine were not cordial. The reasons for this are not clear. Beach's life after 1855 seems to have been uneventful, and his personal influence faded out almost completely. Both mental despondency, brought about by a tragedy in his family, and the inability to maintain his former leadership forced him first into partial obscurity and then into complete retirement, until his death in 1868.

AMERICAN ECLECTICISM: A BRIEF HISTORICAL APPRAISAL

The establishment of a teaching institution in Worthington, Ohio, in 1830 by the followers of Beach was to have extremely important repercussions for the future history of the eclectic group. This first chartered sectarian medical school in the United States was the forerunner of the EMI of Cincinnati, the acknowledged fountainhead of American eclecticism. For a few years, the school, despite its share of vicissitudes, made modest progress. In 1836, the professors of the institution began publishing a monthly journal titled *The Western Medical Reformer.*

It was to be expected that the new school at Worthington would be subjected to derision and harassment at the hands of its rivals, the numerically superior regulars and Thomsonians. Thomson himself treated the institution with cold contempt. "I am, therefore, satisfied," he wrote, "that if my medicine were taken from them, their

Institution would not be worth a cent. . . . But to have bought the right," he added sarcastically, "would have been too mean for such dignitaries; but, to steal it from a *quack,* was, perhaps, in their estimation more honorable!!!"[4]

Intensely embarrassed by the community's inability to distinguish between the genteel professors of Worthington and the numerous uncouth, fanatical disciples of Thomson who had overrun the area, the "reformed" faculty scoffed at the Thomsonian patent system that "has been so industriously puffed by interested agents" and called their pretensions to medical reform a "slanderous" attempt "to deceive and misguide the public mind."[5]

The Medical Department of Worthington College, as the school was known, ceased to exist in 1839. It had been seriously affected by the nationwide depression of 1837. The blow that sealed the school's fate, however, was struck when a mob, infuriated by reports of "resurrectionist" activities at the college, looted and sacked the building. Although eclectic historian Alexander Wilder discounted the grave-robbing accusations as the product of "exaggerated stories,"[6] Harvey Wickes Felter gives a surprisingly frank account of this colorful episode.[7] According to Felter, the trouble all started when a Mrs. Cramm died at the State Insane Asylum, whereupon she was buried in a potter's field. When Mrs. Cramm's relatives arrived to claim the body, they found, to their astonishment, no Mrs. Cramm. Suspicions were directed at the most obvious source, Worthington Medical College. Passions were again inflamed when it was discovered that two other graves had been disturbed. Soon the irate citizens of Worthington and elsewhere organized a party to attack the college building. Gaining word of the impending assault, students and faculty stood firm with pistols and shotguns to defend the school. Battering rams were constructed to demolish the building, but before the destruction began, the mob received keys to the college. At this point, Dr. Morrow saw nothing further to be gained by resistance and he surrendered, provided that the college's property would be spared, a condition that was granted. The crowd's suspicions of grave robbing were confirmed when what was believed to be Mrs. Cramm's body was subsequently found upon a dissecting table within the school. Despite its inglorious end, eighty-eight practitioners had been graduated from the Worthington school during its brief existence.[8]

If Wooster Beach was the founder of eclecticism, then surely Thomas Vaughan Morrow (1804-1850) must be considered its missionary apostle. It was Morrow who had been the guiding spirit at Worthington, and, as we have seen, who bravely defended it against all odds. Realizing the futility of remaining in Worthington, he and his "Beachite" colleagues managed to secure a charter in 1845 for the EMI in Cincinnati, over the strong opposition of the regulars. In many ways, the history of this medical college, the most important of the sect, illustrates the vagaries of American eclectism. During its very first session (1845-1846), the school catalogue announced that the "theory and practice of Homeopathy, and also Hydropathy, will not only be discussed by the professors . . . but will be specially illustrated by a brief course of lectures from gentlemen well acquainted with those methods of practice."[9] Joseph R. Buchanan (1814-1899) lectured for a number of years on "phrenology, anthropology, and kindred topics."[10] In 1849, a strange coalition with the homeopaths took place when the first chair in Principles and Practice of Homeopathy in the West was established at the institute. The popularity of this course so alarmed Dr. Morrow and his associates that the chair was summarily abolished, but not before six students had graduated from the institute with joint degrees in homeopathic and eclectic medicine.[11]

Speaking of the confused state of teaching at the institute, Pickard and Buley write, "Drawing for ideas and materials as the faculty did upon the whole field of Botanic practice as well as that of the regulars, each instructor was inclined to become a system unto himself. One can imagine the complications which might result from using Eberle's *On the Theory and Practice of Medicine,* a standby of the regulars, and at the same time including lectures on the elements of homeopathy."[12] The eclectics, however, had their own reasons for maintaining such catholic notions of the healing arts. "Eclectic reformers considered themselves medical protestants," writes Haller, "deliberately casting themselves adrift from the authority of allopathic medicine. As medical iconoclasts," he continues, "they chafed at the boundaries set by medical orthodoxy and proposed instead that each physician seek authority within his own convictions."[13]

The nineteenth century was certainly not lacking in strange healing cults whose tenets, no matter how bizarre, were at least consistent. But the feverish borrowing and the tortuous policies of the eclectics never ceased to amaze the devotees of other schools of medicine. Alva Curtis, spokesman for the physio-medical practitioners, accused the eclectics of "becoming all things to all men."[14] He apologized to his readers for his inability to give a lucid account of the principles of eclecticism on the grounds that "we should not expect order in a description of the inmates and operatives of bedlam."[15] The homeopaths described eclecticism as "merely a general and indiscriminate appropriation of the intellectual property of others—bringing together a heterogenous mass of borrowed matter, destitute of all originality."[16] As for the regulars, their sarcasm knew no bounds, argued *The Medical and Surgical Reporter:*

> All the *"ics," "lics," "isms," "cisms," "ists,"* and *"pathies"* are said to be compounded into what is called Eclectic, which is therefore the most comprehensive of them all, and at the same time the least original. Most other fallacies spring up at once, create a great sensation and often stagger and stun the intelligent, by the startling novelty of their propositions, bewilder the unwary by the immensity of their premises, and then die out. But the Eclectics keep themselves alive by swallowing everything which happens to turn up, until they have become like Macbeth's caldron, an extraordinary conglomeration of such incompatibles as Injun doctoring, Dutch homeopathy, watercure, electropathy, physio-medicalism, etc.[17]

For the first ten years of its existence, the EMI prospered. Its graduates, numbering 593,[18] went out into the world to spread the nebulous doctrine of selecting and adopting "whatever is most beneficial." Indeed, by the 1850s, Cincinnati's eclectic citadel had graduated over one-fourth of all Ohio physicians.[19] In 1856, however, the college was torn by violent dissension, which took three years to mend. By 1861, the institute as well as the eclectic profession in general were confronted with a serious crisis involving their entire medical status. The loss of faith in the efficacy of concentrated remedies, on which the eclectics had pinned such great hopes a decade before, contributed heavily to the demoralization that set in. John Milton Scudder, one of the outstanding eclectic leaders of the period, remembered this near catastrophe years later. The Eclectic Medical Institute was so badly managed that it could barely meet expenses, and the *Eclectic Medical Journal* fell from 1,800 subscribers to a mere 500. "We were overweighted with men who, whilst claiming to be Eclectics, talked and acted something else," admitted Scudder, "with a lot of miserable 'concentrated medicines,' with a poor pharmacy, and druggists that sought to make things cheap rather than good . . . and worse than all, our profession had lost faith and was badly demoralized."[20]

It was John Milton Scudder, "the most conspicuous man in modern Eclecticism,"[21] who is generally conceded to have lifted the institute and his profession out of the morass into which it had sunk. His efforts were greatly aided by John King, whose forte was the eclectic materia medica, and Andrew Jackson Howe (1825-1892), the most prominent of the eclectic practitioners and teachers of surgery. The triumvirate of Scudder, King, and Howe virtually dominated the eclectic world after the Civil War.[22]

Scudder's great influence after 1869 was in therapeutics. His doctrine of "specific medication," first formally enunciated in 1869,[23] was quickly accepted by the eclectic profession and continued to be popular with the sect's practitioners well into the twentieth century. "We use the term *specific* with relation to definite pathological conditions, and propose to say that certain well-determined deviations from the healthy state will always be corrected by specific medicines."[24]

No sooner had this doctrine been announced than the adversaries of the eclectics, as usual, were quick to cry, "Plagiarism!" Wilder admits that the homeopathic influence on "specific medication" was strong.[25] Although it is true that Scudder did not employ infinitesimal dosing, nor subscribe to Hahnemann's *similia similibus curantur* (the doctrine of like cures like), he did advocate fairly high dilutions. In this connection, it is interesting to note that more than four decades later, a prominent eclectic leader urged a coalition of the eclectic and homeopathic practices on the grounds that homeopaths and eclectics practiced specific medication and both practiced forms of drug attenuation whose differences he believed were "tri-fling."[26]

The doctrine of "specific medication" supplied a definite need for the eclectics, coming as it did on the heels of the great disillusionment with concentrated remedies. Scudder wrote, in 1879, that many eclectic physicians had concluded, by the time of the Civil War, that the majority of the concentrated medicines were worthless and not as effective as the crude plant drugs. "But having dropped them [the crude plant medicinals]," he added, "they were loath to take them up again, and so many gradually drifted into the habit of using a routine of podophyllin, quinine, and morphia, as many of their competitors [the regulars] used calomel, quinine, and morphia. It was a poor practice, and it was no wonder that those who pursued it thought there was little in maintaining a distinct organization."[27]

Although the specific issues involving the eclectic concentrate controversy will be discussed later, suffice it to say that the essential problems with the so-called concentrated remedies were the hodge-podge nature of their preparations, with little or no real attempt to examine the active principles of the plant materials being concentrated, and the fact that patients found them bitter and unpalatable. The problems of taste could, perhaps, be surmounted with sugar and/or pungent exipients, but standards of preparation affecting quality were serious. Chemist E. S. Wayne issued a four-page critique of the B. Keith and Company concentrates and found them without merit. Subsequent analysis of other eclectic concentrates yielded equally embarrassing results. "To show that these resins, and oleo-resins, are not in all instances the active, or medicinal properties of plants in a concentrated form," Wayne explained, "is the object I have in view, . . . and also, to induce the medical faculty [of the EMI] to investigate this matter a little more attentively than they have done, so as not to be deceived into the use of substances possessing little or none of the active principle of the plant or root that it represents."[28] Wayne's devastating and frank characterization of the eclectic concentrates confirmed calls already issued within the eclectic ranks that these preparations were substandard, if not wholly useless. For example, John King warned, "if we permit such trash to be foisted on them [the regular physicians] as pure agents, they will believe that Eclecticism is indeed quackery and humbug, and it will require years to overcome the effects of such a disgraceful blow."[29]

It should be emphasized, however, that the adoption of concentrated medicines by the eclectics had, in turn, also supplied a need. It had replaced the remedial procedures in vogue under the earlier "doctrine of substitution," when the eclectics, similar to the regulars, had entertained ideas of "phlogosis" and "antiphlogistics" (see "The 'Antiphlogistic Period,' 1830-1850," p. 125). Thus, the evolution of a century of eclectic therapeutic concepts appears to fall into three phases: the "antiphlogistic" period, roughly 1830-1850; the span of years during which the "concentrated preparations" predominated, roughly from 1850 to the Civil War; and, finally, the era of "specific medication," which extended from 1869 into the twentieth century.

Some of the more important aspects of eclectic organizational activity have been mentioned previously.[30] By 1879, ten eclectic medical schools had been chartered in the United States, besides the EMI, and by 1893, as many as eighteen had been incorporated,[31] many of which were short lived. The commencement exercises of the Eclectic Medical College held on June 7, 1939 would mark the end of over 100 years of continuous eclectic education in this country.[32]

Despite its longevity, the eclectic movement was not always grand nor glorious. Two eclectic schools were implicated in a diploma-selling scandal.[33] One medical college, incorporated in Illinois in 1868, called itself The Bennett College of Eclectic Medicine and Surgery, after Dr. John Hughes Bennett of Edinburgh, a pillar of allopathic respectability.[34] The prospectus of this institution stated that "the scientific principle of conservative Eclectic medicine, first enunciated and so ably defended by Professor Bennett, of the University of Edinburgh, some years ago, has established true Eclecticism upon a basis which cannot be controverted."[35] This was undoubtedly news to Dr. Bennett. Dr. John Milton Scudder, amazed at the action of his colleagues, referred to the prospectus of the Bennett College as "a singular statement of faith."[36] Toward the end of the century, the eclectics claimed that they numbered 10,292 practitioners, as compared with 72,028 regular physicians, 9,648 homeopaths, and 1,553 physio-medical doctors.[37]

In evaluating the nature and caliber of eclectic practice in light of what has been presented, its dominant characteristics appear to have been lack of originality, frequently bordering on plagiarism, and an almost all-pervasive mediocrity. Even in the investigation of the indigenous plant materia medica, the eclectics, with few exceptions, evinced a singular lack of scientific acumen.

THE ECLECTIC IMPACT
ON AMERICAN PHARMACY, 1830-1869

As mentioned earlier, from the beginning, eclectics and the other botanics had claimed that the regulars were killing their patients with depletive treatments, such as bloodletting and the administration of massive doses of injurious minerals, such as calomel and antimony. For botanics, the answer to health and healing resided primarily in America's field and forests. Apart from that, little difference existed between many botanics and regulars. John Milton Scudder admitted that "[t]he anatomy, the physiology, the chemistry, the art of obstetrics, the art of surgery, the preventive medicine, are the same in all [schools of medical practice]. . . . The points of differences, then, are in materia medica, and the administration of remedies for cure."[38] Even so stalwart a regular as William Osler knew it too. "Anatomy, physiology, chemistry, histology, embryology [sic], medicine, surgery, obstetrics, gynæcology, and medical jurisprudence know no 'isms.' The differences only become glaring when we touch the subject of therapeutics," he once stated, "a subject in which among members of each so-called schools [sic] the greatest of individual opinions exist."[39] However, this caused problems for maintaining identity within a public besieged by "different" medical systems and less attuned to the recondite debates on therapeutic theory raging among medical pundits. "From the patient's perspective," writes historian William Rothstein, "there was little to choose between eclectic physicians and their competitors in the other sects" because their differing therapeutic beliefs did not represent distinctions between scientifically valid and invalid systems.[40]

THE "ANTIPHLOGISTIC" PERIOD, 1830-1850

It has already been pointed out how the "Beachites" attempted to ape the "antiphlogistic" treatment of the regulars by administering their own distinctive remedies.[41] Powerful depletion with plant purgatives and emetic medicinals was strongly advocated and practiced by Beach as a substitute for calomel and bloodletting.[42] In addition, chemical ingredients were utilized in moderation in some of the early eclectic pharmaceutical preparations,[43] and this continued to be the policy with later practitioners as well.

The vast majority of the early eclectic physicians compounded their own medicines from their saddlebags and home stock. Ingredients were obtained in several ways, for example, through wholesale botanic houses, from the Shakers and their agents, by personally gathering plant medicinals in the field (i.e., wildcrafting), or through regular drug channels. By the 1840s, it is fairly commonplace to find Beach's remedies advertised with those of Thomson and Horton Howard in the botanic "depots" and Shaker agencies of the period. Thus, for example, A. Warner, agent for the Shakers in New York City, advertised in 1848 that "we keep on hand a general assortment of the various preparations introduced by Beach, Thomson, Howard, Smith and others."[44]

Although Beach's remedies were frequently prescribed by "reformed" and early eclectic physicians, a serious drawback to their wide public acceptance was their foul, nauseating taste and large crude dosage forms. In this respect, Beach's medicines were similar to those of Thomson. Typical remedies prescribed by Beach included a "Pulmonary Balsam" of spikenard root *(Aralia racemosa),* horehound *(Marrubium vulgare),* and elecampane *(Inula helenium);* "Anti-Choleric and Anti-Spasmotic Mixture" of camphor, peppermint, capsicum, and ginger; and "Syrup for Dysentery" made up of "a handful" of rhubarb and wild cherry bark with four tablespoons of sugar.[45] Among these remedies was his "neutralizing cordial" composed of rhubarb, peppermint, and saleratus (sodium bicarbonate), which, in somewhat revised form, later found a place in the *United States Pharmacopeia* (USP),[46] and, subsequently, in the *National Formulary* (NF). Many of Beach's recipes eventually turned up in King's *American Dispensatory* and "thence into pharmaceutical literature generally."[47]

THE "CONCENTRATED PREPARATIONS,"
1847 TO THE CIVIL WAR

In 1835, John King made a strong alcoholic extract of podophyllum. Filtering this solution, he added an equal amount of water, and upon distilling off the alcohol, the resinous material of the plant was precipitated. Attempting to evaluate this substance clinically, King rashly administered between twelve and fifteen grains of the medication to one of his patients, who promptly became violently ill and almost died.[48] Subsequently, King produced in a similar fashion the resins of macrotys *(Cimicifuga racemosa),* and the resins and oleoresins of iris, leptandra, and several other plants.[49] Some years later, an argument ensued concerning the priority of the discovery of resin of podophyllum, with a number of writers crediting W. Hodgson for making the discovery in 1831, and John R. Lewis for verifying Hodgson's findings in an inaugural dissertation published in the *American Journal of Pharmacy* in 1847.[50] Procter specifically stated that Lewis's claims "are entirely scientific, and refer to the chemical nature of the active principle of podophyllin, its activity being substantiated by experiments on himself."[51] This assertion was ably controverted by John Uri Lloyd, who, crediting John King with the discovery, pointed out that both Hodgson and Lewis had used strong chemical reagents, with the result that their yields were essentially decomposition products of podophyllum, rather than the actual resin.[52]

Manufacture and marketing of the resin of podophyllum, along with the other "resinoid"[53] plant medicinals, were first begun in 1847 by William S. Merrell and Company of Cincinnati. In 1850, Merrell boasted, before a gathering of eclectic physicians, "It is often asked with respect to Podophyllin, Leptandrin, and other analogous preparations, am I the discoverer of these? I am so in the same sense that Fulton invented the steamboat and Morse the electric telegraph."[54] This statement was disingenuous in view of King's prior work.[55]

The generic ending *in,* first utilized by Merrell to designate the eclectic resinoid medicinals, was quickly adopted by virtually all subsequent manufacturers of these concentrations. In due course, severe criticism was leveled at this nomenclature, notably by Procter and Squibb. Merrell stated that the name "podophyllin" had been suggested to him by George B. Wood, influential co-editor of the *United States Dispensatory*.[56] "Even when the preparation became official in the *United States Pharmacopeia* (1860) as *Resina Podophylli*," wrote Lloyd, "the title of the commercial drug remained unchanged."[57]

By 1853, William S. Merrell and Company was advertising two classes of resinoids:[58] (1) *Powdered resinoids*,[59] which were described as "the Medicinal Principles of the Indigenous roots from which they are obtained and named, in a state of proximate, if not absolute purity. They are mostly of a *Resinoid* character, in form of a Powder, more or less colored, and generally Amorphous. Their medical strength is from 12 to 24 times that of the powdered root which yields them. . . . For uses and Doses, see Eclectic Dispensatory"; and (2) *Soft resinoids and oleoresins*,[60] which were stated to be "like those of the first class, [which] are precipitated by water from their alcoholic solutions and are of nearly the same degree of medical power and purity. But they are soft or semifluid in their character, and cannot be presented in the powdered form without decomposing, by strong Acids or Alkalies. . . . We have obtained dry powders from several of them, but not such as appear to us to possess fully the medical virtues of the plants. We may yet succeed in doing so satisfactorily, and shall then transfer them to the first class. At present we present them in form of soft extracts, or thick oils, put up in 1 oz. vials."

Merrell's advertisement was prefaced by a very revealing statement, bringing into sharp focus a basic weakness of the eclectic pharmaceutical manufacturers of this period: "Our efforts are directed, not to the improvement of Chemistry but of Medicine; not to make scientific analyses of plants, but to present their Medicinal Principles in a concentrated, definite, and economical form, as articles of the Materia Medica. Therefore," he admitted, "we do not aim so much at the chemical purity of these preparations, as to retain their medical virtues unimpaired."

It is precisely this reluctance to pursue phytochemical work along the lines of the Philadelphia College of Pharmacy, or to emulate the work of the distinguished continental pharmacist-chemists, that doomed so much of eclectic pharmacy to scientific sterility and gross empiricism.

The psychological impact of these concentrated remedies on eclectic practitioners was tremendous. According to Wilder, there had been nothing like it since the repeal of restrictive medical regulatory acts "to fire the heart of Eclectic physicians with such glowing hope."[61] The physios attempted to climb aboard the eclectic bandwagon and to claim a share of the glory (see pp. 110-113). Now, for the first time, the eclectics believed they could match the alkaloidal pharmacy of the regulars with concentrated medicines of their own. Moreover, it was claimed by a number of eclectics and physio-medicals that the new concentrated preparations represented the therapeutic effects of whole plants and, thus, were superior to the "old school" products that violated "the integrity of nature's combination of proximate principles" in their isolation of separate plant constituents.[62] Furthermore, many of the bulky and nauseating plant medications could now be replaced with "new school" remedies, which would take up little space in the physician's saddlebags, and which would be far more agreeable for the patient to take.[63] The fashionable clientele, hitherto attracted by the palatable infinitesimal dosing of the homeopaths, would now flock to the eclectic practitioners. The prospects for the future were indeed alluring.

In the meantime, Merrell's successful venture into the manufacture of eclectic concentrates was the signal for many other firms to enter the field.[64] The manufacture and sale of eclectic concentrated remedies became a large-scale and lucrative industry. The new resins, resinoids, oleoresins, and alkaloids were soon distributed and sold through all regular drug channels. In 1857, the *Eclectic Medical Journal* announced that the sale of concentrated remedies had gained so much ground that "the sales of the firm of B. Keith & Co., to the Allopathic profession is about as great as those to the Eclectic."[65]

The distinction between eclectic and regular pharmaceutical establishments became increasingly difficult to discern as the nineteenth century progressed. Indeed, in Rothstein's words, "The problem of therapeutic distinctiveness haunted eclectic physicians throughout the nineteenth century."[66] Even at an early date (1853),

Merrell advertised that he kept for sale "the usual assortment of Foreign Medicine and Allopathic Preparations."[67] It is interesting to note also that no one saw the incongruity involved when Merrell, a man highly influential in eclectic circles,[68] advertised his products (eclectic and allopathic) in regular medical journals that were violently hostile to eclecticism.

Merrell had begun to manufacture the "essential tinctures" alluded to in the previous advertisement in 1858. These tinctures were concentrated alcoholic extractions of crude plant drugs and were described as "containing . . . all the virtues of the plant separated from extraneous matter, and being of definite and known strength, may readily be diluted by alcohol into *officinal* tinctures, or be added to simple syrup to form beautiful . . . *medicinal syrups,* or be evaporated to the pilular consistence, and thus form most permanent and reliable *alcoholic extracts.*"[69] That same year, Merrell read a paper at the annual meeting of the American Pharmaceutical Association, in which he expounded his theories on alcohol as a solvent in plant extraction and expressed his views on essential tinctures.[70]

As stated earlier, profound disillusionment with concentrated remedies had set in among large segments of eclectic practitioners by the time of the Civil War. If Scudder's report is accurate, then certainly many eclectics had by then lapsed supinely "into the habit of using a routine of podophyllin, quinine, and morphia." The lucrative business of making and selling concentrated medicines nevertheless continued throughout the nineteenth and into the beginning of the twentieth centuries. Nostrum manufacturers and other unscrupulous persons reaped huge profits from their sale. According to Lloyd, "A heterogeneous collection was that which was finally included in the commercial lists of resins, resinoids, alkaloids, and concentrations, a list that stands yet in current catalogues [written 1909]. . . . The odium of it all rested, unfortunately, on the Eclectic school of medicine, by reason of the origin of the first of these products . . . as well as from the fact that many over-enthusiastic Eclectic physicians had been entrapped in the craze."[71] "Out of it all," concluded Lloyd, "came the introduction of a few resins and a few alkaloidal salts of American plants, but yet these few, introduced into the Eclectic school over a century ago, comprise all of any importance whatever that are today used by any class of physicians [written 1910]."[72]

Despite their limitations, the concentrated remedies created quite a stir. As would be expected, the introduction of an eclectic pharmacy of such wide scope immediately interested a number of outstanding leaders in nineteenth-century pharmacy, such as Edward S. Wayne, Edward Parrish, and William Procter Jr. Their authoritative views give us an important insight into the eclectic pharmacy of the 1850s and 1860s.

E. S. WAYNE VERSUS B. KEITH AND COMPANY

Encouraged by the success of William S. Merrell and Company, B. Keith of New Hampshire came to New York City in the early 1850s and proceeded to manufacture concentrated remedies. Keith employed Dr. Grover Coe, an ex-president of the National Eclectic Medical Association[73] to work in his laboratory and act as publicity man for the firm. Soon after the organization of this company, it was announced that the concern would be known not only by the name of B. Keith and Company but also as the American Chemical Institute. "The object of this Institute," it was stated, "is to prepare the active principles of Indigenous and Foreign Medical Plants. . . . All the articles manufactured at our laboratory will be put up in vials of flint glass, be hermetically sealed and stamped 'American Chemical Institute, N.Y.'"[74] Fourteen wholesale agents were listed by B. Keith and Company as distributors of the products of the American Chemical Institute, among which were such establishments as Coolidge, Adams and Bond, Law and Boyd, and McKesson and Robbins of New York City.[75]

In 1855, B. Keith and Company sponsored the publication of an anonymous book of 300 pages titled *Positive Medical Agents: Being a Treatise on the New Alkaloid, Resinoid, and Concentrated Preparations of Indigenous and Foreign Medical Plants*, by authority of the American Chemical Institute.

In his review of this work in the *American Journal of Pharmacy,*[76] Procter pointed out that "[t]he real object of the book is to create a demand for the medicines which, owing to the utter silence of the writer on their mode of preparation can only be had of the

'American Chemical Institute.'"[77] Procter was puzzled by the book. The title, he admitted, suggested "some valuable additions to pharmacy," but a careful search of its pages yielded no contribution to the field whatsoever.[78]

Shortly after Procter's review appeared, Edward S. Wayne (1818-1885), a prominent pharmacist and chemist of Cincinnati, subjected the concentrated medicines of B. Keith and Company to chemical analysis and published his results in the *American Journal of Pharmacy*.[79] His findings showed that many of their products were fraudulently adulterated with magnesium carbonate and were completely at variance with the "high tone" and "boast of superior chemical and pharmaceutical lore" assumed by the American Chemical Institute.[80] Later, Wayne's analysis of the concentrates of William S. Merrell left him similarly unimpressed.[81]

It will be recalled that the faculty of the Eclectic Medical Institute of Cincinnati had been rent by bitter dissension in 1856. One faction that had succeeded in wresting control of the EMI and its publication, the *Eclectic Medical Journal,* warmly supported the products of B. Keith and Company. The defeated portion of the faculty immediately founded a rival medical school in Cincinnati, The Eclectic College of Medicine, and launched an opposition periodical, *The College Journal of Medical Science.* This latter group, of which John King was a member, was extremely critical of the concentrated medicines put out by B. Keith and Company, and it was the request of another member of this ousted opposition group, Dr. C. H. Cleaveland, that had actually induced Wayne to undertake an examination of the products of the American Chemical Institute.[82]

Repercussions from Wayne's report were quick to follow. The *Eclectic Medical Journal,* which had been consistently praising B. Keith and Company and carrying the advertisements of the American Chemical Institute, published a blistering attack on Wayne, written by Dr. Grover Coe.[83] "We do repeat, with all sincerity of purpose," wrote Coe, "that Mr. Wayne has entirely mistaken his vocation, and ought to be seriously advised by some kind friend to stick to his drugs, and not attempt to assume a suit of qualifications which nature never intended he should wear."[84] Simultaneously, Professor L. E. Jones of the EMI defended Keith's remedies against the charge of adulteration and announced that he was convinced "that the 'concentrated remedies' as now prepared by them, are as pure as the present state of organic chemistry will permit."[85]

In the meantime, Wayne published a second article giving additional data on the constituents of Keith's much-publicized preparations. This time his paper was published in *The College Journal of Medical Science*, the publication of the ousted rival group of Eclectic professors. Again his findings showed that Keith's medications were adulterated with magnesium carbonate, iron salts, sodium chloride, and tannic acid.[86] This second article elicited the wrath of the *Eclectic Medical Journal*, which attacked both Wayne and the rival eclectic publication: "[It was] the editors of the College Journal . . . who brought Mr. Wayne before the public with fulsome panegyric. They indited several long paragraphs to this gentleman, and since that time, there are many chemists who question his ability of subjects of even the simplest character."[87]

In the same issue of *The College Journal of Medical Science*, an additional and even more significant paper by Wayne was published, questioning the value of concentrates as commonly manufactured by the pharmaceutical houses of that period.[88] Wayne pointed out that the conventional procedure for producing these substances was to precipitate the resinous or oleoresinous material from a concentrated tincture of the crude plant by the addition of water. The resinous precipitate was then collected, dried, and powdered. When manufacturing on a large scale, the alcohol was recovered by distillation and subsequently used for other operations. Wayne conceded that this method was effective in extracting the therapeutic resin from such plants as jalap and podophyllum, but he added, "It does not follow that gentian, cinchona, opium, hydrastis, prunus, sanguinaria, should yield . . . [their therapeutic principles] by the same mode of treatment."[89] He further argued that valuable water-soluble principles of many plants are lost in this process and concluded, "These resins have been claimed as an advance in pharmacy. For my part, I cannot perceive it. . . . A good extract is in many instances the best form of concentrated remedies, and contains when well made, all the medicinal properties of the substance it was made of."[90]

A vigorous but unconvincing rejoinder by William S. Merrell followed Wayne's article. Merrell emphatically denied that all eclectic concentrated remedies were made in the manner described by Wayne:[91] "Of the articles which I have introduced into the profession as proximate medicinal principles," he wrote, "scarcely any two are prepared by just the same process."[92] Merrell carefully refrained from revealing the important details concerning his methods of manufacture but, moreover, failed to demonstrate that he had subjected any of his products to serious chemical analysis.

It is interesting to note that at least one segment of the eclectic profession was genuinely concerned in obtaining a true picture of the therapeutic and pharmaceutical status of the concentrated medicines that were flooding the market. Between 1856 and 1859, *The College Journal of Medical Science* attempted to alert eclectic practitioners to the adulterated and worthless eclectic concentrations that were being sold widely. John King, who had pioneered in the introduction of these preparations, was among the first to sound the alarm. Calling the mass-manufactured eclectic concentrates "a most stupendous fraud," King pointed out that the eclectics "have sufficient to do in contending for the truth and justice of our cause, without warring against the impositions" of manufacturers more interested in profit than product.[93]

In 1858, Dr. Grover Coe, the publicity man for B. Keith and Company, published a pretentious 445-page book, in which he announced, "We have not sought to charm the sense of elegance of diction, nor aimed to delude the reason by ingeniously wrought hypothesis; but simply to present, in a concise manner, an array of scientific facts which we hope will be of practical utility to the profession."[94] Coe's work was designed to promote the sale of B. Keith and Company's products under the guise of being a scientific treatise. Procter's review of this book was short and to the point: "Our country is deluged with medicines of this class, and it is time that a stand should be taken to discourage their introduction into regular pharmacy, whilst they remain secret preparations.[95]

It might be asked at this point whether Wayne's exposé, along with the sharp criticism of John King, *The College Journal of Medical Science,* and Procter, had any effect in curbing the operations of B. Keith and Company. All evidence points to the contrary. According to Wilder, Keith's business "became very prosperous and lucrative," and, eventually, "the proprietor dropped all relation with the Reformed and Eclectic schools."[96] Interestingly, even as late as the 1920s, Lloyd Brothers, who were never associated with eclectic concentrations, continued to manufacture and sell a line of these products. The continued presence of these concentrations in the Lloyd Brothers inventory was more a testimony to the endurance of lingering physician demand than to Lloyds' belief in their therapeutic value. "These preparations we look upon," they cautioned their customers in 1921, "as a class, as 'hold overs' from the pharmacy of the past."[97] Nonetheless, they acknowledged their historical importance in forming a link between the "crudities of primitive pharmacy" and "the better understood pharmaceutical preparations of the present."[98]

PARRISH'S CRITIQUE OF THE CONCENTRATES

The distinguished nineteenth-century Philadelphia pharmacist Edward Parrish (1822-1872) devoted considerable attention to the new eclectic concentrated remedies. In 1851, Parrish published a critical review of Merrell's preparations, along with observations on eclectic pharmacy.[99] He pointed out that the "so-called resinoids have attained a very considerable sale, and from being used almost exclusively in the West, where they originated, have been introduced into our market [Philadelphia] and into those of New York and Boston."[100] Parrish, among other things, hotly criticized Merrell's method of discussing resinoid medications in the eclectic press as "intimating that they are prepared by a difficult process not conveniently resorted to by pharmaceutists generally," and "intended, rather to discourage any attempts to prepare them, than to invite the co-operation of pharmaceutists by a candid and full detail of the process and results."[101]

When Edward Parrish first published his *Introduction to Practical Pharmacy* in 1856, he devoted barely two pages to "Concentrated or Resinoid Extracts."[102] In his discussion of these preparations and the practitioners who used them, he stated that "they have been instrumental in introducing to notice some obscure medical plants which possess valuable properties," but "their narrow and unscientific system . . . limited their usefulness and excluded them from the pale of the regular profession."[103]

In the second edition of *An Introduction to Practical Pharmacy* (1859), Parrish devoted almost three times as much space to "Concentrated Extracts or Resinoids" than he had in the previous edition (nearly six pages).[104] A significant observation occurs in the second edition not present in the first: "The 'concentrated remedies' of the so-called *eclectics* have within a few years obtained increased popularity, not only with practitioners of that school, but with physicians generally."[105] This statement confirmed the claims of the eclectics that their concentrated medicines were being increasingly used by regular practitioners. In addition to this observation, Parrish also made an interesting deletion of a phrase employed in the text of the first edition. The reference to the eclectic practitioners as pursuing " a narrow and unscientific practice" is discreetly omitted. However, his charge of "pharmaceutical empiricism" leveled against the eclectics in the first edition is reiterated with full force.[106]

It was, however, in the third edition of his textbook, published in 1864, that Parrish presented his most comprehensive analysis of eclectic concentrates, with sixteen pages devoted to the subject.[107] He prefaced his discussion by indicting the eclectic manufacturers for their lack of standardization ("each claiming the superiority of his own preparations over those of his rivals"), their inconsistent nomenclature, and, in many cases, the secrecy of their formulas.[108] Parrish singled out the nomenclature used by eclectic pharmaceutical establishments as particularly problematic. He pointed out that the generic termination *in* was being applied indiscriminately to substances whose true chemical nature was not clear. A serious problem had arisen, he noted, when eclectic products bearing the ending *in* were being confused with the true alkaloids of commerce.[109] More than fifty "Unofficinal Concentrated Remedies" manufactured by various eclectic concerns were discussed by Parrish.[110] Parrish complained that the eclectics relied too heavily upon a single process of precipitation, indicating that it was quite appropriate where the active constituent was resinous, but hardly suitable for many other medicinal plant substances. He also pointed out that "bringing all these concentrated remedies to the condition of powders by the addition of sugar of milk, or other dry material" to "naturally soft or oily" products "has many objections, among which are their unnecessary dilution, and the increased exposure of their particles to oxidation or evaporation." Parrish concluded by objecting to the empirical and idiosyncratic nature of eclectic pharmacy and "its rather unprofessional and business-like character."[111]

PROCTER'S CRITIQUE OF KING
AND THE ECLECTICS REVISITED

William Procter's reviews of King's *American Eclectic Dispensatory* (1854) and the *American Dispensatory* (1859) were discussed at some length from the standpoint of the utilization and investigation of the plant materia medica (see pp. 55-57), but Procter's analysis had an important bearing on eclectic pharmacy of the decade 1850 to 1860, beyond the examination and use of an indigenous materia medica: his analysis pointed out significant problems in the eclectics' pharmaceutical approach and methodology. It was Procter's opinion that the eclectics showed a singular inability to pursue original work in chemical analyses, even though by the 1850s the eclectics were using many chemical preparations. The eclectics were especially vulnerable to criticism for avoiding phytochemical investigations of the indigenous plant materia medica. It will be recalled that Procter berated the eclectics for not emulating the work of students and faculty of the Philadelphia College of Pharmacy in carrying out proximate analyses of plants. Similar to Parrish, Procter criticized the loose nomenclature applied to the concentrated preparations whose chemical nature had not been elucidated.[112]

On the credit side, Procter was pleased to see William S. Merrell, an experienced druggist,[113] contribute his knowledge to King's *American Dispensatory*. He indicates that the eclectics had well-constructed galenical preparations (e.g., syrups, tinctures, extracts, etc.) made from their distinctive plant drugs. Despite the extreme emphasis that the eclectics of the decade 1850 to 1860 put on concentrated medicines, their galenical pharmacy, although minimized in their medical journals of this period, should not be overlooked by the historian. Procter approved of King's critical attitude toward the American Chemical Institute and similar drug companies. An important point stressed by Procter was that despite serious shortcomings of eclecticism, certain aspects of eclectic activity de-

served to be carefully investigated and should not be contemptuously dismissed. This reasonable attitude was characteristic of American pharmacy, as subsequent discussion will show, and contrasted
sharply with the uncompromising hostility directed at the eclectics
by the regular physicians.

When John King, in collaboration with Robert S. Newton, published the first edition of *The Eclectic Dispensatory of the United
States* in 1852, a suit for plagiarism was instituted against this book
by the proprietors George B. Wood and Franklin Bache. The courts
ruled against King, who had to destroy the plates of this work and
forfeit about $6,000 in damages.[114] This accounts for Procter's
criticism that the work included no commentary on the *United
States Dispensatory* or the *United States Pharmacopeia*. Actually,
what Procter apparently did not know was that King, from the very
beginning, could not get permission to use the USP. This would
account for the absence of USP formula from King's *American
Dispensatory.*

THE SHAKERS AND ECLECTIC PHARMACY

Shaker pharmaceutical activity is of considerable interest,[116] but
only two aspects of this activity have a direct bearing on the present
discussion. First, for a good part of the nineteenth century, the Shakers were purveyors of plant medicinals to botanic physicians and
botanic wholesale and retail establishments (see Appendix 8).[117]
Second, to a limited extent, the Shakers manufactured recipes copied
from Thomsonian and early eclectic literature, and for a short time,
the New York Shakers made a brief attempt to compete with their
rival, Tilden and Company of New Lebanon, New York, in the
manufacture of eclectic concentrated preparations.

These conclusions are based upon a thorough search through
Shaker source materials in an attempt to assess the role of this
interesting religious sect in the botanico-medical movement.[118]
Throughout the investigation of Shaker pharmaceutical activity,
particular attention was directed to ascertaining any ideological
influences of Thomsonianism or eclecticism. The conclusion that
botanicism made no significant *ideological* impact on Shaker pharmaceutical and medical views has been confirmed, but this, of

course, does not imply no influence whatsoever. The Shakers' devotion to herbal medicines was strong and enduring, and it would have been remarkable if absolutely no impact was made upon their activities by the botanico-medical movement. Elder Henry Blinn (1824-1905), who oversaw the Canterbury and Enfield Shaker communities in New Hampshire most of his life, indicated that the Shakers adopted a Thomsonian "pepper puke," along with some other remedies, rather early on.[119] Still, such influence was limited. The only allusion that we have seen to the Shaker manufacture of eclectic concentrated remedies is in an editorial written by Procter, in which he alludes to a visit at a Shaker community where he was shown "some crude specimens of some of the 'concentrated preparations' . . . which were in course of preparation."[120]

CONCLUSION OF THE EARLY PERIOD

The eclectic impact on American pharmacy during this early period to 1869 is best characterized as one of groping and uncertainty. True, the eclectics had begun a significant manufacturing enterprise under the leadership of men such as William S. Merrell, B. Keith, and others, but they had also suffered from a lack of quality control and standardization in their preparations. This injured their professional standing and credibility within the medical and pharmaceutical communities. All this was about to change, however, as the eclectics embarked upon their last and greatest therapeutic phase, the era of specific medication. Established by John Milton Scudder, promoted by his colleague John King, and developed by John Uri Lloyd, specific medicines would bring to American eclecticism a measure of recognition and scientific standing that it had thus far found elusive.

A NEW ERA DAWNS— SPECIFIC MEDICATION, 1869-1936

As indicated earlier, the doctrine of specific medication enunciated by John Milton Scudder in 1869 was eagerly accepted by large segments of the eclectic profession. "Small doses and pleasant medicines" became the keynote of the new therapeutic policy.[121] "A series of experiments," stated Scudder, "found that they [specific medicines] could be put in the form of very strong tincture and dispensed in water, and then could be easily carried, and would not offend the palate or stomach."[122]

The monopoly to manufacture specific medicines was given by Scudder to H. M. Merrell and Company, predecessors of the firm of Merrell, Thorp, and Lloyd of Cincinnati. An 1879 advertisement of this pharmaceutical company states that, in accordance with the teachings of specific medication, Scudder "prepared a set of labels and had them copyrighted. He gave upon each the specific use of the remedy, and the dose."[123] Two other advertisements that same year by Merrell, Thorp, and Lloyd illustrate the nature of specific medicines. One of these advertisements informs its readers that specific tinctures are "made from fresh indigenous plants, and represent sixteen troy ounces [of the crude plant drug] to each fluid pint" and that they "stand out distinctly from the officinal tinctures and fluid extracts of the pharmacopoeia, which admits the crude materials found on the market are often worthless from drying and atmospheric action."[124] The second of these advertisements, which is very similarly worded, states, "We prepare these remedies at the request of Prof. John M. Scudder from fresh materials when indigenous to this country." As for foreign plant drugs, this advertisement went on to say that "Belladonna, Hyoscyamus, Arnica, Pulsatilla, Staphysagria, are directly tinctured to our order, in their native country while fresh, and imported direct."[125] In addition to advertising specific medicines, this company also listed nitrous ether, resins, oils, alkaloids, compound syrups, elixirs, fluid extracts, solid extracts, and powdered solid extracts.

As ownership of Merrell, Thorp, and Lloyd changed hands, the monopoly to manufacture medicines using the copyright name of "Specific Medicine" passed successively to Thorp and Lloyd Brothers (1881), to Lloyd Brothers (1885), and finally to Lloyd Brothers Pharmacists, Inc. (1924). In 1932, Lloyd Brothers Pharmacists, Inc., published a *Dose Book* of specific medicines with indications for their therapeutic uses.[126] Nearly 100 specific medicines based on plant medicinals were listed, and minim doses (usually five to fifteen) were directed to be administered well diluted in water. By this time, John Uri Lloyd had developed a colloidal form of specific medicine that he called "Colloidum." The colloidal preparations would mix readily with water, glycerine, diluted alcohol, or syrup without precipitating. This transferred "the natural, desirable, non-crystalline (colloidal) structure of the drugs to liquid solvents . . . without lessening or altering the preparation's therapeutic qualities."[127]

"Specific tinctures" closely resembled the "essential tinctures" that William S. Merrell had put on the market in 1858. In fact, the *California Medical Journal,* an eclectic publication, charged that when "Dr. J. M. Scudder wrote his 'Specific Medication,' it was Wm. S. Merrell, AM, MD, and Albert Merrell, MD, now of St. Louis, who gave to Dr. Scudder the pharmaceutical data upon which was based the formulae for the manufacture of the so-called 'Specific Tinctures.'"[128] The situation was further complicated by the appearance on the market in the 1880s of "normal tinctures," formulated by Albert Merrell and described in *A Digest of Materia Medica and Pharmacy* as tinctures with rated strengths based upon a "normal" standard, expressed as N/1. Thus, a tincture of half strength would be rated at N/2 (i.e., two parts of tincture to one part of the drug). In this way, presumably each tincture could be easily identified as to its relative strength. A tincture marked 3N/10, for example, would indicate "that ten parts of the preparation to the name of which it was affixed contained 3 parts of the 'normal' or drug."[129]

A confusing situation resulted from the publication of Merrell's *Digest of Materia Medica and Pharmacy.* In 1870, the National Eclectic Medical Association had created a committee to prepare a national eclectic pharmacopoeia.[130] Nothing had been done about the matter until Albert Merrell, a member of the Committee on Pharmacopoeia, presented a plan for this work to the association in 1880, which, according to Wilder, "was adopted, and a proposition was accepted from Dr. Merrell to prepare and publish the work at his own expense, he having the copyright."[131] Thus, when the work finally appeared in 1883, it was a one-man job, paid for and copyrighted by Merrell, with the status of having been prepared "under the supervision and with the concurrence of a committee of the

National Eclectic Medical Association," and "the official approval of that body."[132] In the meantime, a resolution had been adopted in 1879, at the convention of the National Eclectic Medical Association, designating the *American Dispensatory* as "the standard authority of the National Eclectic Medical Association."[133] It will be noted that Lloyd, in 1882, advanced certain arguments against the desirability of having an eclectic pharmacopoeia, stating, "Our [eclectic] physicians and students were taught that the Pharmacopoeia of the United States was the authority as far as fundamentals were concerned," but he also added later that the *American Dispensatory* "is really the pharmacopoeial standard of a great section of American [eclectic] medicine." Thus, by the end of the 1800s, eclectic practitioners could consult three "pharmacopoeial" standards.

JOHN URI LLOYD (1849-1936)

The close association of William S. Merrell with the concentrated remedies debacle caused King and Scudder to look elsewhere for someone to research their new line of specific medicines. Thus, when John King was looking for someone to assist his colleague in developing these pharmaceuticals, he passed up the doyen of eclectic pharmacy (Merrell) for a young and conscientious clerk just recently released from apprenticeship: John Uri Lloyd. The choice was fortuitous. Not only did Lloyd expand specific medicines to more than 300 different items, he ultimately became the most important individual working in eclectic pharmacy, and a person of considerable stature in American pharmaceutical circles as well.[134] His contributions in the fields of phytochemistry, colloidal chemistry, and manufacturing pharmacy were of a very high caliber. During his long and productive life, he also found time to teach, write novels and regional studies, publish numerous articles and books, and develop a unique library.

Born in New York State in 1849, Lloyd spent his boyhood in Kentucky, where he received an elementary education largely from his parents, who were themselves college educated and former teachers. Apprenticed at the age of fifteen to pharmacists W. J. M. Gordon and, later, George Eger of Cincinnati, young Lloyd subsequently came under the influence of Drs. King and Scudder, who induced him to work in eclectic pharmacy by securing a position for Lloyd with the eclectic firm of H. M. Merrell in 1871. So capable was the young pharmacist, that in the space of one year, he was made manager of the company's laboratory, and by 1877, Lloyd had become a partner in the company of Merrell, Thorp, and Lloyd. Subsequently, in 1881, Merrell retired; his interest was purchased by John Uri Lloyd, who then brought his younger brother, Nelson Ashley Lloyd (1852-1925), into the firm, at which point the name of the company became Thorp and Lloyd Brothers. Thorp retired in 1885, selling his interest to John and Nelson Lloyd (Lloyd Brothers). In 1886, Curtis (1859-1926), the youngest brother, was admitted to a full partnership but soon thereafter devoted all his time to the study of mycology, in which field he achieved an international reputation.[135] The firm's name underwent another and final change in 1924, becoming Lloyd Brothers Pharmacists, Inc. John Uri Lloyd's death, on April 9, 1936, marked the passing of the last of the three brothers. After some family wrangling in the courts over the disposition of the estate, the company was finally sold to S. B. Penick Company of New York City in 1938.

The foregoing story of an obscure young man rising through ability and hard work to attain financial success is a familiar one in American economic life, and John Uri Lloyd carefully crafted a public persona cast in the idyllic image of Horatio Alger himself—trials and adversity serving to build a character of honest fortitude that eventually surmounted all odds to achieve fame and fortune. As inspiring as this story is, Lloyd had special advantages, not the least of which were well-educated and supportive parents of comfortable means who carefully directed their son into a practical career that particularly suited his interests and abilities. Lloyd's achievements, however, were real and far transcended mere business acumen. What immediately set Lloyd apart from other individuals prominent in eclectic pharmacy, such as William S. Merrell, Henry A. Tilden, F. D. Hill, B. Keith, William H. Baker, and others, was his conviction that chemistry had to be applied to the problems of eclectic pharmacy. It will be recalled that it was the neglect of phytochemistry by eclectic pharmacists that had prompted Procter's severe criticism. Lloyd's policy contrasted sharply with William S. Merrell's announcement in 1853 that "Our efforts are directed, not to the improvement of Chemistry but of Medicine; not to make scientific analyses of plants, but to present their Medicinal Principles in a concentrated, definite and economical form."[136] The difference between Lloyd's approach and that of Merrell was one of the utilization of scientific pharmaceutical chemistry as against reliance on pharmaceutical empiricism. Moreover, Lloyd's interests lay in improving not only eclectic pharmacy, but pharmacy in general.

By the 1880s, Lloyd's work had attracted considerable attention in American pharmaceutical circles. In 1882, he was awarded the Ebert Prize by the American Pharmaceutical Association for his paper on "Precipitates in Fluid Extracts." A second Ebert Prize was awarded him in 1891 for his contribution to alkaloidal assaying ("A Scheme of Assaying"), and in 1916, he received a third Ebert Prize for his paper "Adsorption Powers of Hydrated Siliceous Earths." From 1883 to 1887, Lloyd occupied the chair of professor of chemistry and pharmacy at the Cincinnati College of Pharmacy and, in 1887, was elected president of the American Pharmaceutical Association.

A signal honor befell Lloyd in 1916, when his work in colloid chemistry attracted the attention of the prominent German chemist Wolfgang Ostwald (1883-1943). Ostwald translated a number of Lloyd's essays that had appeared from time to time in the *Proceedings of the American Pharmaceutical Association,* between 1879-1885. These German translations were first published in Ostwald's *Kolloidchemische Beihefte,* and subsequently as a distinct brochure. George Urdang has pointed out that "this quite unusual reprinting and reissuing of old publications means one of the greatest tributes paid to an American scientist by European science."[137] In the preface of the *Kolloidchemische Beihefte* reissue of this pathbreaking work, Ostwald heaped editorial praise on Lloyd, saying that "[he] knows of no more rigorous demonstration of adsorption in capillary analysis than that of J. U. Lloyd" and concluded that his work "constitutes a uniquely original contribution."[138] In the area of pharmaceutical equipment and techniques, Lloyd made noteworthy contributions through his development of the so-called "Cold Still Extractor" and his hydrous aluminum silicate reagent (Lloyd's Reagent) for removing alkaloids in solution by adsorption.

In addition, Lloyd is partly responsible for the development of the *National Formulary* (1888). His book of elixirs, published in 1883, clarified the confusion regarding these liquids, put them into a definite category, and assisted in developing high-quality formulas for their compounding and manufacture. This work, titled *Elixirs: Their History, Formulae and Method of Preparations,* is considered to have been an important stimulus to the issuance of the *National Formulary,*[139] a compendium that was initiated largely out of the need to organize and standardize the elixir dosage form.[140]

When to all these accomplishments are added his other publications, such as *Drugs and Medicines of North America* (1884-1887), in collaboration with Curtis G. Lloyd, *Chemistry of Medicines* (1881), and numerous articles, then one realizes the astounding versatility of Lloyd. In addition, as has already been mentioned, Lloyd's literary productions (six novels and regional studies), as well as the remarkable Lloyd Library of approximately 200,000 volumes sponsored by him in Cincinnati, serve further to perpetuate his name. His receipt of American pharmacy's highest honor, the Remington Medal, in 1920, was a fitting tribute to a man who had given much to his profession at home and abroad. Although the Lloyd Brothers firm would remain in the market under the ownership of S. B. Penick of New York until its final sale to Hoechst in 1960,[141] the passing of its patriarchal leader in 1936 marked the effective end of eclectic pharmaceutical development.

INTERPROFESSIONAL RELATIONS BETWEEN AMERICAN ECLECTICISM AND AMERICAN PHARMACY

In the 1850s, a modus vivendi developed between American eclecticism and American pharmacy that continued throughout the nineteenth century, based on the sale of eclectic remedies through regular drug channels and mutual recognition of positive achievements within each professional group.

There was no gainsaying the economic reality of an eclectic pharmaceutical industry producing concentrated and other remedies, such as Merrell's Essential Tinctures, or Lloyd's Specific Medicines, that were distributed and sold through regular wholesale and retail drug outlets. Eclectic practitioners were quite willing to have their pre-scriptions and remedies prepared by any qualified pharmacists, and even the regular physicians were prescribing eclectic concentrated preparations.

In addition to the economic link between eclecticism and Ameri-can pharmacy, there were certain areas in which both groups could establish professional rapport. The activity of John Uri Lloyd on behalf of eclectic and general pharmacy is an obvious example of this. Similarly, William S. Merrell's membership in the American Pharmaceutical Association helped to cement relations. One can also cite the example of the pharmacist E. S. Wayne working with John King to help solve certain pharmaceutical problems relating to the *American Dispensatory*.[142]

That the eclectics on the whole appreciated and respected the contributions of American pharmacy is clear. In an editorial that appeared in the eclectic press in 1864, the eclectics praised "the vari-ous associations of druggists" and called them "some of the most skillful and persevering investigators in the world." Insisting that the regular pharmacists had withheld "credit that is legitimately our due," the eclectics also admitted that they were as much in debt to mainstream pharmacy for its efforts at creating sound drug standards and tests for adulteration as mainstream pharmacy was in debt to the eclectics for having enlarged their vegetable materia medica.[143]

On the other hand, American pharmaceutical organizations and individuals were frequently critical, and sometimes even hostile, toward eclecticism. For example, it was announced at the Philadel-phia College of Pharmacy in 1863 that "[t]he question as to whether an apprentice in an 'Eclectic' establishment would be eligible to graduate in this College, was decided in the negative."[144] Even John Uri Lloyd, reminiscing in 1924 about his early experiences in eclectic pharmacy, could cast himself as a martyr to the eclectic cause: "In years gone by, when I attended the meeting of the Ameri-can Pharmaceutical Association, I felt as though I were alone. No man knows what I went through in days gone by in behalf of Eclectic pharmacy, and yet I have no ill feeling toward those men who resisted the innovation. . . . Today they stand among the best of my friends."[145] Still, such self-pity rests uneasily upon the shoulders of one who had accomplished so much, both in and outside the eclectic ranks.

The one obvious and fertile meeting ground where the eclectics and representatives of American pharmacy might have met in fruitful cooperation was in the investigation of the indigenous plants employed in eclectic medicine. With the notable exception of Lloyd, the reluctance, or inability, of the eclectics to pursue phytochemical work caused them to suffer a great loss of prestige and made them vulnerable to the charge of pharmaceutical empiricism.

Nevertheless, the eclectic preoccupation with indigenous plant medicinals stimulated the faculty and students of the Philadelphia College of Pharmacy to subject many of the eclectic plant remedies to proximate analysis and pharmaceutical research. In going through the volumes of the *American Journal of Pharmacy,* the evidence of this stimulus can be readily seen.[146] It is also interesting to note that eclectic plant remedies were not infrequently the subjects of graduating student theses at the Philadelphia College of Pharmacy.[147]

Many of the plant drugs used by eclectic practitioners thus passed into the general pharmaceutical literature, with a number also entering the official compendia (USP and NF). One eclectic practitioner, Dr. J. H. Bundy of California, was alone instrumental in introducing three medicinal plants *(Berberis aquifolium, Eriodictyon glutinosum, Rhamnus purshiana)* that, through the cooperation of the manufacturing house of Parke, Davis, and Company, won their way into the general materia medica and subsequently became official in the *United States Pharmacopeia.*[148] Thus, according to the eminent American pharmacist Charles Rice (1841-1900), "Many plants of which the Eclectics alone first availed themselves have ended by becoming the common property of the entire medical profession."[149]

AN EVALUATION

No doubt, much of the eclectic pharmacy during the nineteenth century was weakened, to paraphrase Parrish, by its empiricism and its unprofessional character. On the other hand, a large part of this weakness was later offset by the contributions of John Uri Lloyd.

The rise of an eclectic pharmaceutical industry created a vested interest and economic link with American pharmacy. Professional liaison between eclecticism and American pharmacy was engendered by such men as William S. Merrell and John Uri Lloyd, and rapport was developed through the eclectic promotion and contributions in the field of indigenous plant medicinals.

These significant connections with mainstream pharmacy demonstrate an important difference between the pharmaceutical community and its medical counterparts, namely, that while physicians might posture and inveigh against the sectarian "threat" to the healing art and science, American pharmacy's relationship to the sectarians was much more fluid and, indeed, amicable. There is no better example of this than Lloyd's election to the presidency of the American Pharmaceutical Association. Such an honor was bestowed upon a leading researcher and manufacturer of eclectic pharmaceuticals by professional colleagues representing American pharmacy's best and brightest. The American Medical Association can offer no similar example in its annals. The reason for this profound difference is partly explained in the financial symbiosis that had always existed between druggists and manufacturers, regardless of partisan affiliations, but also in the fact that much of the botanical materia medica was shared largely *without prejudice* by purveyors and compounders of medicaments, wherever they might be, because pharmacists (unlike their medical counterparts) had no professional/political stake in the prescriptions themselves. This allowed men such as William Procter and Edward Parrish, leaders of American pharmacy, to render tough but honest and objective appraisals of the sectarian materia medica. No doubt, the eclectic impact on American pharmaceutical activity of the nineteenth century is of considerable practical and historical import.

Chapter 7

Where Have All the Botanics Gone?

That eclectics had made an impact upon nineteenth-century American pharmacy is undeniable. Nevertheless, by century's end, the immediate future of medicine and pharmacy resided not in medicinal plant inquiry but in wholly new classes of drugs based upon equally new paradigms of medical science. The twentieth century would see the gradual decline of both the eclectics and the neo-Thomsonians, whether they were physio-medicals or some other brand of Thomsonian healer, in favor of a pharmaceutical armamentarium not based upon empirical observation but upon laboratory analysis and clinical trial. As this new pharmacy emerged, the first great botanico-medical movement came to a close in America. Ironically, just as medicinal plant inquiry reached its lowest ebb in American history in the 1960s, a new group emerged to pick up and carry the botanical standard forward.

THE END, 1910 AND AFTER

Nothing showed the appreciable link between the eclectic materia medica and mainstream pharmacy more than an interesting survey conducted by John Uri Lloyd in 1917.[1] In it, Lloyd questioned over 6,000 physicians (eclectic and regular) regarding the botanical drugs they prescribed in their practices. Somewhat surprisingly, the regular physicians named echinacea, a plant wholly associated with eclectic practice, as their number-one botanical medicine of choice. Other top-ranking plants among regulars included many often associated with homeopathic practice, such as aconite, macrotys, and bryonia. Among eclectics, Lloyd noted that "the main remedies . . . are substantially the same [as the regulars]" and that a comparison of both respondents' lists led him to determine that "many old-time Pharmacopoeial drugs have been abandoned by their former friends, and replaced by newer Eclectic remedies."[2] The results led Lloyd to conclude "that the majority of physicians are guided in their uses of remedies by their own judgment, based upon clinical observation and professional necessity. It is evident that physicians in actual practice generally prescribe as they see fit, regardless of whether a drug is mentioned in the Pharmacopoeia or has been recommended by therapeutic instructors, or whether it be advocated or not by leaders now in authoritative positions."[3]

What Lloyd's survey did *not* reveal, however, was the fact that by 1917, whole plant drugs had become passé. In 1910, three signal events heralded fundamental changes in medicine and pharmacy. One of the first clear indications that something truly revolutionary was taking place—something that was changing not only research and laboratory work but daily practice—was in the ninth decennial edition of the USP for that year. For the first time in U.S. pharmacopoeial history (since 1820) botanicals no longer represented a majority of official substances.[4]

The changes in the 1910 USP were more symptomatic than causative, however. That year, a second event occurred which indicated more fundamental changes afoot. This was when Paul Ehrlich (1859-1915) realized the Paracelsian dream of developing demonstrably effective chemotherapeutic agents with his arsphenamine compound, shown in clinical trials to be effective against encephalitis and syphilis.[5] Ehrlich announced his discovery in April at the Congress for Internal Medicine held at Wiesbaden, Germany.[6] Ehrlich's work represented the culmination of innovations in organic chemistry and laboratory synthesis, largely in Germany, that had taken place during the last quarter of the nineteenth century. Ehrlich's discovery became a sensation. Presented with the technology and expertise to discover *patentable* synthetic compounds, drug companies rushed to develop this potentially profitable class of pharmaceuticals to add to their inventory. In contrast, there was little economic incentive to continue a line of plant-based drugs. As botanical houses closed down across the country in the first half of the twentieth century, so did phytomedicinal research and development. Reflecting this trend, the percentage of botanicals in the USP witnessed a precipitous decline (see chart).

Official Phytomedicines in the United States: Percentage of Total USP

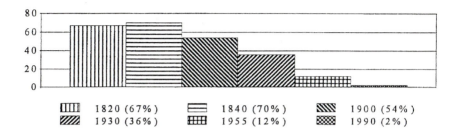

Source: Adapted from Wade Boyle, *Official Herbs* (New Palestine, OH: Buckeye Naturopathic Press, 1991).

The third development did not directly impact the vegetable materia medica itself but significantly affected the botanical sectarians. It occurred with the publication of *Medical Education in the United States and Canada* by Abraham Flexner (1866-1959).[7] The now-famous Flexner Report surveyed the condition of medical education throughout America and, in short, found it severely wanting. The chief complaint was against the large number of substandard proprietary schools that were flooding the health care scene with ill-prepared physicians. The American Medical College Association had already been working to reduce the number of these kinds of schools, but Flexner's report caused closures to accelerate. Flexner's standard was Johns Hopkins University at Baltimore, a school that was leading the way in promoting modern clinical and research-based education, imported largely from Germany. Historian Paul Starr has characterized Flexner's work as "the manifesto of a program that by 1936 guided 91 million dollars from Rockefeller's General Education Board (plus millions from other foundations) to a select group of medical schools."[8] Not surprisingly, the sectarian schools, unable to equip laboratories and weak in virtually all aspects of clinical instruction, were *not* among Flexner's "select group." Interestingly, Flexner praised some aspects of the newly refurbished Eclectic Medical Institute when he visited, but Flexner added a damning aside when he stated that all eclectics were "drug mad."[9]

Irrespective of Flexner's opinion of the eclectics, his report had the more far-reaching effect of spelling the end of botanico-medical education in America.

The twentieth century ushered in more than just the end of the original botanico-medical movement; it also saw research into phytomedicines virtually cease in America. While pharmacology was making great strides in developing new classes of drugs (including whole ranges of antibiotic agents), the one science that might have saved medicinal plant inquiry in this country (pharmacognosy) found itself unable to set a clear research agenda through much of the period. As noted pharmacognosist Varro E. Tyler has observed:

> During the first half of this century, pharmacognosy was almost obliterated by a group of well-intentioned but highly specialized educators and practitioners who approached the subject from an extremely limited viewpoint. As an examination of the most popular textbook of the period indicated [Youngken's *Textbook of Pharmacognosy* (1921-1948)], they considered the subject only as a botanical science and became obsessed with the taxonomy, morphology, anatomy, and histology of the plant that produced the active constituent rather than the chemistry, biochemistry, pharmacology, and therapeutics of that constituent. In other words, they emphasized the nature of the container rather than its contents.[10]

Unfortunately, this deficit was corrected in the latter half of this century by overcompensating in the other direction. "The science rapidly disowned the botanical emphasis that had cost it so dearly," writes Tyler, "and concentrated instead on the isolation and structure determination of organic compounds contained in plants. While a few other aspects were prominent during the early part of the period, by the 1980s American pharmacognosy had settled down to isolation and structure determination and little else."[11] Medical botany had, in effect, been replaced with phytochemistry.

Still, Ehrlich's arsphenamine (marketed under the name Salvarsan) did not turn out to be the medical savior that everyone expected. Arsphenamine, an arsenic-based compound, was unstable, and its activity on the human body unpredictable. Also, Salvarsan's ability to kill other pathogens was extremely limited, and efforts to find other "magic bullets" met with failure and a "period of pessimism."[12] Not until the development of the sulfa drugs would chemotherapeutics be greeted with renewed optimism.

At the same time that pharmacognosists were examining plants as containers, a new group of pharmacologic researchers, under the lead of Dr. Bernard "Steve" Brodie, began performing important studies in the postwar 1940s on drugs as chemicals that worked pharmacokinetically, both on and by the human body. Robert Kanigel points out that even before Brodie, "organic chemistry had progressed to a point that made the synthesis of new drugs possible. But," he adds, "before Brodie, there was so little *basis* for synthesizing them. How, with as pitiful a knowledge of drug metabolism as then existed, could you synthesize a new drug and expect it to work any better than the old? Over the next decade, Brodie and his coworkers changed all that."[13]

Faced with these innovations, by mid-twentieth century, the botanico-medical movement was all but dead. The Eclectic Medical Association would continue to meet into the 1960s,[14] although its substantive work was unmistakably over. Its proceedings read more like reunions of old war horses getting together to reminisce about the "glory days" than the meetings of active professionals exchanging research and ideas. There was no sense in discussing opportunities for advancement or charting new directions for the association; this was an organization without a future. Botanicism was in its death throes; but if this was *how* the botanico-medical movement died, it does not exactly explain *why* it died.

CAUSES FOR DECLINE— SCIENCE AND CULTURE

Historians have advanced numerous reasons for the decline of the American botanico-medical movement. Specific answers to the decline of just one aspect of this uniquely American phenomenon, the Thomsonians, even lack consensus. Joseph Kett has suggested that the decline of the sociopolitical environment so conducive to this grassroots medical movement coincided with the end of the Jacksonian egalitarian spirit of the age.[15] Daniel J. Wallace disagrees, stating that "the sect was not transitional in nature, and could have outlasted Jacksonian America had the sect not professionalized itself."[16]

Both conclusions are incomplete. Wallace fails to understand that the professionalization that took place under the physio-medicals and other neo-Thomsonians was fundamentally the inevitable and inexorable maturation of American social life that was replacing the previous generation of untamed Jacksonians. "In the nineteenth century," writes one analyst of the age, "as refinement spread downward and the middling orders assimilated a diluted refinement of their own, the great divide between polite and coarse isolated the lower orders on the margins of American society."[17] If there was one thing *every* medical sect wanted to avoid, it was being relegated to the margins of public life. After Jacksonian America spent itself in an orgy of egalitarian rhetoric, an ever-enlarging "polite society" demanded not common men but credentialed men, not self-taught healers but educated physicians, and all the major sectarians were ready to provide the necessary accoutrements.

Kett, however, believes that all this is moot. He insists that, by the 1860s, allopathic physicians had solidified their hold on the medical profession due to the proliferation of medical schools that had resulted in the medical degree becoming the clear distinguishing mark of the regular from the empiric practitioner. "The medical profession on the eve of the Civil War," he concludes, "was thus better regulated than it had been at any other time in American history, not because of institutions but in spite of them."[18] Perhaps. But even if it *was* better regulated than ever before, it surely had a long way to go before asserting its hegemony over an entire profession that itself was inundated in the 1860s with sectarian schools in all regions of the nation. Kett seems a bit Whiggish, giving too much too soon to the ultimate victors in a struggle that was hardly settled until the opening decades of the twentieth century.

Clearly the botanics lived on well after Thomson and continued to be a source of contention within American medicine throughout the nineteenth century, so neither Wallace's professionalization thesis nor Kett's assertion of Jacksonian decline and allopathic professional predominance are particularly convincing.

The advances that took place during and after 1910 seem suggestive of a stronger reason for the demise of the botanico-medical movement: medicine was becoming scientific. Innovations in the etiology of disease heralded in by discoveries in microbiology, cytology, and pharmacology forced permanent transformations in the healing arts by the opening decades of the twentieth century. "For the first time," writes historian Richard H. Shryock, "the medical sciences were coming to the aid of the healing arts in a rational and systematic manner."[19] No longer did physicians talk about "miasmas" and "night vapors" but about bacterial infection; no longer were attending physicians encouraged by "laudable pus" but instead became concerned over the effects of necrotic tissue and progressive cytolisis; no longer did members of the medical profession talk about therapeutic specificity defined by climate and place but rather about the universal application of diagnostic and therapeutic principles; no longer was empirical observation at the bedside the benchmark of efficacy, but instead in vitro and in vivo laboratory research supported by clear methodological protocols became the standard of therapeutic development. All this was accompanied by the growth of a formidable pharmaceutical industry producing synthetic organic drugs, antibiotics, and biologicals. Yes, medicine had changed dramatically since the days of Samuel Thomson, and the remaining botanical sects contemporaneous with the Thomsonian era had difficulty in coping with these changes. "Thus while traditional medicine tended to divide physicians," writes William Rothstein, "scientific medicine tended to unify them."[20] For the first time, it was possible to objectively assess the competence of physicians, and these objective standards allowed for the accreditation of medical schools upon a more uniform and certain basis.

The specific demise of each botanic group was unique, but the overriding factors causing their end were essentially the same. Haller points out that the physio-medicals eked out an existence in rural America and among the poor urban working classes of the nineteenth century. They attempted to remain true to Thomsonian practice and tried to buttress their botanical armamentarium with a vague "vital force" doctrine. But this was increasingly anachronistic in the new century.[21] Similarly, the eclectics served in countless small towns in the countryside and in many working-class communities of industrial America. The eclectics, however, were a group without a creed, and as a consequence, as Haller has suggested, "only a minority of eclectics acquired the scientific habits of mind that allowed them to live the disinterested life science demanded. Most merely acquired odds and ends of information that, because they rejected the authority of inherited medical systems, fit into no plan and supported no consistent view of health and disease." In the end, the eclectics became their own worst enemies. "At best," concludes Haller, "they represented a heterogeneous group of practitioners who believed in all and in nothing and failed ultimately to provide meaning to their medical art. By the late nineteenth century, they held such a strong sentimental attachment to their earlier botanic ideas and to specific medication that they were never really able to accept germ theory without wondering if it would bring censure from their colleagues."[22]

The rise of scientific medicine helps to explain the end of the movement, but it is not a totally self-sufficient model. If so, why did the concomitant rise of scientific medicine in Europe (especially in Germany) also not completely obliterate herbal medicine? The answer, it seems to us, is that medicine is indeed a science, but one that exists within a social context as well. The particular culture of medical practice in Germany, for example, allowed for herbal drugs to be incorporated into the modern armamentarium, with the fortunate result that Germany ranks today as the leader in methodologically sound phytomedicinal research. While Germany marched forward in the twentieth century with medicinal plants well established within the *regular* medical armamentarium, America actually retreated. By 1960, for example, America knew *less* about echinacea than it did in Lloyd's day, while Germany continued to pursue serious research into the therapeutic uses of a wide range of echinacea dosage forms. What is true of a popular herb such as echinacea is true of hundreds of other phytomedicinals that grace the pages of German scientific journals such as *Planta Medica, Arzneimittelforschung, Deutsche Apotheker Zeitung,* and others. In contrast, America came to view medicinal plants as part of *alternative* or *complementary* medicine, even though, historically, plant-based drugs had dominated regular therapeutics.

The dramatically different status of phytomedicines in Europe and America is not surprising. Lynn Payer has convincingly demonstrated that diagnostic and therapeutic concepts vary widely among Western countries that are all supposed to practice the latest "scientific" medicine. "World travelers who have had to see a doctor in a foreign country [such as Great Britain, France, or Germany]," writes Payer, "have usually discovered that medicine is not quite the international science that the medical profession would like us to believe. Not only do ways of delivering medical care differ from country to country; so does the medicine that is delivered."[23] An international survey of approaches to health and healing demonstrates differences, and at times ambiguity, in the parameters of "acceptable" treatments. "What I think I have discovered," concludes Payer, "is that the range of 'acceptable' treatments for most diseases is much wider than that admitted in any one country, and a wider view of such acceptable treatments would better serve both doctors and patients."[24]

Medicine is indeed culture dependent. In a twist of irony, the unique development of a strong botanico-medical movement in nineteenth-century America may have tended to more easily cast herbal drugs as part of an alternative practice that was viewed by the majority of practitioners as distinctly unscientific and a challenge to "reputable" medical authority. In Western Europe, where herbal healing has always been an accepted part of health care, botanicals were (and are) more easily incorporated into the corpus of medical practice.

In the end, the demise of the botanico-medical movement was the result of scientific advance and a medical culture that viewed their vegetable materia medica as the product of a bygone era. In contrast, the new synthetic drugs were considered state-of-the-art products of the new sciences of pharmacology, microbiology, and laboratory research. By the early twentieth century, the regular medical profession was glad to abandon its old plant products for a new order of drugs that had no taint of empricism, no hint of sectarian eccentricity.

THE BOTANIC LEGACY

The end of eclecticism marked the last botanic group directly spawned as a response to nineteenth-century heroic therapeutics and the egalitarian spirit of Jacksonian democracy. Variant forms of the sect would, however, carry on. Most notable is naturopathy, a holistic health and healing system originally opposed to all drug therapies and devoted to the water treatments of Father Sebastian Kneipp, supplemented with lifestyle regimens and attention to proper diet.[25] Founded by Benedict Lust (1872-1945), a German immigrant who established a sanitarium and magazine *(Amerika-nische Kneipp-Blätter)* in New York, naturopathy would eventually adopt much of eclectic pharmacy as its therapeutic mainstay. Lust received a medical degree from the Eclectic Medical College of New York in 1914 and soon garnered a comparatively small but devoted following. Although early naturopaths were opposed to the eclectics' isolation of active plant constituents, as time went on, the eclectic impress made itself evident. Two years after Lust's death, the American Naturopathic Association appointed a committee in April of 1947 "to investigate, compile, and edit a compendium of natural remedies common in naturopathic practice."[26] The committee's work culminated in the publication of *Naturae Medicina* in 1953, a compendium of 310 botanicals covering their composition, preparation, actions and therapeutic uses, and toxicology.[27] For naturopaths, this became a landmark publication "destined to be the Magna Carta of the profession."[28] Significantly, *Naturae Medicina* included many botanicals once popular among eclectics. "Opposed in the beginning to all varieties of drugs," writes Francis Brinker, "naturopaths eventually found themselves to be beneficiaries of the Eclectic physicians as the major professional prescribers of botanical medicine in America."[29]

Even postmortem, eclecticism lives on in modified forms in American naturopathy. Today, naturopathic medicine is best exemplified in Bastyr University, a fully accredited institution in Seattle, Washington. In addition, naturopathic schools are located in Portland, Oregon (National College of Naturopathic Medicine); Scottsdale, Arizona (Southwest College of Naturopathic Medicine and Health Sciences); and Etobicoke, Ontario (The Canadian College of Naturopathic Medicine). Students receive 150 to 175 classroom hours in herbal medicine instruction and also cover pharmacology, clinical conditions, and toxicology. Alaska, Arizona, Connecticut, Hawaii, Montana, New Hampshire, Oregon, and Washington—all have state licensing laws for naturopathic physicians. In Florida and Utah, naturopaths can practice under older legal provisions.[30]

It would be wrong, however, to assume that naturopathy has anything near the cohesive strength of the antebellum botanico-medical movement. Earnest in their convictions and dedicated to their own brand of healing, naturopaths are finding increased support and interest in their doctrines; nonetheless, it pales in comparison to the grassroots fervor that greeted the Thomsonians and eclectics. This is not to say that herbal medicine is not growing in America. It is not, however, growing in response to any specific group of practitioners or healers.

THE CURRENT BOTANICISM

At present, this country is in the midst of what many are calling an herbal renaissance. It was sparked not by any organized medical movement but by an activist-advocate laity promoting natural health and healing, many of whom came out of the counterculture of the 1960s.[31] Many were influenced by Jethro Kloss's *Back to Eden* (1939) and embarked upon herbal healing with a passion that matched Samuel Thomson's. Intelligent, self-taught, productive, and earnest in their beliefs, these so-called "Green People" have raised public awareness of medicinal herbs in America through their books, journal publications, organizations (see "A Note on Resources," pp. 207-209), and mass media exposure.[32]

With a receptive audience and committed proponents, the stage was set to secure "protections" for herbs, a class of products that did not fit in well with America's existing pharmaceutical regulations and drug control laws. By the mid-1990s, the political power had shifted in favor of botanicals.

The 1994 Dietary Supplement Health and Education Act (DSHEA) allows herbal products to be sold as "dietary supplements," placing the burden of proof that a particular supplement is unsafe squarely with the Food and Drug Administration (FDA).[33] This legislation provides the legal underpinning for the increasing sales of botanical products, driven by the herb industry and consumer demand. Critics, however, have pointed out that "natural" does not always mean "safe" and have called for mandatory manufacturing standards and

practices as well as stronger adverse reaction reporting requirements.[34] The example of ephedra does show that the FDA can
remove herb products from sale when safety becomes a demonstrable issue, but this agency cannot regulate herbals in the same
way that it regulates over-the-counter drugs. Bill Richardson, repre-
sentative of New Mexico and cosponsor of the bill with Utah's
Senator Orrin Hatch, believes that "[t]he current $200 million-dollar,
twelve-year-long drug approval process simply does not work for
non-patentable products like dietary supplements."[35] In a sense, the
law is reminiscent of the relaxation of regulatory controls witnessed
during the Thomsonian period. Although DSHEA clearly offers
legal protection for herbal products in this country, it represents, in
many cases, what the FDA can*not* do in the supplement market.
True, the relaxations witnessed during the Thomsonian period applied to medical practice only, but in an age that did not clearly
distinguish medicine from pharmacy, the legislative environments
in both cases affected *what* and *how* products were dispensed.

Because of DSHEA, one must be cautious in making compari-
sons with the nineteenth-century botanics. This new wave of interest in botanical medicine has, in its most recent incarnation, adopted
a face quite different from its sectarian predecessors. Although
naturopaths, homeopaths, and other holistic healers are part of this
herbal movement, they are clearly unable to serve as its driving
force in the same way that neo-Thomsonians or eclectics did because they lack the significant organizational structure necessary to
direct such a movement. This makes the current botanicism un-
structured and more diffuse than its nineteenth-century counterpart.
Another distinguishing feature is that, in general, the attempts to
develop various whole-plant supplements by large-scale manufacturers are not based upon some specific medical theory but, rather,
promoted on the basis of "good science" that is presented as acceptable to the mainstream medical community. Few major herbal
manufacturers would rest their reputations upon a particular system,
theory, or group. In this sense, herbals are not being represented as
an organized challenge to medical orthodoxy but as therapeutic
agents coexisting with mainstream regimens. As mentioned before,
the fact that they have not been fully accepted in medicine in this
country is more a reflection of the particular American culture of

health and healing than it is of anything else. In this sense, Varro Tyler is absolutely correct: "Rational herbal medicine is conventional medicine."[36]

Since the Nutrition Labeling and Education Act (NLEA) of 1990 sparked debate and concern over what many viewed as their right to therapeutic choice, Congress has received more mail on this subject than *any* other issue.[37] The American people have clearly indicated an interest in herbs by voting with their dollars in favor of dietary supplements. Since DSHEA, herb sales have been the fastest-growing component of the dietary supplement market; a recent Harvard University study concluded that Americans have spent $5.1 billion on such products.[38] A sense of the increase is suggested by a 1996 study which indicated that as many as 60 million adults spent $3.24 billion on herbs.[39] The point is clear: interest in medicinal herbs is growing in this country because the public is demanding them. Contributing factors are increased marketing of herb products by manufacturers, adverse reactions to conventional drugs, dissatisfaction with the current health care system, and the high cost of pharmaceuticals.

The tremendous popularity of these dietary supplements has caused pharmacy schools to respond within the context of alternative health care education. This fact was summarized in a recent pamphlet issued by the American Association of Colleges of Pharmacy listing programs and courses responding to the increasing interest in alternative therapies.[40] Included are twenty-nine schools from across the country with various programs, courses, and rotations devoted to herbal medicine, homeopathy, naturopathy, and related topics. All indications suggest that herbal medicine may have reached a turning point in America, as scientific attentions are directed toward these once-forgotten products.

Beyond the popular demand for more serious attention to herbal medicines is the fact that the limitations of an overreliance upon synthetic pharmaceuticals is becoming increasingly evident. Even the former enthusiasm of the medical profession for the sophisticated antibiotic drugs of the post–World War II years has waned in the face of newly resistant strains of all too familiar pathogens. By the 1980s, the fight against infectious disease seemed to take an ominous turn. "Underfunded prevention programs and drug resistance," write researchers Donna Hoel and David N. Williams, "were allowing diseases like yellow fever, cholera, malaria, meningitis, dengue fever, tuberculosis, and even plague to spring back with renewed vengeance. By the 1990s, panicky investigators were realizing they had very few resources to combat these stronger, smarter foes."[41] In their search for new therapeutic agents, researchers have begun to look more seriously at plants with suspected immunostimulant, bactericidal, and bacteriostatic properties.[42]

CONCLUSION

It cannot be said with any degree of certainty exactly what the future holds for botanicals in this country. That it will be distinctly different from the path adopted earlier in this century is almost certain. Yet there is a sense of déjà vu. Thomson's strident call for a medicine of the people in the early nineteenth century attacked the pretensions of the medical establishment and asserted itself against the regulars' monopoly on the healing arts. More recently, Orrin Hatch echoed Thomson's egalitarian spirit and attacked the bureaucratic elite as the enemy of therapeutic democracy. In his support of the Health Freedom Act of 1992, Hatch boldly stated, "In our free market system, consumers should be able to purchase dietary supplements, and companies should be free to sell these products so long as the labeling and advertising is truthful and nonmisleading and there exists a reasonable scientific basis for product claims. . . . In our free society consumers should be able to purchase any food they want—whether it is an egg, ice cream, a steak, coffee, potato chips, or a dietary supplement—regardless of whether some of those in the Federal Government approve. Unfortunately, however," concluded Hatch, "some people in the government including some people at the U.S. Food and Drug Administration (FDA) appear to have unfairly treated dietary supplements and have tried to establish unreasonable regulatory burdens on such products."[43] Hatch ended his presentation by asserting the support of the American people for the Health Freedom Act, a claim endorsed by its favorable public reception.

More recent developments, however, suggest that perhaps this brand of medical egalitarianism may be yielding to governmental and professional pressures to more fully mainstream botanicals into the American armamentarium. The U.S. pharmacopeial convention has launched an ambitious botanical monograph development project. At this writing, herbs such as chamomile, cranberry, feverfew, powdered garlic, powdered ginger, ginkgo, oriental ginseng, milk thistle, saw palmetto, and St. John's wort have already received official USP status.[44] Cognizant of this important shift in the status of many medicinal plants, the American Medical Association has called upon Congress to revise DSHEA "to require that dietary supplements and herbal remedies, including the products already in the marketplace, meet USP standards for identity, strength, quality, purity, packaging, and labeling."[45] The mainstreaming of herbal health care products is further enhanced by the FDA's "Ten Year Plan," an extensive policy agenda that sets forth its comprehensive "dietary supplement strategy."[46] Issued in January 2000, the FDA's goal is to have a science-based regulatory program by 2010 that establishes standards for labeling; safety; good manufacturing practices; structure/function claims; legal definitions, including the role of dietary supplements within the larger over-the-counter and prescription drug environment; and specific enforcement mechanisms.

It is difficult to speculate upon the future of botanicals in this country during such a time of dynamic change. Although it is true that few of the significant issues surrounding the decline of herbal use in America concerned the efficacy or effectiveness of the products involved (although some were and are undoubtedly of questionable therapeutic value), other issues relating to the larger principles of herb use continue to be problematic. For example, one of the herbalist's most distinctive and persistent claims, namely, that plants possess synergistic properties—i.e., the idea that the whole plant is therapeutically greater than the sum of its constituents—remains to be scientifically verified.[47] Also, Senator Hatch's equating herbal "dietary supplements" with coffee and potato chips is a reductio ad absurdum. Although legislation in the 1990s has, on the whole, served to protect the availability of herbs to the consumer, the decade appeared to close with a retreat from such reductionist thinking that belies the use of these substances as remedial agents and exposes the obvious difficulties surrounding DSHEA. Science and market demand can often be mutually exclusive, but the popularity of herbals among American consumers suggests that this issue will continue to dominate public discourse for some time to come. Indeed, the increasing use of these dietary supplements, in part, resides in the products themselves: their multiple-constituent nature makes herbals generally less prone to serious side effects than many highly potent chemotherapeutic agents. Thus, at present, the role of dietary supplements in American therapeutics is unclear but certainly not over. Although botanicism exists in a different social and medical context, as one contemplates the long and some-times tortuous history of medicinal herbs in this country, the call "vox populi" still lingers on.

APPENDIXES

Appendix 1

Materia Medica of Dr. Samuel Thomson's Guide and Narrative, Being a Correct Catalogue of all the Plants Recommended by Him, in His Practice of Medicine

1. LOBELIA INFLATA, VEL THOMSONIA
   Emetic Plant, Puke of Asthma Weed, Indian or Wild Tobacco, Eye-bright.

2. CAPSICUM ANNUUM
   Cayenne Pepper.

3. MYRICA CERIFERA
   Bayberry, Myrtle, Candle or Wax Berry.

4. NYMPHOEA ODORATA
   Sweet Water Lilly, White Pond, or Toad, or Cow Lilly—
   Cow or Water Cabbage.

5. ABIES, VEL PINUS CANADENSIS
   Hemlock Spruce.

6. STATICE CAROLINIANA
   Marsh Rosemary, American or Sea-Side Thrift, Sea Lavender, Ink Root.

7. RHUS GLABRUM
   Smooth Sumach.

Source: The Thomsonian Recorder (Columbus, Ohio) 2, 22 (August 2, 1834).

8. HAMAMELIS VIRGINICA
Winter Witch-Hazle, Snapping Hazle, Winter Bloom.

9. RUBUS STRIGOSUS
Wild Red Raspberry.

10. POPULUS TRIPIDA, VEL TREMULOIDES
Aspen or Poplar.

11. ERIGERON PURPUREUM
Cocash or Squaw Weed, Skevish or Scabish.

12. CHELONE GLABRA
Balmony, Snake or Turtle Head, or Bloom Shell Flower.

13. BERBERIS VULGARIS
Barberry.

14. AMYGDALUS PERSICA
Peach Tree, kernels used.

15. APOCYNUM ANDROSEMIFOLIUM
Bitter Root, Wandering Milk Weed, Honey Bloom, Catch-Fly
or Trap, Ipecac.

16. FRASERA VERTICILLATA
Ohio Kercuma, Golden Seal, Meadow Pride, Columbo Root,
Pyramid, Indian Lettuce, Yellow Gentian.

17. HYDRASTIS CANADENSIS
Yellow Root, Ground Raspberry, Eye Balm, Puccoon, Orange
or Tumeric Root.

18. PRUNUS VIRGINIANA
Wild Cherry Tree, kernels used.

19. CYPRIPEDIUM PUBESCENS, VEL PARVIFLORUM, VEL
LUTEUM ET HUMILE, VEL ACAULE
Umbil or Nervine, Noah's Ark, Moccasin Flower, Lady Slipper,
Bleeding Heart, or American Valerian, and Indian Shoe.

20. AMYRIS KATAF, VEL MYRRHA
Myrrh.

21. ZINGIBER AMONUM
    Ginger.

22. PIPER NIGRUM
    Black Pepper.

23. LAURUS CAMPHORA
    Gum Camphor.

24. OLEUM TEREBINTHINAE
    Spirits of Turpentine.

25. MENTHA PEPERITA
    Peppermint.

26. MENTHA VERIDIS
    Spear or Water Mint.

27. SATURCIAE HORTENSIS, VEL SATUREJA HORTENSIS
    Summer Savory.

28. HEDLOMA PULEGIOIDES
    Pennyroyal, Squaw Mint, Stinking Balm, Tickweed.

29. MARRUBIUM VULGARE
    Hoarhound.

30. INULA HELENIUM
    Elecampane.

31. ANTHEMIS COTULA
    Mayweed, Wild Chamolile, Dillweed or Dilly, Dog's Fennel.

32. ATIMISEA ABSYMTHIUM
    Wormwood.

33. TANACETUM VULGATE
    Tanzey.

34. ANTHEMIS NOBILIS
    Chamomile.

35. VERBASCUM THAPSUS
    Mullen.

36. ARCTIUM LAPP
    Burdock.

37. MATRICARIA VULGARIS, VEL CHRYSANTHEMUM
    PARTHENICUM
    Feverfew or Featherfew.

38. BETULA LENTA
    Black Birch.

39. CELASTRUS SCANDENS
    Bittersweet, Fevertwig, or Staff Vine.

40. ICOTODES FOETIDA,VEL SPATHYENE FOETIDA
    Skunk Cabbage or Weed, Collard, Itchweed, Skoka.

41. ARUM TRIPHYLLUM
    Indian Turnip, Wake Robin, DragonRoot or Turnip, Pepper Turnip.

42. EUPITORIUM PERFOLIATUM
    Boneset, Thoroughwort or Stem, Indian Sage, Sweating Plant, Ague
    Weed or Crosswort, Feverwort, Vegetable Antimony, Jocpye.

43. GEUM VIRGINIANUM
    Evan Root or White Avens, Chocolate or Throat Root, Bennet,
    or Cure-All.

44. GALIUM VERUM ET APARINE
    Cleavers or Cilvers, Goose Grass, Yellow Bedstraw, Cleavewort,
    Savoyan, Milk Sweet, Poor Robin, Clabber Grass, Gravel Grass, etc.

45. ABIES, VEL PINUS BALSAMEA
    Balsam Fir.

46. UIMUS FULVA
    Red Slippery or Sweet Elm.

47. ARISTOLOCHIA SERPENTARIA
    Virginia Snake Root, Birthwort, Snagrel.

48. SINAPIS ALBA, ET NIGRA
Mustard.

49. COCHLEARIA ARMORACIA
Horse Raddish.

50. JUGLANS CINEREA
Butternut.

51. VERBENA HASTATA
Blue Vervain or Purvain.

52. VERBENA URTICIFOLIA
White or Nettle-leafed Vervain.

53. SOLIDAGO ODORA
Sweet Golden Rod.

54. PYROLA UMBELLATA
Pipsissawa or Greenleaf, Ground Holly, King's Oure, Rheumatism
Weed.

55. PYROLA MACULATA
Pipsissawa or White Leaf, etc., etc.

56. CNICUS OFFICINALIS
Bitter Thistle, cultivated in gardens, for medical use.

57. RUMEX CRISPUS
Yellow Dock.

58. CARDUUS BENEDICTUS, VEL CENTAUREA BENEDICTA
Blessed or Lovely Thistle.

59. ZANTHOXYLON FRAXINEUM
Prickly Ash, Toothache Bush, Yellow Wood, or Suterberry,
or Pellitory.

60. PYROLA ROTUNDIFOLIA
Wild Lettuce, Round Leaf Consumption Weed.

61. ALETRIS FARINOSA
True Unicorn Root, Star Grass, Blazing Star, Aloe Root, Bitter Grass,
Star Root, Devil's Bit.

62. HELONIAS DIOICA
    False Unicorn Root, Colic Root, Devil's Bit, Drooping Starwort.

63. COPTIS TRIFOLIA
    Gold Thread, Yellow Root, Mouth Root.

64. LYCOPUS VIRGINICUS—VAR: RUBER
    American Archangel, Bugle Weed, Water Hoarhound, Paul's Betony,
    Gipsy.

65. LYCOPUS VULGARIS, VEL EUROPEUS
    Green Archangel, Bugle Weed, etc.

66. POPULUS BASLAMIFERA
    Balsam Poplar—Indian name, Tackamahaka.

67. POPULUS CANDICANS
    Balm of Gilead Poplar.

68. PANAX QUINQUEFOLIA
    Ginseng.

69. MYRICA GALE
    Meadow Fern, Sweet Gale, Bog or Dutch Myrtle.

70. TRIFOLIUM PRATENSE
    Red Clover.

Appendix 2

Platform of Principles
Adopted by the National Convention
at Baltimore, October 1852

Whereas, There have arisen in different ages and countries, and of every sect in medicine, men of noble minds and benevolent hearts, who exerted all their energies to reform the errors and abuses of what was called the science and practice of medicine;

And whereas, The men of this description of the Allopathic school are still compelled to pronounce their principles an "incoherent assemblage of incoherent ideas;" and their most efficient medication "horrid, unwarrantable, murderous, quackery;"

And whereas, Many modern New School reformers of the same honest intentions, have few fixed principles of practice in which they can agree, and no firm bond of union in effort for the promotion of Reform;

Therefore, It appeared to be the first and most important duty of this convention, to point out the generative errors of all the popular systems of the day, and to lay down in clear and unmistakable terms the fundamental principles of true Medical Science and practice, as guides to all who may desire to attain to perfection in the knowledge of the Healing Art, and as a common creed, which all can advocate and defend, and as a bond of union in effort for the promotion of this most glorious cause of science and humanity; Therefore

Resolved, By the Reformed Medical Association of the United States, that medical science pertaining altogether to natural subjects, must be in itself as fixed and definite as any other natural science.

Resolved, That the reason why medical men have not learned it, is they have attempted to base it upon the violation of physical laws, which are

Source: The Physio-Medical Recorder or Impartial Advocate of Sanative Medicine 18 (1852-1853): 155-156.

immutable: they have built their system on what they call pathology—or rather they have pronounced that pathology which is only deranged physiology, and built upon this error.

Resolved, That the Reformers of past times have failed to perfect their practice, because of the impossibility of doing it while they retain the false notion that the science is based on pathology, or the doctrine that physiological derangements are disease.

Resolved, That the fundamental principles of true medical science are not pathological but physiological.

Resolved, That the disease is not vital action deranged, or obstructed, increased or diminished, but any condition of the organs in which they are unable to perform their natural functions: a condition that permanently deranges, obstructs or diminishes vital action, and in this sense is a unit.

Resolved, That irritation, fever, inflammation—terms used to signify increased, deranged, obstructed, or accumulated vital action in the nervous or vascular systems, are not disease, but physiological symptoms of disease; and are not to be directly subdued, but always to be aided in their ultimate design and intention in removing obstructions and restoring the nervous and circulatory equilibrium.

Resolved, That suppuration is to be encouraged and promoted whenever there is accumulated morbific matter to be removed; that gangrene, being no part of inflammation, but a purely chemical process in opposition to all vital action, and occurring only when vital action has wholly ceased, the associating of it with inflammation, and treating the latter as tending to terminate in the former, has been a source of immense mischief in medication.

Resolved, That it is the duty of the practitioner to reject in toto every means and process, which, in its nature and tendency, in authorized medicinal quantities, degrees or modes of application, has been known to have directly destroyed human life, or permanently injured the tissue or deranged the physiological action, and use those only, which have a direct tendency to aid the vital organs in the removal of causes of disease and the restoration of health and vigor.

Resolved, The agents of this character are not confined to the vegetable kingdom, but are found in every department of nature, and to be "seized upon wherever found."

Resolved, That though we shall exercise charity toward the ignorance and prejudices of all men, we can count no one a true medical reformer who rejects the doctrines of the foregoing resolutions.

[The Report was received and adopted with but *two* dissenting voices, Drs. P. John and H. F. Johnson.]

Appendix 3

Union Platform of Principles
(Subscribed to by the Middle States
Reformed Medical Society
and the Faculty of the Eclectic
Medical College of Pennsylvania)

Whereas divisions have occurred among medical reformers, and various parties have arisen entertaining different views only upon some of the minor points of true medical science and practice: and whereas these divisions have greatly retarded the progress of scientific medicine: we the members of the Middle States Society of Medical Reform, do agree to unite with our Eclectic friends upon the following platform of principles.

1st. The fundamental principles of true medical sciences are not Pathological but physiological.

2nd. Disease is not vital action deranged or obstructed, increased or diminished, but disease we understand to be that condition of a part which disqualifies it for the performance of its function in a normal manner.

3rd. Fever is a manifestation of an effort of the system to remove disease, a physiological action under the circumstances—a general or constitutional indication of disease.

4th. Inflammation is an evidence of local disease—an action produced for the restoration of a diseased part—an effort of the vital force to remove disease.

5th. Physiology is the science of life in its modes of being, but is now usually restricted to life in a state of health.

6th. Pathology is the science of life in a state of disease. It is physiology under abnormal circumstances.

Source: The Middle States Medical Reformer and Advocate of Innocuous Medication (Dover, Delaware) 1 (1855): 52 ff.

7th. Holding these views, which are legitimate teachings of physiological science, we reject from our materia medica every article,
means or process of cure which . . . is directly antagonistic to the
laws of vitality, and use those and those only which have a direct
tendency to aid the vital organs in the removal of the causes of
disease and the restoration of health and vigor.

8th. We cordially invite all medical reformers in the United States to
unite with us upon the platform . . .

9th. Upon these principles, as the basis of the science of medicine, as
taught in the Eclectic Medical College of Pennsylvania, the society herein agrees to use all its influence to sustain said institution.

10th. We recognize all who stand upon this platform as true medical
reformers.

In Witness Whereof, we, the committee representing the Middle States
Reformed Medical Society, and the Eclectic Medical College of Pennsylvania respectively, this 18th day of May, 1854.

For the Middles States Reformed
Medical Society

John Palemon, MD
John S. Prettyman, MD
Wm. J. Williams, MD
Wm. Fields, MD
Wm. Armstrong, MD

For the Trustees and Faculty
of the Eclectic Medical
College of Pennsylvania

John Foney, MD
John Sites, MD
Henry Hollemback, MD

Appendix 4

Platform, Constitution, and By-Laws of the American Physio-Medical Association

PLATFORM OF PRINCIPLES

1. The Science of Medicine, like all other sciences, is based upon the laws of Nature; and Medical Art can be true and reliable only when it is in harmony with those laws.

2. Disease is that condition of bodily structures in which they are unable to perform their functions in a natural manner, which condition disturbs the harmony of equilibrium of the system; and the object of medical science is the restoration of diseased structures to their normal state, as far as possible, that they may be enabled again to perform their offices.

3. Physiological actions are always resistive to the causes of disease, and tend to the restoration of health when it is disturbed; and remedial treatment should harmonize with these physiological efforts, conserving and assisting the inherent curative powers of the system.

4. Observing this physiological standard as the only true guide in the Curative Art, no article should be used in the cure of disease that by its nature tends to damage the integrity of structures, or impair the vitality of tissues; hence all measures that are injurious, and all agents that are poisonous, are to be rejected from medical practice, as being in themselves causes of disease and not promoters of health.

CONSTITUTION

1. The name of this organization shall be THE AMERICAN ASSOCIATION OF PHYSIO-MEDICAL PHYSICIANS AND SURGEONS.

Source: The Cincinnati Medical Recorder (Cincinnati, Ohio) 51, 6 (May 15, 1883).

2. Among the objects of this Association shall be: (1) The promotion of the principles of Physio-Medical Science, as enunciated in the Platform of Principles adopted by this organization; (2) The enlightenment of public sentiment upon these principles; (3) The encouragement of all measures that will advance professional education; (4) The mutual benefit of the members of this Association, and resistance to all unjust laws against Physio-Medical Science.

3. Members of this Association shall conform their sentiments and their practice to its Platform of Principles, and their professional life and conduct shall comport with the honor and dignity of this humane calling.

4. The officers of this Association shall consist of a President, two Vice-Presidents, a Secretary, and a Treasurer; to be elected annually, and to remain in office till their successors are chosen.

5. The Association, at each annual meeting, shall elect three members, who, with the above-mentioned officers, shall constitute the Executive Committee.

. . .

7. The membership fee shall be two dollars a year, and thereafter such an amount as may be annually determined upon by the Executive Committee.

8. This Constitution may be altered or amended by a vote of two-thirds of the members present, at any regular meeting of the Association, one year's notice of the proposition to alter or amend having been publicly given to the Association.

BY-LAWS

1. A Board of Censors shall be appointed by the President, and confirmed by the Executive Committee, who shall examine all applicants for membership of this organization.

2. Gentlemen and ladies who are graduates of a medical college in good standing, or licentiates of a regularly organized Physio-Medical Society, or shall pass an examination before the Board of Censors, may become members of this Association by subscribing to its Constitution, agreeing therein to submit to its principles and by-laws.

3. Applicants for membership in this Association shall make application to the Board of Censors, accompanying the application with a fee of two dollars, and be recommended by two members of the Association.

4. The Board of Censors shall be guided in the examination of applicants for membership by the Platform of Principles, and shall take such measures as said Board may deem best calculated to elucidate facts bearing on the application, and shall present the conclusions arrived at to the Association; and pending the action of the Association any decision of the Censors shall stand as the decision of the Association.

. . .

6. This Association shall be divided into sections, as follows: Theory and Practice, Materia Medica, Surgery, Physiology, Obstetrics, Gynecology, Chemistry, Hygiene, Microscopy, Pathology, and Histology. The President of the Association shall appoint the Chairmen of the above committees on sciences, and these shall report at the next annual meeting.

7. All papers read before this Association shall belong to the Association. The following are the charter members of the American Association of Physio-Medical Physicians and Surgeons:

Indiana:	24	Ohio:	11	Illinois:	5	Iowa:	2
Minnesota:	1	Texas:	1	Nebraska:	1	New York:	2
California:	1						

TOTAL: 48

AN ADDRESS TO THE PUBLIC

Physio-Medicalism, as a distinct school in medical practice, asks from the public a calm hearing and a just judgment. It should not be judged by the statements of those who do not understand it. Persons not informed on a matter may condemn or deride it, because their interests or their prejudices are served thereby; but such partisan statements may be very bold and bitter, and yet not be at all true. Americans love fair play and justice, and Physio-Medicalism asks nothing more.

Physio-Medicalism claims to be able to treat disease on principles that are more truly scientific, and by means that are more decidedly effectual, than those of any other school. Its advocates pursue it for conscience sake, convinced that it has far greater power than any other system of medicine to preserve health and prolong life; and health and life are too sacred to be submitted to inferior and uncertain methods, when superior and reliable ones are at command. If these claims are correct, the fact can be determined by fair examination; and the people have such a profound interest in claims that promise such rich advantages, which touch the dearest interests of man on earth—that no passion or prejudice should be allowed to prevent the public from understanding what Physio-Medicalism really is.

First—Physio-Medicalism looks to Nature as its parent and guide; for all science is a knowledge of Nature's rules and laws, and he alone is learned who understands those laws, and is skilled in their application. Whatever is contrary to Nature's laws, or at variance with them, or not fully in harmony with them, is not true. And whatever is not true can not be scientific, and can not be depended on. Man may put forth glittering speculations; but they are imaginative and worthless, unstable and shifting as the quicksands, unless founded upon the immutable laws of Nature. Physio-Medicalism accepts no assertions of men, bows to no human dictation, admits nothing as authority except the laws fixed in all created things by Nature's God. Herein is the foundation for the one and only true Science of Medicine. It includes every department of knowledge that has a bearing upon human life, or that conduces to human health. It embraces every fact and principle that is true and good. It is a science as broad, as comprehensive, and as perfect, as the other sciences established by Heaven for the benefit of Man.

Second—The Life Power of Vital Principle in every human being resists the causes of disease, and promotes a return to health as far as possible. It repairs injuries, heals wounds, mends fractures, restores strength, and frequently of itself overcomes the most severe diseases. No cure and no repair is ever possible except by this Life Power. It is the duty of the physician to assist this Power, to obey its laws of cure, and to use only such measures as are in perfect harmony with these laws. He must cooperate with Nature, aid her curative intentions, favor her healing processes, and advance her every effort to restore the diseased body to a healthy condition. Physio-Medicalism is the one true Medical Science in being the constant friend and helper of the curative power of Nature.

Third—Physio-Medicalism rejects all poisons, whether obtained from the mineral, vegetable, or the animal kingdom. Any article to which human experience attaches the term *poison,* is dangerous to the human frame and at war with vitality. Such articles can cause disease. Their use in disease is in opposition to Nature's curative efforts, and adds more burdens to the afflicted body; hence by their action they delay recovery, do violence to the constitution, and may even turn the scale suddenly against struggling Nature and in favor of death. Physio-Medicalism rejects every article of that character, uses only such articles as will harmonize with Nature, will favor the return of a healthy condition. Such agents are the *only true remedies.* Physio-Medical remedies are powerful for good, but never for mischief. They never do damage to the structures, even of the most delicate lady or most tender babe. They help to shorten the duration of disease, but never leave in the body a disease of their own making, nor damage a constitution by their dangerous properties.

Such are the fundamental doctrines of the Physio-Medical school. All reasonable and thinking people must approve of them, for they harmonize with our best judgment, and commend themselves as fulfilling the true purposes of Medical Art. Founded in the purest and most exact science, builded deeply and solidly upon Nature, they permeate every branch of medical study, and possess capabilities of enlargement that will terminate only when science is terminated. A system of philosophy and of cure thus established in the laws of Nature and of Life is fraught with blessings and benefits that can not be measured.

During the century it has existed, this system has grown from quite humble beginnings to national proportions. With fewer than twelve disciples at first, its educated practitioners now number thousands. It has published journals, developed literature, and established several colleges. Its growth has not been favored by wealth or other circumstance, but has been due wholly to its own superior successes.

When all other systems have failed, it has saved life; when others have declared patients to be beyond the reach of man, and have given them over to the grasp of death, it has interposed its higher philosophy and its grander means of cure, and has restored health.

When all others were appalled by the cholera of 1832, and subsequently, and turned helplessly from medicine to medicine, and lost half their patients, this system calmly met the monster and saved ninety per cent or more.

In such dread maladies as pneumonia, diphtheria, typhus, scarlatina, yellow fever, and similar diseases, it has reduced the death rate to three or four per cent, when other systems lose from twenty to twenty-eight per cent.

Where others have decided that limbs must be amputated, it has saved those limbs by a superior surgery.

Where others have hurried to the use of instruments—mangling helpless mothers, crushing innocent babes, entailing months and years of suffering upon woman—it has shown such methods to be a lack of true science, has proven such instruments to be absolutely needless, and has saved those sufferings and those lives.

Such triumphs are not occasional, accidental, nor isolated. They are numbered by hundreds of thousands, are uniform with thousands of practitioners, and extend through an hundred years. Put to the unjust test of having thrust upon it the abandoned patients of others, it has saved thousands of these. By such abounding evidences has Physio-Medicalism proven itself to be, not the whim of a few men, or an accident of favorable circumstances, but a *new* and *complete system* of medicine, founded in accurate science, and superior to all others at the bedside. Through its success it has won the confidence and respect of the public wherever it has been known.

The people, afflicted with disease, and broken with the use of poisons, have great need that this system should be established as the only school of medical practice known among men. Nothing should deprive them of its superior benefits; nothing should hinder any one from employing it if he desire to; nothing should prevent the poorest person in the land from saving his life by it, if he wish to.

Physio-Medicalism, in the name of justice and humanity, now respectfully but firmly demands the following rights:

That it shall be accorded the same governmental recognition as is accorded to any other school of medicine in this free government, which is not designed to sustain any school or sect by special favors.

That it shall have equal opportunities with any other school, in the army, navy, hospitals, asylums, and other institutions supported by the public treasury, and where the poor are now denied all right of choice among medical systems.

That it shall have equal privileges with any other school in all medical laws, and enjoy an equal representation on all State Medical Boards; and not be ruled without being allowed representation and not be placed under the control of another school having power to oppress Physio-Medicalism.

These rights it asks from the people and through the people, as rights accorded by the Constitution to every American citizen, and rights that are for the benefit of science and humanity.

WM. H. COOK, MD
G. N. DAVIDSON, MD
A. F. ELLIOTT, MD
Committee National P.-M. Association

Appendix 5

Specification of a Patent Granted for "Fever Medicine." To SAMUEL THOMSON, of Surrey, County of Cheshire, New Hampshire, March 2, 1813

A specification for preparing and using certain medicines in fevers, colics, dysenteries, and rheumatisms.

No. 1. The emetic herb, or Lowbela [Lobelia?] medica, a plant that grows about twelve or fifteen inches high, with leaves of the size of mint leaves, bearing a pod the size of a white bean, of a sharp taste, like that of tobacco, creating nausea. It must be gathered when the leaves and pods are a little yellow; dried, pounded fine, and sifted, when it forms a powerful emetic. Dose, in powder, from 4 to 12 grains, with or without an equal quantity of No. 2.

No. 2. Cayenne, or red pepper, pulverized.

No. 3. Marsh rosemary, two parts, the bark of bayberry, or candleberry (the myrtle from which wax is obtained from the berry) roots, one part, pulverized, or sumach bark, leaves, or berries, or raspberry leaves, may be substituted. A tea made with one ounce of the above powder (No. 3) in a pint of boiling water. Dose, wine-glassful, occasionally, sweetened.

No. 4. Bitters for correcting the bile; take the bitter herb, or *balmony,* barberry bark, and poplar bark, equal parts, pulverized. One ounce to half a pound of wine, or spirit, and hot water. Dose, half a wine-glassful, and for hot bitters, add half a drachm to the ounce.

No. 5. A sirop. Take one ounce of peach kernels, or cherry stones; half an ounce of gum myrrh, made fine; add three half pints of hot water, two ounces of white sugar, half a pint of brandy. Half a wine-glassful to be used three times a day.

Rheumatic drops. Take one gallon high wines, one pound gum myrrh, put into a stone jug, and boil it in a kettle of water for half an hour; when settled, pour it off; add four ounces camphor, half an ounce of cayenne pepper in powder, one quart of spirits of turpentine, then bottle it, and it is prepared for bathing in rheumatisms, any swellings, or external pains.

No. 1, is used to cleanse the stomach, overpower the cold, and promote a free perspiration. No. 2, to raise the inward heat. No. 3, to scour the stomach, promote perspiration, and repel the cold. No. 4, to correct the bile, and quicken the appetite. No. 5, to strengthen the stomach, and restore the digestive powers, after cases of dysentery, or other weakening disorders. The three first numbers may be used in any other case, to promote perspiration, or as an emetic.

SAMUEL THOMSON

Specification of a patent granted for a mode of preparing, mixing, compounding, administering, and using, the medicine therein described, to SAMUEL THOMSON, of Boston, Suffolk County, Massachusetts, January 18, 1823.

First. The mode of preparing and compounding medicine for an emetic, to be administered in diseases caused by cold and obstructed perspiration, such as fevers, colic, rheumatism, dysentery, asthma, numb-palsy, dropsy, and consumption, and various others.

Take the emetic herb *Lobelia Inflata* of Linnaeus, dry the pods and leaves, or the leaves only, and reduce them to a fine powder in a mortar; sift and keep it from the air. For a dose, take from ten to twenty grains, steeped in warm water, sweetened. This emetic is called by the patentee, *number one,* in his system of practice in medicine.

The emetic herb, or *Lobelia,* above-mentioned, is a biennial plant, grows about twelve or fifteen inches high, with leaves of the size of mint leaves, and pods about the size of a white bean, containing very small seeds; is of a sharp taste, like tobacco, exciting the glands of the throat, and producing nausea. It should be gathered when the leaves and pods are turned a little yellow, but is good in any stage of its growth: when perfectly dry, the seeds should be shaken from the pods, and preserved separate.

Another mode of preparing the emetic, number one, from this herb, is as follows, to wit: take the green herb, pound it in a mortar, and put it in an equal quantity of spirit; after being well steeped, strain off the liquor, and keep it, close stopped, in a bottle for use. Prepared in this manner, and adding *cayenne,* as hereinafter mentioned in *number two,* two drachms to a pint of the liquor. Dose, one teaspoonful. This is an effectual remedy in removing the effects caused by poison, either taken internally, or by bathing the part affected. The seeds of this plant are more powerful than the leaves, and one half the quantity pounded fine, and steeped as above described, is of sufficient power for an emetic.

Secondly. To attain the internal vital heat of the system, and cause a free perspiration. Take cayenne, *(capsicum)* or red pepper, ground fine; dose, from ten to twenty grains, in hot water, sweetened, or to be combined with the other medicine hereinafter described. This is called by the patentee, *number two.*

Thirdly. To scour the stomach and bowels, and remove the canker. Take bayberry, or candle berry, *(Myrica certifera* L.) (the myrtle from which wax is obtained from the berries) the bark of the root dried and pulverized; the inner bark of the hemlock tree (*Pinus canadensis,* L.) pulverized, equal parts of each, steep one ounce of the powder in a pint of boiling water, and give, for a dose, a common wine-glassful, sweetened.

When the above cannot be had, take, as a substitute, red sumach bark, leaves, or berries, *(Rhus glabrum,* L.) red raspberries *(Rubus streorsus of Michaux)* or witch hazel leaves (*Hamamelis virginica,* L.) marsh rosemary, *(Statice lemonium,* L.) and white pond lily roots (*Nymphoea odarata* Ait.) or either of them: let them be dried, rounded and steeped, as above mentioned. This is called by the patentee, *number three.*

When the violence of the disease requires a course of medicine, take an ounce of the foregoing medicine, *number three,* steeped in a pint of hot water, strain off a wine-glassful when hot, and add ten or twenty grains of *number one,* and an equal quantity of *nerve powder,* hereafter described, to quiet the nerves. Let this compound be administered three times, at intervals of fifteen minutes, and let the same compound be given by injection once, and, if the case requires it, again be repeated.

When mortification is apprehended, a tea-spoonful of medicine, *number six,* as hereinafter described, may be added to each dose, and, from these applications, which is usually within two or three hours, let the mode of raising perspiration by steam, as hereinafter described, be applied.

Fourthly. To make bitters for correcting the bile. Take the bitter herb, *(Balmony)* Barberry bark (*Barberis vulgaris,* L.) and poplar bark, *(Populus trepida)* in equal parts, pulverized. One ounce to a pint of hot water, and half a pint of spirit. For a dose, take half a wine-glassful; for hot bitters, add a teaspoonful of *number two;* this is called, by the patentee, *number four.*

Fifthly. To make a sirop for dysentery, to promote digestion, and strengthen weak patients. Take poplar bark, the bark of the root of bayberry, each one pound, boil them in two gallons of water, strain it off, and add seven pounds of good sugar, then scald and skim it, and add half a pound of peach meats, or cherry stone meats, pounded fine; when cool, add a gallon of good brandy. Bottle it up, and keep it for use. Take half a wine-glassful, two or three times a day. This is called by the patentee, *number five.*

Sixthly. To make rheumatic drops, to be used to remove pain, and to prevent mortification, given inwardly, or to be added to the injections, or to be applied externally.

Take one gallon of any kind of high wines, one pound of gum myrrh, one ounce of cayenne, *number two,* put into a stone jug, the jug being unstopped; boil it a few minutes in a kettle of water; when settled, bottle it up for use. Or it may be prepared without boiling, by letting it stand for five or six days, shaking it well every day, when it will be fit for use.

For bathing, in rheumatism, itch, or other humours, or in angry swelling or external pain, add one-quarter pint of spirits of turpentine. One or two teaspoonfuls of these drops, without the spirits of turpentine, may be given alone, and, also, may be used to bathe with; or, one tea-spoonful may be added to a dose of either of the medicines before mentioned. This is called by the patentee, *number six.*

In the earlier stages, and in less violent attacks of disease, a composition or vegetable powder may be administered, prepared as follows, to wit: take two pounds of the bark of the root of bayberry, one pound of the inner bark of the *hemlock tree,* one pound of ginger, two ounces of cayenne, *number two,* two ounces of cloves, all pounded fine, sifted through a fine sieve, and well mixed together. For a dose, take one tea-spoonful of this powder with a tea-spoonful of sugar, in a wine-glassful of boiling water, as soon as sufficiently cool, the patient being in bed, or covered with a blanket by the fire.

The medicine, *number one,* and, also, the nerve powder, hereinafter described, may be used with this compound, and will be proper in more violent cases.

In all cases of symptoms of nervous affection, a nerve powder must be used, which is prepared as follows, to wit. Take ladies slipper *(Cypripedium pubescens,)* dig the roots when done growing, wash them clean, dry and reduce them to a fine powder. For a dose, take half a tea-spoonful in hot water, sweetened, or the same quantity may be given mixed with either of the other medicines, in all nervous cases.

When the above described medicine, or such part thereof as may be deemed proper to administer, shall have produced the intended effect, a copious perspiration should be produced by applying heat to the body, by the aid of steam, in the following manner, to wit. Let several stones of different sizes be made hot, then put one (the smallest first) into a pan, or kettle, of hot water about half immersed; place the patient over it undressed, covered with a blanket to shield him from the cold air; change the stones as often as they grow cool and keep the patient in this situation as long as he can conveniently bear it; then he may be rubbed all over with a cloth wet with spirits, or cold water, and either dress or go to bed.

When the patient is too weak to sit, or stand, over the steam, take three hot stones, quench them a little in water, and wrap them in several thicknesses of cloths well wet with water, place one at his feet, and one on each side as he lies in bed, which will produce a lively steam, and with a dose of medicine, *number two,* taken inwardly, will cause a free perspiration.

The preparing and compounding the foregoing vegetable medicines, in the manner herein described, and the administering them, to cure diseases, as herein mentioned, together with the use of steam to produce perspiration, the said Samuel Thomson claims as his own invention.

SAMUEL THOMSON

Appendix 6

An Attack Made by Morris Mattson Against the Alva Curtis Faction That Seceded During the Seventh National Thomsonian Convention in 1838

The enemies of Dr. Thomson have stated that he urged a dissolution of the old convention, from a desire to monopolize the sale of medicines. It was his principle aim to propose such measures as were calculated to keep his system in the hands of the *people,* and to prevent them from being imposed upon by a junto of designing knaves, who have used every effort to trample Dr. Thomson in the dust.

The individuals composing this *scarecrow* faction were headed by that ineffable nuisance, that notorious drunken sot, Dr. Draper, who had probably procured a short respite from Moyamensing for that important service. After the old convention had dissolved, and the mongrels discovered the impossibility of hanging on any longer by the skirts of the Thomsonians, Dr. Draper interrupted the assembly with one of his billingsgate speeches, in which he proposed that his followers should adjourn to a tavern in Chestnut Street (Philadelphia), and there organize an "Independent" convention. The suggestion was carried into effect, and after a two days' session, they had matured a constitution, passed sundry resolutions, and adjourned to meet within a year, in New York City.

Now this was all well enough, with the exception that they should not have christened themselves the "Thomsonian" society. . . . If they can do without Dr. Thomson's system, they can certainly do without his *name.* They should have styled themselves the "butternut society," or the "purify-

---

Source: The Boston Thomsonian Manual and Lady's Companion 5 (1838): 8-11.

ing syrup society." Either of these would have been far more appropriate than the one selected.

This tavern convention, we perceive, consisted of about thirty members. Ephraim Larabee of Baltimore, a notorious vender of secret nostrums, was the president. We find the names, also, of John A. Brown of Providence, R.I., one of the most noted of the mongrels; B. W. Sperry of New Haven, Conn., a man who, unless very much belied, uses opium and laudanum in his practice in disguise, and engaged in printing a *counterfeit* edition of the New Guide; A. C. Draper, of almshouse and Moyamensing notoriety; William Armstrong, a vender of Jewett's liniments; William Burton and Samuel Ross of Philadelphia, well known in that city for their abominable quackery, and sale of secret compounds; James Thorn (called, par excellence, doctor), the Pennsylvania agent for the sale of Howard's *improved* system of medicine; and last, though not least, Dr. Curtis of Columbus, Ohio. . . .

Appendix 7

Preamble and Constitution of the New York Thomsonian Medical Society

The Convention met according to adjournment, after which the Committee appointed to frame a Constitution for a State Botanic Society, reported the following *preamble* and Articles of the *constitution*, which were read and adopted.

PREAMBLE

WHEREAS, The great success that has attended the exhibition of the philosophical principles, and the administration of the healing remedies of the Thomsonian System of Medical Practice since its introduction into this state, has enlisted a respectable portion of this community in its favor by inspiring a confidence in its general utility, in consequence of its simple but efficacious means in removing disease and restoring health; as well as to excite in another portion, feelings of the most implacable hostility to its doctrines; and to institute necessary, proper and just regulations respecting the natural capacities and acquired abilities of those who assume the arduous and responsible stations as public practitioners; to resist the malignity of our enemies, increase the confidence of our friends, preserve the purity and perpetuate the benificent designs of the illustrious founder whose name we bear, we do each and all hereby agree to be governed by the following:

Source: The Thomsonian Manual 1.2 (December 1835). Proceedings of the Botanic State Convention held at Geddes, Onondaga County, New York, September 28, 1835.

CONSTITUTION

Art. 1. This society shall be known and called by name of the *Thomso-nian* Medical Society of the State of New York.

Art. 2. This society shall consist of two degrees of Membership.

Art. 3. Any person who shall have attained to the age of twenty-one years, is a citizen of the United States, who possesses a good moral character and certificate for the right of practice secured to Dr. Samuel Thomson by letters patent from the President of the United States, may become a member of the first degree, by subscribing to this constitution and paying the sum of one dollar into the Treasury.

Art. 4. Any member of the first degree may become a member of the second degree by exhibiting such testimonials of ability, under-standing, and other necessary qualifications, as shall secure to him a diploma from the officers of this society inducting him into general practice.

Art. 5. The officers of this society shall consist of a President, Vice-President, Secretary and Treasurer, and five Censors.

Art. 6. It shall be the duty of the President to preside at each and every meeting of the Society, and to preserve and keep good order therein.

Art. 7. It shall be the duty of the Vice-President to preside at any and every meeting of the Society in the absence of the President, and by his request at all times, to officiate in his stead.

Art. 8. It shall be the duty of the Secretary to make and preserve a record of all the proceedings of this society. Also to keep a record of the names of all the members of this society with their residences, and make a true and faithful report at the annual meeting.

Art. 9. It shall be the duty of the Treasurer to receive and keep all the moneys or funds that may belong to this society, and render an exact account of the State of the Treasury at every regular meet-ing of this Society, and pay the necessary expenses by order of the President, Secretary or Censors; when sanctioned by a vote of the majority of the Society, and furthermore he shall, if required, give good and sufficient security for the faithful performance of his duty.

Art. 10. It shall be the duty of the Censors to criticise and examine all such members of the first degree that shall apply to them, as it respects their knowledge of the *Thomsonian* system of medicine, of the symptoms and nature of the various diseases incident to the human frame, of the general principles of midwifery and the relative position of the organs and functions of the human body, and as to their natural and acquired abilities for becoming physicians, and shall also present them with a certificate from some regular authorised practitioner of this society, certifying that he sustains a good moral character, and has studied the *Thomsonian* System of Medicine for the term of at least one year; and if they find said applicant well qualified to practice medicine they shall grant him a Diploma to that effect, for which he shall pay into the Treasury the sum of five dollars.

Art. 11. The officers of the society shall serve for the term of one year, or until the annual meeting when all the officers of the society shall be chosen.

Art. 12. This Society shall hold a meeting on the second Tuesday of June annually, at such place as it may previously appoint.

Art. 13. A majority of all the members present shall rule in the transaction of any business before the Society, and in case of a tie, the President shall give the casting vote.

Art. 14. If any member of the second degree, or that has a diploma, does, by will, neglect or bad management in practice, violate, or does not conform to the rules and regulations of this society, shall, on conviction before this society, be expelled by a vote of two thirds of all the members then present, and a notice of the same shall be published in one or more of the newspapers in the county where he resides.

Art. 15. No members of this society shall practice phlebotomy, or use as medicine any mineral, animal or vegetable poison, or any deleterious drug whatever.

Art. 16. No person shall be fellowshipped by this society as a practitioner except he shall obtain a diploma from the Board of Censors.

Art. 17. No member of the second degree, or that has received a diploma from this society, shall withhold any knowledge in medicine that he may possess, from a brother member of the same degree, it shall be his duty, if required, to make a written description of all such preparations, compounds or simples, together with the usual quantum of dose and the time of administering the same, to his brother members of the same degree; and said members shall not expose a knowledge of said medicine to another person or persons, on penalty of being forever debarred from the privileges of this society.

Art. 18. This Constitution may be altered or revised, on concurrence of two thirds of all the members present at the annual meeting of this society, and it shall be proper to make such by-laws and regulations as shall be found necessary for the government thereof.

Art. 19. This society shall have power at each and every stated meeting to fill all vacant seats of office, by an election pro tempore.

Art. 20. Twelve members of this society shall constitute a quorum to transact any business therein.

Appendix 8

Advertisement in Samuel Emmons' Book
The Vegetable Family Physician,
Boston, 1842

NEW ENGLAND THOMSONIAN DEPOT
D. L. HALE
At His Establishment
79 & 81 Blackstone St.
Boston, Mass.
Offers for Sale, Wholesale and Retail,
An Extensive Stock of Superior
Vegetable Medicines, Among Which Are
The Following, Viz.

African Cayenne	Beth Root
Nerve Powder	Strengthening Plaster
Goldenseal	Adhesive do.
Ginger	Cancer do.
Green Lobelia	Meadow Fern Ointment
Brown do.	Stimulating Liniment
Slippery Elm	Nipple Shields
Poplar Bark	Raspberry Leaves
Fine Bayberry	Witch Hazel
Coarse do.	Headache Snuff
Unicorn Root	Healing Salve
Composition	Cough Balsam

Spiced Bitters	Eye Water
Female Restorative	Volatile Liniment
Anti Dyspeptic Bread	Nerve Ointment
Injection Powder	Sumach Leaves
Cough do.	do. Berries
Lobelia Pills	Tincture of Lobelia
Cayenne do.	do. Meadow Fern
Sumach do.	do. Fir Balsam
Rheumatic Drops	do. Scullcap
Dysentery Syrup	do. Cayenne
Wine Bitters	do. Myrrh
Antispasmodic Tincture	Essences
Nursing Bottles	Volatile Oils
Respirators	Alternative Mixture
Cough Syrup	Ramadge's Tubes

This establishment is the largest, and has a more extensive trade than any one of the kind in America. Medicines are sent from it into all the States, to Mexico, the British provinces, Europe, Asia, and Africa.

For sale also as above, a large, and extensive assortment of Shaker's Herbs, embracing all those kinds used in the Botanic Practice, at a great discount from Shaker's prices, all warranted fresh, and of a superior quality.

D. L. Hale's assortment of Syringes is the most extensive in New England, embracing every variety of approved pattern in use. He is now selling at low prices, a splendid article, manufactured expressly for his establishment, which takes the place of the common syringe and is fully equal to the patent, at half the price.

Also a general assortment of Dental instruments, Trusses, &c. The business at this Depot being now conducted entirely on the cash principle, the Proprietor is enabled to sell at such prices, as cannot fail to give entire satisfaction. Every article warranted pure, and free from adulteration.

Mattson's American Vegetable Practice, Curtis's Obstetrics, and other Botanic Works.

Appendix 9

Notice for an Alleged Libel Against the Impositions of Paine D. Badger, Boston, 1839

THOMSONIAN BOTANIC INFIRMARY
No. 554 Washington-street, Boston
(Opposite the Worcester Rail-road Ticket Office)

The subscriber having purchased the interest of Dr. Brown, his late partner, in that large and spacious Infirmary above named, and lately occupied by them as partners, and has fitted it up in a style not surpassed by any other in the State for convenience and comfort; and would now inform his friends and the public that he is not only ready to accommodate them when sick with the most assiduous attention and medical treatment, after the Botanic System of Practice, but also with large and airy rooms commanding a fine prospect of the Worcester and Providence Rail-roads, and surrounding country, on the west; Boston Harbor, its islands, shipping, light-houses, etc. on the east; and so situated as to enjoy as good air as the city affords.

The subscriber is also determined that nothing shall be wanted through every department of this Infirmary as to neatness and regularity; good order, the best of nursing and attention, to make everyone who favors him with their patronage, happy and contented. He has also a valuable library of the best selected books for the instruction and amusement of his patients. He has also in readiness clean changes of linen for all patients who

Source: This notice appeared in the *Boston Daily Advocate* and is reproduced in *The Report of The Trial of Dr. Samuel Thomson* (Boston: Printed by Henry P. Lewis, 1839).

come to take single courses of medicine, and India Rubber coverings for the mattresses and beds, he always uses to prevent contagion—his steam-boxes have windows and curtains, so that patients who are feeble can at any time put out their heads and breathe the fresh air—boilers are so constructed that he can at any moment graduate the steam to suit their wish or ability to bear—so that there is not the least danger to the most feeble constitution, nor even for an infant of a month old. The shower of two quarts of cold water is delicious, though we never insist on it, as it is always a matter of choice with the patients, and a person who has once taken it, will never after be denied, but will frequently call for more.

The subscriber has owned Dr. Samuel Thomson's Family Right nearly three years—has given strict attention to its precept, and for the five last months has administered pure Thomsonian Medicine to over two hundred persons, many of whom suffered under the most desperate complaints, and have been given over to die by the regular physician; and such has been his success, that out of the whole number, every individual except two persons, have been relieved, and more than three-fourths cured who have left his Infirmary. He will still continue to administer Thomsonian Medicines in their purity, at his Infirmary, assisted by Dr. Darling, of No. 52 Salem-street, in all difficult cases, who has been a regular practitioner of the Thomsonian System, for more than fourteen years in this city. Mrs. Badger will attend to the ladies department at all times—she having been an experienced nurse over eighteen years—a part of which time she was nurse in the Massachusetts General Hospital;—since in private families, and for the last two years a strict Thomsonian nurse. The subscriber would invite the afflicted of all descriptions to call and examine for themselves, and if they should see fit to put themselves under his care, let their disease be what it may, if timely application be made, he will ensure a speedy relief.

P. D. BADGER, Botanic Physician

N.B. For sale at the above establishment, a general assortment of pure Thomsonian Medicines, done up with directions for use, at wholesale or retail.

October 28, 1835

Appendix 10

Some Typical Remedies
Compounded and Sold
in Thomsonian Establishments

The following recipes are typical of the many medications compounded and sold in Thomsonian stores, depots, and infirmaries. Recipes numbered from 1 through 8 are taken from Colby's *A Guide to Health;* numbers 9 and 10 from *The Thomsonian Materia Medica,* Thirteenth Edition; and numbers 11 through 15 from Luken's *The Sick Man's Guide.*

1. Spiced Bitters

Poplar bark	2 lbs.
Golden seal	8 oz.
Prickly ash bark	12 oz.
Ginger	8 oz.
Cloves	8 oz.
Balmony	8 oz.
Cinnamon	4 oz.
Cayenne	6 oz.
White sugar	5 lbs.

The whole finely pulverized, sifted, and well mixed. This is an excellent tonic compound. . . .

DOSE: Take a tea-spoonful of the powder, in half a cupful of hot water, three times a day, before eating; or take the same quantity into the mouth dry, and wash down with cold water.

2. Female Restoratives

Poplar bark	5 lbs.
Cloves	8 oz.
Cinnamon	8 oz.
Bethroot	1 lb.
Witch hazel leaves	1 lb.
Loaf sugar	8 lbs.
Cayenne	6 oz.

All finely pulverized, sifted and well mixed.

DOSE: A teaspoonful in half a cupful of hot water, three times a day.

3. Head-Ache Snuff

Bayberry	1 oz.
Blood root	½ oz.
Sassafras bark	1 oz.

Finely pulverized and mixed.

4. Anti-Spasmodic Tincture

Lobelia seed, pulverized	1 lb.
Valerian	4 oz.
Holland gin	1 gallon

Infuse for ten days in a closely-stopped vessel, shaking it every day; then strain off for use.

This preparation is valuable in violent attacks of any form of disease, such as lock-jaw, fits, hydrophobia, suspended animation, to expel poison of any kind from the system; as an external application it is useful in sprains, bruises, rheumatic pains, etc.

DOSE: A teaspoonful, repeated as often as the nature of the case requires, in some warming tea.

5. Dysentery or Cholera Syrup

White pond lily, root	4 oz.
Green peppermint	8 oz.
Bayberry	4 oz.

Boil in one and a half gallons of water down to one gallon, strain and add:

Gum myrrh	1 oz.
Cayenne	¼ oz.
Rhubarb	4 oz.
Saleratus	½ oz.
Loaf sugar	1 lb.
Fourth Proof brandy	1 pt.

DOSE: Half a wine-glass once in two hours. This syrup is an invaluable remedy for diarrhoea, dysentery, cholera morbus, and the summer complaint of children.

6. Emetic Powder

Lobelia, herb	4 oz.
Lobelia, seed	4 oz.
Bayberry	2 oz.
Cayenne	4 oz.
Valerian	2 oz.

All finely pulverized, and well mixed.

DOSE: Put four teaspoonfuls in a cup of hot water, and give four teaspoonfuls, after the sediment settles, once in ten minutes until it operates freely as an emetic.

Note: An asterisk (*) indicates that the recipe was at variance with the materia medica of Samuel Thomson.

7. Cough Drops

Lobelia Herb	4 oz.
Hoarhound	2 oz.
Comfrey	2 oz.
Elecampane	2 oz.
Boneset	4 oz.

Boil in three quarts of water to three pints, strain and add two pounds of white sugar and one pint of Holland gin.

DOSE: Two or three teaspoonfuls once an hour; for asthma, croup, cough, whooping cough, consumption, etc.

8. Compound Tincture of Myrrh or Hot Drops

Put them into a jug or glass demi-john, and shake them several times a day for a week, when the liquor may be poured off and bottled for use. This preparation is useful for bathing in cases of debility or a relaxed state of the surface, as in night sweats—to check diarrhoea, relieve pain in the stomach or bowels, and also for the toothache.

DOSE: From one to two teaspoonfuls in hot water. For the toothache, wet a piece of cotton in it, and put it into the tooth.

9. Wine Bitters

Take five pounds of poplar bark and one of balmony, boil them in fifteen gallons of water, then add while hot, twenty pounds of sugar and one pound of nerve powder. Strain off and add four gallons of fourth proof Jamaica rum or brandy, twenty gallons of best Malaga wine, and one gallon each of tincture of meadow fern and prickly ash bark. When cool put it into a barrel and it is fit for use.

DOSE: From half to a wineglassful three times a day.

*10. No. 2 Antiscorbutic Syrup— A Valuable Article

Take of the yellow or narrow dock and burdock roots, each one pound; burdock seeds and American senna of each one half pound;

pulverize and mix them well together, and then boil in ten quarts of water for half an hour; strain off, and add half a gallon of brandy and the same quantity of molasses. Keep it bottled close for use. This is one of the best antiscorbutic syrups I have ever made, for all humors of the body.

DOSE: From a fourth to half glass, three times a day, or less or more, according to the circumstances of the case.

*11. Embrocation for Sprains, etc.

Sal Ammonia	1 oz.
Spts. Hartshorne	4 drachms
Spts. Lavender	4 drachms
Oil Spike	½ pint
Oil Turpentine	½ pint

Mixed.

12. Tonic and Alternative Pills

Green Lobelia	½ oz.
Nerve Powder	1 oz.
Cayenne	½ oz.
Gum Myrrh	½ oz.

Add no. 6, make into Pills with Gum Arabic.

*13. Ointment for the Itch

Hog's lard	1 lb.
Sulphur	1 lb.
Sal ammoniac	1 oz.
White hellebore	1 oz.
Essence lemon	1 drachm

*14. Cathartic Pills

May-apple root	6 oz.
Black root	4 oz.
Camboge	8 oz.
Lobelia seed	4 oz.
Cayenne	½ oz.

DOSE: 3-6 pills

*15. Elixir of Health

Senna	3 oz.
Jalap	1 oz.
Coriander seeds	½ oz.
Caraway seeds	½ oz.
Diluted Alcohol	3 lbs.

Digest and filter through paper.

RESOURCES

A Note on Resources

Anyone initiating a study of sectarian medicine immediately confronts a mass of diffused and, at times, very ephemeral literature. So daunting a task is made more manageable by honing the subject down to a particular group, aspect, or phase of the movement, but as the bibliography (pp. 259-274) demonstrates, even then the body of material can be substantial. The works listed on the following pages (more than 300 in all) represent those utilized in the present study. The authors were aided significantly by finding the vast majority of resources at one repository: the Lloyd Library and Museum, 917 Plum Street, Cincinnati, Ohio 45202. Established by the Lloyd brothers and carefully managed by leading eclectic researcher and pharmaceutical manufacturer John Uri Lloyd, this facility remains at some 200,000 volumes, the single largest collection devoted to pharmacy, botany, and, especially, the American botanico-medical movement. The Lloyd Library not only holds a large collection of published botanico-medical material but also has all of the extant records of the Eclectic Medical Institute, the largest and most enduring botanico-medical school in America.

In the preface and in our historiographical analysis, we mentioned those historians and their works which have been most helpful in developing our approach to the subject. One aspect we did not pursue, however, was the impact of the Thomsonians on Canada. Those interested in this fascinating facet of the movement should consult Jennifer J. Connor's "Thomsonian Medical Books and the Culture of Dissent in Upper Canada," *Bulletin of Canadian History of Medicine* 12 (1995): 289-311, and, with J. T. H. Connor, "Thomsonian Medical Literature and Reformist Discourse in Upper Canada," *Canadian Literature* 131 (1991): 140-155.

Of all the various components of the botanico-medical literature, clearly the most complex are found in its many and disparate serial publications. Printed in virtually every section of the country, numerous editors, agents, colleges, societies, and associations started journals and magazines, some, such as the *Eclectic Medical Journal,* lasting nearly 100 years, others, surviving no more than a single issue. John Haller has provided a great service to future scholars of the Thomsonian movement by listing "United States: Botanic Medical Journals From 1822 to 1860" (pp. 271-284) in his

The People's Doctors. Haller painstakingly listed eighty-five Thomsonian journals, their years and places of publication, their editors, and any pertinent comments, such as their frequency, scope and content, and final disposition. We know of no other more complete or in-depth survey of Thomsonian journal literature available. For eclectic journals, the collection located at the Lloyd Library offers the most comprehensive selection. Two of the most prominent eclectic serials, the *Eclectic Medical Journal* (1849-1937) and *Eclectic Medical Gleaner* (1894-1912), are available at the library in complete runs. In addition, the Lloyd Library has earlier eclectic journals, such as the *Eclectic Medical Reformer* and *Western Medical Recorder,* which cover 1836 to 1848. These materials taken together cover the broad history of American eclecticism and are essential to understanding the many practical and professional issues and concerns that formed the discourse of nineteenth-century botanic practitioners.

For a better sense of what we have called "the current botanicism," a number of sources should be consulted, much of which can be found on the Internet. The National Center for Complementary and Alternative Medicine (formerly the Office of Alternative Medicine), operated by congressional mandate under the aegis of the National Institutes of Health, keeps the public continually updated on its research activities related to herbal medicine via its home page <http://altmed.od.nih.gov/oam/>. Also, the American Herbalists Guild is the largest and most important organization of its kind in the United States. It describes itself as "founded in 1989 as a nonprofit, educational organization to represent the goals and voices of herbalists. It is the only peer-reviewed organization for professional herbalists specializing in the medicinal use of plants. AHG membership consists of professionals, general members (including students) and benefactors." Their Web site address is <http//:www.healthy.net/herbalists/Intro.htm>; their mailing address is P.O. Box 70, Roosevelt, UT 84066. Also very active in the current botanical movement is the American Botanical Council (ABC). The ABC is an educational organization headed by Executive Director Mark Blumenthal, who publishes the most widely circulated peer-reviewed journal on herbal medicine in the United States, *HerbalGram.* Located at the Case Mill Homestead in Austin, Texas, their mailing address is P.O. Box 144345, Austin, TX 78714; their Web site is <http://www.herbalgram.org/>. Finally, is the Herb Research Foundation (HRF). HRF's Web site (<http://www.herbs.org/>) states that it is "dedicated to responsible informed self-care with medicinal plants." A sister organization to ABC, the Foundation, under Rob McCaleb's direction, conducts research, provides information, and maintains an herbal resource center that contains over 150,000 scientific articles. Although not historical in content, these leaders of the current botanical movement demonstrate the tenacity of herbal medicine in the American health care market.

We do not represent these notes and bibliography as an exhaustive survey of the literature related to the American botanico-medical movements, but we do believe that it contains significant primary and secondary materials related to the subject, particularly in those areas pertaining to its influence upon American pharmacy and the materia medica. We offer it in the hope that it might be useful to future researchers pursuing new and different aspects of this important and colorful tradition in American health and healing.

Notes

Preface

1. William G. Rothstein, "The Botanical Movements and Orthodox Medicine," in *Other Healers: Unorthodox Medicine in America,* edited by Norman Gevitz (Baltimore, MD: Johns Hopkins University Press, 1988), p. 31.

2. See Alex Berman's "The Thomsonian Movement and Its Relation to American Pharmacy and Medicine," *Bulletin of the History of Medicine* 25 (1951): 405-428, 518-538; "Neo-Thomsonianism in the United States," *Journal of the History of Medicine and Allied Sciences* 11 (1956): 133-155; and "Wooster Beach and the Early Eclectics," *University of Michigan Medical Bulletin* 24 (1958): 277-286.

3. Norman Gevitz (Ed.), *Other Healers: Unorthodox Medicine in America* (Baltimore, MD: Johns Hopkins University Press, 1988), p. 26.

4. See, for example, David L. Cowen and William H. Helfand, *Pharmacy: An Illustrated History* (New York: Harry N. Abrams, 1991), pp. 134-135; John Duffy, *From Humors to Medical Science: A History of American Medicine,* Second Edition (Urbana, IL: University of Illinois Press, 1993), p. 87; and Barbara Griggs, *Green Pharmacy: The History and Evolution of Western Herbal Medicine,* Second Edition (Rochester, VT: Healing Arts Press, 1997), p. 220. The term *neo-Thomsonians* is retained in this book because it offers a useful descriptive label for *all* botanics who came out of the Thomsonian tradition *regardless* of their specific sectarian affiliation. Thus, when neo-Thomsonian is used in this book, it is intended as an umbrella term referring to independent Thomsonians, physio-medicals, and Coffinites. In places where specific groups are referred to, the appropriate designation—e.g., independent Thomsonian, physio-medical, or Coffinite—is used.

5. Joseph F. Kett, *The Formation of the American Medical Profession: The Role of Institutions, 1780-1860* (New Haven, CT: Yale University Press, 1968).

6. Ibid., pp. 130-131.

7. William G. Rothstein, *American Physicians in the Nineteenth Century* (Baltimore, MD: Johns Hopkins University Press, 1972), pp. 125-128, 177.

8. Abraham Flexner, *Medical Education in the United States and Canada: A Report to the Carnegie Foundation for the Advancement of Teaching,* Bulletin no. 4 (New York: Carnegie Foundation, 1910), p. 156.

9. Lamar Riley Murphy, *Enter the Physician: The Transformation of Domestic Medicine, 1760-1860* (Tuscaloosa, AL: University of Alabama Press, 1991), p. 71.

10. In particular, see Alex Berman's "Heroic Approach in 19th Century Medical Practice," *Bulletin of the American Society of Hospital Pharmacists* 11 (1954): 321-327; and "Social Roots of the 19th Century Botanico-Medical Movement in the United States," *Actes du VIIIe Congrès International d'Histoire des Sciences,* Florence (September 3-9, 1954): 561-565.

11. John Harley Warner, *The Therapeutic Perspective: Medical Practice, Knowledge, and Identity in America, 1820-1885,* Reprint Edition (Princeton, NJ: Princeton University Press, 1997), p. 220.

12. Berman's essay "Heroic Approach" was reprinted in the first edition of *Sickness and Health in America: Readings in the History of Medicine and Public Health,* edited by Judith Walzer Leavitt and Ronald L. Numbers (Madison, WI: University of Wisconsin Press, 1978), pp. 77-86. John Harley Warner's "From Specifity to Universalism in Medical Therapeutics: Transformation in the 19th-Century United States" can be found in *Sickness and Health in America,* Second Edition (1997), pp. 87-101.

13. See, for example, Daniel J. Wallace, "Thomsonians: The People's Doctors," *Clio Medica* 14 (1980): 169-186; James O. Breeden, "Thomsonianism in Virginia," *Virginia Magazine of History and Biography* 82 (1974): 150-180; Ronald L. Numbers, "The Making of an Eclectic Physician: Joseph M. McElhinney and the Eclectic Medical Institute of Cincinnati," *Bulletin of the History of Medicine* 47 (1973): 155-166; and Ronald L. Numbers, "Do-It-Yourself the Sectarian Way," in *Medicine Without Doctors: Home Health Care in American History,* edited by Guenter B. Risse, Ronald L. Numbers, and Judith Walzer Leavitt (New York: Science Publications, 1977), pp. 49-72.

14. John S. Haller Jr., *Medical Protestants: The Eclectics in American Medicine, 1825-1939* (Carbondale, IL: Southern Illinois University Press, 1994).

15. John S. Haller Jr., *Kindly Medicine: Physio-Medicalism in America, 1836-1911* (Kent, OH: Kent State University Press, 1997).

16. John S. Haller Jr., *A Profile in Alternative Medicine: The Eclectic College of Medicine, 1845-1942* (Kent, OH: Kent State University Press, 1999).

17. John S. Haller Jr., *The People's Doctors: Samuel Thomson and the American Botanical Movement, 1790-1860* (Carbondale, IL: Southern Illinois University Press, in press).

Chapter 1

1. Roy Porter, *The Greatest Benefit to Mankind: A Medical History of Humanity* (New York: W.W. Norton, 1997), pp. 282-283; and Barbara Griggs, *Green Pharmacy: The History and Evolution of Western Herbal Medicine,* Second Edition (Rochester, VT: Healing Arts Press, 1997), pp. 109-110.

2. Quoted in Porter, *The Greatest Benefit,* pp. 288-289.

3. David L. Cowen, *America's Pre-pharmacopoeial Literature* (Madision, WI: American Institute of the History of Pharmacy, 1961), p. 19; see also Mary Rhinelander McCarl, "Publishing the Works of Nicholas Culpeper, Astrological Herbalist and Translator of Latin Medical Works in Seventeenth-Century London," *Canadian Bulletin of Medical History* 13 (1996): 225-276.

4. I.K. Steele, "A London Trader and the Atlantic Empire: Joseph Cruttenden, Apothecary, 1710 to 1717," *William and Mary Quarterly*, Third Series, 34 (1977): 281-297.

5. G.S.B. Hempstead, "Reminiscences of the Physicians of the First Quarter of the Present Century, with a Review of Some Features of Their Practice," *The Cincinnati Lancet and Clinic* 40 (1878): 54.

6. Will H. Blackwell, *Poisonous and Medicinal Plants* (Englewood Cliffs, NJ: Prentice Hall, 1990), p. 28.

7. This statement was made by the famous polemicist and pamphleteer, William Cobbett (1763-1835) in *The Rush-Light* (New York), February 28, 1800, p. 49; cited by R.H. Shryock, *Dictionary of American Biography*, s.v. "Rush, Benjamin."

8. Worthington Hooker, "Rational Therapeutics; A Prize Essay," *Publications of the Massachusetts Medical Society* 1.2 (1857): 157-160.

9. Ibid., p. 160. James Hamilton, the younger (d. 1839), professor of midwifery at the University of Edinburgh, was one of the few men of his day who criticized the universal practice of indiscriminate, massive dosing with calomel. In the introduction to his book, *Observations on the Use and Abuse of Mercurial Medicines in Various Diseases* (1820), he wrote of the dangerous properties of mercury: "for some ages after mercury became an article of the *Materia Medica,* physicians recommended it only on the most urgent occasions—but within these few years British practitioners seem to have overlooked the necessity for such caution, and to exhibit that medicine with very little scruple" (American Edition, [New York: Bliss and White], 1821).

10. For example, in his work on the history of malaria in the upper Mississippi valley, Professor Ackerknecht has observed that "the decline of . . . 'active' treatment assumed considerable proportions only in the '50's and even then was slow enough"; Erwin H. Ackerknecht, *Malaria in the Upper Mississippi Valley* (Baltimore, MD: Johns Hopkins Press, 1945), p. 118.

11. H.C. Wood, "The Heroic Treatment of Idiopathic Peritonitis," *Boston Medical and Surgical Journal,* 98 (1878): 556; cited by J.J. Woodward, in *The Medical and Surgical History of the War of the Rebellion,* Volume 1, Part 2, *Medical History* (Washington, DC: Government Printing Office, 1879), p. 687. A good example of George B. Wood's reactionary views is to be found in his *Treatise on Therapeutics and Pharmacology; or Materia Medica,* Volumes 1 and 2, Third Edition (Philadelphia: J.B. Lippincott, 1868). He wrote on bloodletting, "As an antiphlogistic measure, the loss of blood holds a position far above any other agent; and it is in this capacity, moreover, that it exercises the most beneficial therapeutic influence" (Volume 2, p. 40). For historical accounts of heroic therapeutics see Alex Berman, "The Heroic Approach in 19th Century Medical Practice," *Bulletin of the American Society of Hospital Pharmacists* 11 (1954): 321-327; Leon S. Bryan Jr., "Blood-Letting in American Medicine, 1830-1892," *Bulletin of the History of Medicine* 38 (1964): 516-529; and John Harley Warner, *The Therapeutic Perspective: Medical Practice, Knowledge, and Identity in*

America, 1820-1885, Reprint Edition (Princeton, NJ: Princeton University Press, 1997).

12. B.J. Stern, *Society and Medical Progress* (Princeton, NJ: Princeton University Press, 1941), pp. 29-30.

13. See Benjamin Rush's "A Defense of Blood-Letting As a Remedy for Certain Diseases," *Medical Inquiries and Observation,* Volume 4 (Philadelphia: Thomas Dobson, 1796), pp. 244-255.

14. Ibid. Interestingly enough, Samuel Thomson saw nothing inconsistent in visiting Dr. Barton and Dr. Rush, the great exponent of bloodletting in Philadelphia, where, as he stated, "I remained several days . . . to confer with them upon the subject of introducing my system of practice to the world." The deaths of Rush in 1813 and Barton in 1815 were regarded by Thomson as a great misfortune, and he wrote, "I was deprived of the influence of these two men, which I was confident would have been exerted in my favor"; see Samuel Thomson, *New Guide to Health; or, Botanic Family Physician, to which is Prefixed the Life and Medical Discoveries of the Author* (Boston: J.Q. Adams, 1835), pp. 124-125.

15. Elisha Bartlett, *An Essay on the Philosophy of Medical Science* (Philadelphia: Lea and Blachard, 1844), pp. 224-244.

16. The term allopathic comes from the Greek words *allos* (different) and *pathos* (illness), meaning to cure a disease by prescribing remedies different from the symptoms presented. The term was coined by Samuel Hahnemann (1755-1845), founder of homeopathy, to distinguish his *similia similibus curantur* (like cures like) principle from the regular or orthodox profession's *contraria contrariis* (cure by contraries). The term quickly lost Hahnemann's original connotation and was soon generally applied to any regular practitioner.

17. See Charles E. Rosenberg, *The Cholera Years: The United States in 1832, 1849, and 1866* (Chicago: University of Chicago Press, 1962), pp. 70-72.

18. Quoted in J.S. Chambers, *The Conquest of Cholera* (New York: Macmillan, 1938), p. 170.

19. Ibid.

20. Cited by *The Thomsonian Recorder* 2 (1833): 14. Daniel Drake was not averse to prescribing calomel, but in doses that were considered small at that time. As part of the treatment for cholera, he prescribed ten grains of calomel and one grain of opium. See his "Proclamation to Citizens of Cincinnati," reproduced from the *Cincinnati Chronicle,* in Chambers, *The Conquest of Cholera,* p. 106.

21. *The Thomsonian Recorder,* 2, p. 15.

22. Norwood describes Caldwell as "perhaps the most spectacular character to adorn the Transylvania Medical Faculty. For consummate conceit, he stood without a peer"; see W.F. Norwood, *Medical Education in the United States Before the Civil War* (Philadelphia: University of Pennsylvania Press, 1944), p. 293; see also Rosenberg, *The Cholera Years,* p. 152.

23. Cited by *The Boston Medical and Surgical Journal,* 15 (1836): 158-159.

24. Thomas D. Mitchell, "Calomel Considered As a Poison," *New Orleans Medical and Surgical Journal,* 1 (1844-1845): 28 ff.

25. Ibid., p. 30.

26. Alexander Means, "Calomel—Its Chemical Characteristics and Mineral Origin Considered, in View of its Curative Claims," *Southern Medical and Surgical Journal* (March 1845); cited in the *New Orleans Medical Journal* 1 (1845): 588.

27. *New Orleans Medical Journal,* 1, p. 589.

28. Ibid., p. 591.

29. Charles W. Wilder, "Pulmonary Consumption, Its Causes, Symptoms & Treatment," *Medical Communications of the Massachusetts Medical Society,* Second Series, Volume 3 (Boston: The Society, 1848), pp. 112-120. Read at the Annual Meeting, May 31, 1843.

30. Ibid., p. 116.

31. The independent Thomsonians and physio-medicals came to the fore after Thomson's death. They abandoned the name "Thomsonian," attempted to strip the system of its more blatant crudities, and at the same time continued to pay homage to the original founder. For a detailed discussion of the neo-Thomsonian trend, see Chapter 5. See also John S. Haller Jr., *Kindly Medicine: Physio-Medicalism in America, 1836-1911* (Kent, OH: Kent State University Press, 1997).

32. A typical "course" of Thomsonian medication was described in great detail (about thirty-eight pages) in Morris Mattson, *The American Vegetable Practice, or, A New and Improved Guide to Health* (Boston: D.L. Hale, 1841), pp. 392-425. John Uri Lloyd and Curtis Gates Lloyd have made the following able condensation of Mattson's exposition in their monograph on lobelia; see *Drugs and Medicines of North America* 2 (1884-1887): 85-86.

33. Samuel Thomson viewed *Lobelia inflata* (Indian tobacco) as a virtual cure-all. The current assessment of the plant's medicinal value is less enthusiastic. Lobelia contains several alkaloids, the most prominent being lobeline. Modern research has confirmed lobeline's expectorant properties and its ability to relax the smooth muscles of the body, thus verifying its use in upper respiratory complaints and asthmatic conditions. However, lobelia is considered unsafe by the FDA, and it can have many side effects, including nausea, vomiting, diarrhea, and tremors. If "safe" dosages are exceeded, profuse sweating and rapid heartbeat, "possibly followed by depression of the central nervous system with attendant hypothermia, convulsions, low blood pressure, suppressed and irregular breathing, coma, and death," can occur. Such demonstrated activities leave the historian guessing as to the results achieved by Thomson and his followers. For current analysis of lobelia, see Andrea Peirce, *The American Pharmaceutical Association Practical Guide to Natural Medicines* (New York: William Morrow, 1999), pp. 406-408.

34. John William Fyfe, *Specific Diagnosis and Specific Medication* (Cincinnati, OH: Scudder, 1909), pp. 5-8. John William Fyfe was an eclectic teacher and pracititioner. See also John Milton Scudder's "Doctrine of Substitution" in his *Eclectic Practice of Medicine,* Eighth Edition, Revised (Cincinnati, OH: Medical Publishing Company, 1877), pp. 289-291.

35. Fyfe, *Specific Diagnosis and Medication,* p. 7. The examples of eclectic substitution are taken from Fyfe's work and from Scudder. The latter vigorously attacked the "Doctrine of Substitution" in the early 1870s.

36. Fyfe, *Specific Diagnosis and Medicaiton,* p. 7.

37. Others have concurred. Ronald L. Numbers wrote, "it may well be that the eclectic physicians sent out from Cincinnati in the 1840s and 1850s did their patients less harm than many doctors who proudly displayed the most orthodox credentials"; see his "The Making of an Eclectic Physician: Joseph M. McElhinney and the Eclectic Medical Institute of Cincinnati," *Bulletin of the History of Medicine* 47 (1973): 166.

38. John Dawson, "Dr. Dawson's Address," in *Proceedings of the Medical Convention of Ohio Held at Columbus on the 5th, 6th, and 7th of May, 1841* (Columbus, OH: Wright and Legg, 1841), pp. 80-84.

39. Some historians, most notably John Harley Warner in *The Therapeutic Perspective,* insist that the use of calomel was greatly diminished by the 1880s. Warner's conclusion is not supported by recent research, nor did he take into account the valuable prescription surveys listed in E.N. Gathercoal's *Prescription Ingredient Survey* (see note 78). Thorough examination of the available data suggests that calomel remained a popular item in the armamentarium until well into the twentieth century. For a complete discussion, see Michael A. Flannery, "What Did Doctors Really Do? In Search of a Therapeutic Perspective of American Medicine," *Journal of Clinical Pharmacy and Therapeutics* 24 (1999): 151-156.

40. Citied by *The Medical and Surgical Reporter* 5 (1860): 320.

41. The "modest place for science" in early nineteenth-century American medicine is discussed in James H. Cassedy, *Medicine in America: A Short History* (Baltimore, MD: Johns Hopkins University Press, 1991), pp. 34-44. For a broader discussion of science in medicine for the period, see W.F. Bynum, *Science and the Practice of Medicine in the Nineteenth Century* (New York: Cambridge University Press, 1994), especially, pp. 114-117.

42. Henry I. Bowditch, "Venesection, Its Former Abuse and Present Neglect." *Publications of the Massachusetts Medical Society,* 3,3 (1871): 223-249.

43. Bowditch recommended venesection in the following cases: (a) "the heart . . . becomes distended with blood"; (b) during "very acute pain in any part of the thorax, for example, from inflammation of the pleura, causing orthopnoea and distress"; (c) "in violent acute cephalic symptoms . . . when the head is hot, the face flushed, and the pulse full and hard"; and (d) "in certain cases of threatened miscarriage" (Ibid., p. 249).

44. Ibid., p. 223.

45. Samuel D. Gross, "A Discourse on Bloodletting Considered As a Therapeutic Agent," *Transactions of the American Medical Association,* 26 (1875): 421-433.

46. Ibid., p. 421.

47. See *The Medical and Surgical Reporter* 3 (1860): 495-521; and *The Medical and Surgical Reporter* 4 (1860): 35.

48. *The Medical and Surgical Reporter* 3, p. 500.

49. Ibid., p. 518.

50. Ibid., p. 519.

51. Ibid., p. 499.

52. Ibid., p. 521.

53. *The Medical and Surgical Reporter* 4, p. 35. Louis's "numerical system" refers to Pierre Charles Alexandre Louis (1787-1872), who was influential in the introduction of statistics in medicine with his *Recherches sur les effects de la saignée dans quelques maladies inflammatoires* . . . (Paris, 1835), translated into English in 1836.

54. *The Medical and Surgical Reporter* 3, p. 496.

55. Jacob Bigelow, "Discourse on Self-Limited Disease," *Medical Communications of the Massachusetts Medical Society* (Boston: The Society, 1836): 319-358. Bigelow defined self-limited disease as follows: "By a self-limited disease, I would be understood to express one which receives limits from its own nature and not from foreign influences; one which, after it has attained foothold in the system, cannot, in the present state of our knowledge, be eradicated, or abridged, by art,— but to which there is due a certain succession of processes, to be completed in a certain time; which time and processes may vary with the constitution and condition of the patient and may tend to death, or recovery, but are not known to be shortened, or greatly changed, by medical treatment" (p. 322).

56. John Forbes, "Homeopathy, Allopathy, and 'Young Physic,'" *British and Foreign Medical Review* 21 (1846): 225-265.

57. Ibid., p. 257.

58. Oliver Wendell Holmes, "Currents and Counter-Currents in Medical Science," an address delivered before the Massachusetts Medical Society at the annual meeting, May 30, 1860, published in *Medical Essays, 1842-1882* (Boston: Houghton Mifflin, 1883), pp. 173-208. Bigelow's influence was reflected in the following essays: A.A. Gould, "Search Out the Secrets of Nature," read at the annual meeting of the Massachusetts Medical Society, 1855; Hooker, "Rational Therapeutics"; and W.J. Walker, "On the Treatment of Compound and Complicated Fractures," read at the annual meeting of the Massachusetts Medical Society, 1845; all cited by Holmes, p. 182.

59. Holmes, "Currents and Counter-Currents," p. 183. The Bigelow influence was still active in Massachusetts in 1868. Three prizes were awarded that year to physicians for essays dealing with "the part performed by nature and time in the cure of diseases."

60. Ibid., p. 204.

61. Gross, "Discourse on Bloodletting," p. 426.

62. Lois N. Magner, *A History of Medicine* (New York: Marcel Dekker, 1992), p. 206.

63. *The Medical and Surgical Reporter* 5, p. 321.

64. Gross considered "Toddism" as having "exercised the most perverse and baneful effects upon civilized society. Ensconsing itself behind a false position, it has literally enslaved the medical world, entrapping alike the wise and foolish, and sweeping over human life with a force equal to that of the most destructive hurricane" ("Discourse on Bloodletting," p. 423). Elsewhere, Gross wrote that he thought "Toddism" was responsible for having "slain millions of human beings by

the indiscriminate manner in which it has been employed" (*Autobiography of Samuel Gross, M.D.,* Volume 1 [Philadelphia: G. Barrie, 1887], p. 380.

65. Roberts Bartholow, *Annual Oration on the Degree of Certainty in Therapeutics* (Baltimore, MD: np, 1876), p. 2. Bartholow (1831-1904) was a professor at the Medical College of Ohio and the author of a very popular textbook on materia medica and therapeutics.

66. For example, Ackerknecht has shown how quinine, which for a time "was only one element in the treatment of malaria, and often the least important," replaced the old prostrating methods when it was empirically observed that large doses of quinine were very effective (Ackerknecht, *Malaria in Mississippi,* p. 115). The same is true of other diseases, e.g., the empirical substitution of aconite and veratrum viride as "antiphlogistic" agents in the treatment of "inflammatory affections" in place of bloodletting (Gross, "Discourse on Bloodletting," p. 426).

67. See P.C.A. Louis, *Researches on the Effects of Blood-letting in Some Inflammatory Diseases and on the Influence of Tartarized Antimony and Vesication in Pneumonitis,* translated by C.G. Putnam, with preface and appendix by James Jackson (Boston: Hilliard, Gray, 1836). For an able discussion of Louis's "numerical method," see Richard Harrison Shryock, *The Development of Modern Medicine,* Reprint Edition (Madison, WI: University of Wisconsin Press, 1979), pp. 157-160, 165-166. Louis's "numerical method" had its zealous advocates in this country (Bartlett, Holmes, and others) and its detractors (Hooker and others). See also Erwin H. Ackerknecht, *Medicine at the Paris Hospital, 1794-1848* (Baltimore, MD: Johns Hopkins Press, 1967), pp. 102-104.

68. The complete Circular no. 6 is reprinted in Woodward, *Medical and Surgical History of the Rebellion,* Volume 1, Part 2, p. 719.

69. Ibid., Part 2, p. 719 ff. Woodward mentioned several regular medical journals that approved Hammond's action. He also cited a letter on file in the surgeon general's office, from the Massachusetts Eclectic Medical Society, tendering "heart-felt congratulations to Surgeon General Hammond for the liberal and independent position assumed in this matter" (p. 720).

70. Ibid., p. 719.

71. *Transactions of the American Medical Association* 14 (1864): 29-33.

72. Woodward, *Medical and Surgical History of the Rebellion,* Volume 1, Part 2, p. 720.

73. Ibid. Although Hammond's order struck calomel from the supply table, it did not affect the following mercurial preparations on the list: *Hydrargyri chloridum corrosivum; Hydrargyri iodidum falvum; Hydrargyri oxidum rubrum; Hydrargyri pilulae; Hydrargyri unguentum;* and *Pilulae catharticae compositae.* Woodward reports that calomel was available in plentiful supply, with 140,169 ounces of calomel and 488,447 dozen compound cathartic pills issued by the Union Army during the war.

74. For a typical botanic reaction to Hammond's order, see the editorial "A Home-Thrust at Regular Medicine by the Surgeon General," *Eclectic Medical Journal* 22 (1863): 294-295. "We should judge," stated the editor, "that this would

fall like a thunderbolt among those who have so strenuously contended that disease could not be treated without mercury." On the role of sectarians during the Civil War, see Michael A. Flannery, "Another House Divided: Union Medical Service and Sectarians During the Civil War," *Journal of the History of Medicine and Allied Sciences,* 60 (1999): 478-510.

75. William A. Hammond, *A Statement of the Causes which Led to the Dismissal of Surgeon General William A. Hammond from the Army* (New York: np, 1864). For a thorough discussion of the trial, see Louis C. Duncan, "The Strange Case of Surgeon General Hammond," *The Military Surgeon* 64 (1929): 98-110, 252-262; and Harvey C. Greisman, "William Hammond and His Enemies," *Medical Heritage* 2 (1986): 322-331.

76. Woodward, *Medical and Surgical History of the Rebellion,* Volume 1, Part 2, p. 722.

77. "Report of Edinburgh Committee on Action of Mercury, Podophylline and Taraxacum on the Biliary Secretion," *The British Medical Journal,* 1868-1869; W. Rutherford and M. Vignal, "Experiments on the Biliary Secretion of the Dog," *Journal of Anatomy and Physiology* (1876). For a complete summary of the calomel investigations, see Edward John Waring, *Bibliotheca Therapeutica, or Bibliography of Therapeutics,* Volume 2 (London: The New Sydenham Society, 1879), pp. 485-486.

78. E.N. Gathercoal, *The Prescription Ingredient Survey: Consisting of The Ebert Survey of 1885, The Hallberg Survey of 1895, The Hallberg-Snow Survey of 1907, The Charters Survey of 1926, The Cook Survey of 1930, The Gathercoal Survey of 1930, The U.S.P.-N.F. Survey of 1931-32* (Washington, DC: American Pharmaceutical Association, 1933), p. 94. Other research confirms that there was little therapeutic change in the use of calomel. Comparative analysis of 958 prescriptions of a Burlington, New Jersey, apothecary written in 1854 with 800 prescriptions of Kentucky physicians written in 1887 shows that opium/morphine and mercury remained the remedies of choice. See David L. Cowen and Donald F. Kent, "Medical and Pharmaceutical Practice in 1854," *Pharmacy in History* 39 (1997): 91-100.

79. Alfred Stillé, *Therapeutics and Materia Medica,* Volume 1, Fourth Edition (Philadelphia: H.C. Lea, 1874), p. 31.

80. Stillé had been in close association with two of Louis's students, Gerhard and Pennock, and had himself gone to study in Paris. See Bartlett, *Essay on Philosophy of Medical Science;* and Erwin H. Ackerknecht, "Elisha Bartlett and the Philosophy of the Paris Clinical School," *Bulletin of the History of Medicine* 24 (1950): 43-60.

81. Pharmacology in this country had its beginnings when John J. Abel (1857-1938) was appointed professor of pharmacology at the University of Michigan in 1890. In France, experimental pharmacology started with Magendie in 1809 (J.M.D. Olmsted, *Francois Magendie, Pioneer in Experimental Physiology and Scientific Medicine in XIX Century France* [New York: Schuman's, 1944], p. 44), who was sui generis, and his illustrious pupil Claude Bernard; in Germany, it was closely related to the growth of what Ackerknecht has called "laboratory

medicine." For a complete discussion of the development of pharmacology in the United States, see John Parascandola, *The Development of American Pharmacology: John J. Abel and the Shaping of a Discipline* (Baltimore, MD: Johns Hopkins University Press, 1992).

82. On the physiological action of calomel, see Louis Goodman and Alfred Gilman, *The Pharmacological Basis of Therapeutics: A Textbook of Pharmacology, Toxicology and Therapeutics for Physicians and Medical Students* (New York: MacMillan, 1941), p. 804.

83. Bartholow, *Annual Oration on Certainty in Therapeutics,* pp. 12-14.

84. Richard H. Shryock, "Empiricism versus Rationalism in American Medicine, 1650-1950," *Proceedings of the American Antiquarian Society* (April 1969): 99-150.

85. William H. Cook, "Leaving First Principles," *Physio-Medical Recorder,* 29 (1865): 69-75.

86. On the persistent use of calomel and antimony after the war, see Guenter B. Risse, "Calomel and the American Medical Sects During the Nineteenth Century," *Mayo Clinic Proceedings,* 48 (1973): 57-64; and John S. Haller Jr., "The Use and Abuse of Tartar Emetic in the 19th-Century Materia Medica," *Bulletin of the History of Medicine* 49 (1975): 235-257.

87. Alex Berman, "A Striving for Scientific Respectability: Some American Botanics and the Nineteenth-Century Plant Materia Medica," *Bulletin of the History of Medicine* 30 (1956): 7-29.

88. Both the eclectics and neo-Thomsonians lasted throughout the nineteenth and into the twentieth centuries.

Chapter 2

1. Thomas Jefferson, *The Life and Selected Writings of Thomas Jefferson,* edited, with an introduction, by Adrienne Koch and William Peden (New York: Modern Library, 1998), p. 259.

2. Jefferson, letter to Jean Baptiste Say, February 1, 1804, in *Life and Selected Writings,* p. 526.

3. Jefferson, *Life and Selected Writings,* p. 260.

4. This theme is discussed at length in the now-classic John William Ward, *Andrew Jackson: Symbol for an Age* (New York: Oxford University Press, 1955).

5. See Frederick Jackson Turner, "Significance of the Frontier in American History," reprinted in his *Frontier in American History* (Tuscon, AZ: University of Arizona Press, 1986), p. 37.

6. Ward, *Andrew Jackson,* pp. 73-74.

7. Jefferson, letter to Doctor Casper Wistar, June 21, 1807, in *Life and Selected Writings,* pp. 534-535.

8. On Jackson's cause of death, see Robert V. Remini, *The Life of Andrew Jackson,* Reprint Edition (New York: Penguin Books, 1990), pp. 358-359. Suffering from a hemorrhagic cough and chills and fever, Jackson said, "[between] the lancet to correct the first, and calomel to check the second, I am greatly debilitated" (quoted in Remini, p. 352).

9. Worthington Hooker, *Physician and Patient; or, A Practical View of the Mutual Duties, Relations, and Interests of the Medical Profession and the Community* (New York: Baker and Scribner, 1849), p. 112. Note: Thomson's name was frequently misspelled by writers, usually adding a *p* after the *m*.

10. *American Journal of Pharmacy* 26 (1854): 570.

11. Oliver Wendell Holmes, *The Position and Prospects of the Medical Student.* An address delivered before the Boylston Medical Society of Harvard University, January 12, 1844; cited by Elisha Bartlett in *An Essay on the Philosophy of Medical Science* (Philadelphia: Lea and Blanchard, 1844), p. 114.

12. "Thompsonianism [sic] . . . like certain forms of religion—Mormonism, Millerism—finds the greatest number of adherents amongst the least educated portions of the people," observed Bartlett, "while homeopathy, on the other hand, is received with especial unction and favor by the more intelligent and better educated classes; and particularly by persons the tendencies of whose minds are toward ultra and abstract principles in politics and morals, and rational mysticism in religion. A non-resistant, transcendentalist, and Grahamite makes the most devoted disciple, and the staunchest advocates of homeopathy" (Bartlett, *Essay on Medical Science,* pp. 244-245).

Homeopathy, according to Hooker, won converts "among the refined, the learned, and the wealthy for the most part" while Thomsonianism depended for support on "the uneducated and the poor, or those who are in moderate circumstances" (Worthington Hooker, *Lessons from the History of Medical Delusions* [New York: Baker and Scribner, 1850], p. 79).

13. Introduced into New York in 1825 by Hans B. Gram, who became converted in Copenhagen, homeopathy soon acquired increased acceptance through the activities of Charles Hering and his associates in Pennsylvania. A sizeable influx of homeopathic physicians began in the Midwest in the late 1830s and assumed large proportions after 1840; see Madge E. Pickard and R. Carlyle Buley, *The Midwest Pioneer: His Ills, Cures and Doctors* (H. Schuman, 1946), pp. 208ff.; and Martin Kaufman, *Homeopathy in America: The Rise and Fall of a Medical Heresy* (Baltimore, MD: Johns Hopkins University Press, 1971).

14. Daniel Drake, "The People's Doctors," *The Western Journal of the Medical and Physical Sciences* 3 (1829): 407.

15. Contrasting the fees of the Thomsonian with the homeopathic physician, Hooker stated, "While the Thompsonian [sic] is satisfied with a small compensation for his liberal dosing, the infinitesimal doses of the Homeopathist are generally paid with fees very Allopathic, sometimes fairly 'heroic'" (Hooker, *Lessons,* p. 79).

16. Cited in *The Boston Thomsonian Medical Journal* 1 (1845): 69.

17. Elias Smith, *The Life, Conversion, Preaching, Travels and Sufferings of Elias Smith* (Boston: np, 1840), p. 362. Originally issued: Portsmouth, NH: Beck and Foster, 1816.

18. This religious journal was published under the editorship of Wooster Beach in the 1820s.

19. *The Telescope* 2.1 (June 4, 1825): 4.

20. Frightened by this episode, Alva Curtis, who had at one time evinced abolitionist sentiments himself, denounced the Thomsonian participants of the uprising. In a statement published in the *The Thomsonian Recorder* 3 (1835): 352, he wrote, "from what we have now learned, we greatly fear a number of botanic practitioners of Mississippi, have been led by blind fatuity to embark with other misguided citizens in a scheme of folly and madness, that has not only called down the vengeance of an exasperated community upon their heads, but will justly cover their names and memories with execrations and infamy." In a personal communication to Alex Berman, Professor David L. Cowen of Rutgers University indicated that the incident is described in Clement Eaton's *Freedom of Thought in the Old South* (Durham, NC: Duke University Press, 1940), p. 97.

21. Harvey Wickes Felter, *History of the Eclectic Medical Institute, Cincinnati, Ohio, 1845-1902* (Cincinnati, OH: Alumnal Association, 1902), p. 86; see also Michael A. Flannery, "Thomas Vaughan Morrow, 1804-1850: The Apostle of Eclecticism," *Transactions of the Kentucky Academy of Science* 57 (1997): 113-119.

22. See *Utah Historical Bulletin* 10.4 (1942). This reference source was called to Berman's attention by Professor G.E. Osborne of the University of Utah College of Pharmacy.

23. Cited in *The Boston True Thomsonian* 2 (1842): 27.

24. Curtis formally rejected Thomson's leadership in 1838, subsequently becoming the chief organizer of the neo-Thomsonian trend.

25. Alva Curtis, *Discussions Between Several Members of the Regular Medical Faculty and the Thomsonian Botanic Physicians on the Comparative Merits of Their Respective Systems* (Columbus, OH: A. Curtis, 1836), pp. 226-227.

26. Curtis, *Discussions,* p. 267.

27. Cited by the *Physio-Medical Recorder* 30 (1860): 134-135.

28. Daniel Drake, *Practical Essays on Medical Education and the Medical Profession in the United States* (1832), with an introduction by David A. Tucker Jr. (Baltimore, MD: The Johns Hopkins Press, 1952).

29. Ibid., pp. 12-13.

30. Henry Burnell Shafer, *The American Medical Profession (1783-1850)* (New York: Columbia University Press, 1936).

31. Ibid., pp. 35-36.

32. William Frederick Norwood, *Medical Education in the United States Before the Civil War* (Philadelphia: University of Pennsylvania Press, 1944), p. 379.

33. William G. Rothstein, *American Physicians in the Nineteenth Century: From Sects to Science* (Baltimore, MD: Johns Hopkins University Press, 1972), p. 227.

34. The medical activity and resources in Paris in the year 1830 were impressive. No fewer than thirty hospitals cared for the needs of 20,000 patients and offered instruction to 5,000 medical students residing in the city at that time. Of the larger hospitals in Paris, the Hôtel-Dieu alone possessed 1,000 beds. See Richard H. Shryock *The Development of Modern Medicine* (Philadelphia: University of Pennsylvania Press, 1936), pp. 150-51; Erwin Ackerknecht, *Medicine at the Paris Hospital, 1794-1848* (Baltimore, MD: The Johns Hopkins Press, 1967).

35. Richard H. Shryock, *American Medical Research, Past and Present* (New York: Columbia University Press, 1947), p. 30.

36. Shafer, *American Medical Profession,* p. 36.

37. P.J. Buckner, "Address," in *Constitution, By-Laws and Proceedings of the Medical Association of Adams, Brown, and Clermont Counties, Ohio* (May 1847), pp. 9-10.

38. Ibid., p. 10.

39. Charles Warren, "Medical Education in the United States," in *Annual Report of the Commissioner of Education Made to the Secretary of the Interior for the Year 1870* (Washington, DC: Government Printing Office, 1870), p. 384.

40. Ibid., p. 385.

41. Ibid.

42. Medical Historical Research Project of the Works Projects Administration, *Medicine and Its Development in Kentucky* (Louisville, KY: Standard Printing, 1940), p. 215.

43. Warren, "Medical Education," p. 385.

44. Ibid.

45. Ibid., pp. 385-386.

46. Ibid., p. 386.

47. Ibid.

48. Ibid.

49. N.S. Davis, *Contributions to the History of Medical Education and Medical Institutions in the United States of America, 1776-1876. Special Report Prepared for the United States Bureau of Education* (Washington, DC: Government Printing Office, 1877), p. 45.

50. Ibid.

51. Ibid., p. 46.

52. In Otto Juettner, *Daniel Drake and His Followers* (Cincinnati, OH: Harvey Publishing Company, 1909), pp. 192-193.

53. Pickard and Buley, *Midwest Pioneer,* pp. 123-124. The authors, in describing a fracas that occurred in 1844 at the Transylvania Medical School, during which such choice epithets as "snarling emissaries of a bastard aristocracy" and "gross impudent upstart" were employed, state that similar spectacles were not unusual at other medical schools of the period.

54. Felter, *History of the Eclectic Medical Institute,* pp. 41-42.

55. Ibid., p. 42.

56. Linden F. Edwards, "Resurrection Riots During the Heroic Age of Anatomy in America," *Bulletin of the History of Medicine* 25 (1951): 178-184.

57. Pickard and Buley, *Midwest Pioneer,* p. 250.

58. This is shown in Edwards, "Resurrection Riots," pp. 180-184.

59. Richard H. Shryock, "Public Relations of the Medical Profession in Great Britain and the United States: 1600-1870," *Annals of Medical History,* New Series, 2 (1930): 319. Shryock cites numerous examples in the public press in which the medical profession was attacked on the grounds of quackery, low standards, therapeutic incompetence, and for its alleged monopolistic designs.

60. Worthington Hooker, *Dissertation on the Respect Due to the Medical Profession and the Reasons That It Is Not Awarded by the Community* (Norwich: J.G. Cooley, 1844), p. 8.

61. Ibid., pp. 8-9.

62. Ibid., p. 22.

63. Cedric Larson, "Patent-Medicine Advertising and the Early American Press," *Journalism Quarterly* 14 (1937): 333-341.

64. Hooker, *Lessons*, p. 72.

65. Larson, "Patent-Medicine Advertising," p. 338. The author writes, "The Indian was a useful creature to the copy-writer of medicinal advertisements, for his savage and untamed figure was a synonym for virility and health and a certain nobility of nature in the popular mind. Indian specifics . . . had their merits flaunted before newspaper readers from the Atlantic to the Mississippi."

How economically important the sale of these nostrums was for the pharmacists of this period is graphically illustrated in the decision of the American Pharmaceutical Association, in 1855, to delete as unrealistic the original statement in its Code of Ethics that condemned the vending of such nostrums. See Glenn Sonnedecker, *Kremers and Urdang's History of Pharmacy*, Fourth Edition, Revised and reprinted (Madison, WI: American Institute of the History of Pharmacy, 1986), pp. 200-201.

66. For treatments of the popular nineteenth-century domestic health guides and their promoters, see the essays collected in *Medicine Without Doctors: Home Health Care in American History*, edited by Guenter B. Risse, Ronald L. Numbers, and Judith Walzer Leavitt (New York: Science History Publications, 1977); and Lamar Riley Murphy, *Enter the Physician: The Transformation of Domestic Medicine, 1760-1860* (Tuscaloosa, AL: University of Alabama Press, 1991).

67. According to Pickard and Buley, this work "was topping the field in sales in the 1850's and after the Civil War; with active agents all over the West it reached its two hundred thirteenth 'edition' in 1885" (*Midwest Pioneer*, p. 93).

68. John C. Gunn, *Domestic Medicine, or, Poor Man's Friend in the Hours of Afflication, Pain and Sickness* (Xenia, OH: J.H. Purdy, 1838), title page.

69. Ibid., p. 133.

70. Ibid., p. 134.

71. Ibid., p. 135.

72. Ibid., p. 137.

73. Ibid., p. 247.

74. Philip D. Jordan, "The Eclectic of St. Clairsville," *Ohio State Archæological and Historical Quarterly* 56 (1947): 388.

75. Shryock, in his article on the public relations of the medical profession during this period, writes, " 'The Present Position of the Medical Profession' was a common theme in medical literature. After some years of professional soul-searching, it reappeared under such pessimistic captions as: 'To What Causes Are We to Attribute the Diminishing Respectability of the Medical Profession in the Estimation of the American Public?' " ("Public Relations," p. 324).

76. *Boston Medical and Surgical Journal* 49 (1854): 96-97.

77. Buckner, "Address," p. 6.

78. Benjamin Rush, "Observations on the Duties of a Physician and the Meth ods of Improving Medicine. Accommodated to the Present State of Society and Manners in the United Sates," in *Medical Inquiries and Observations*, Volume 1, Second Edition (Philadelphia: J. Conrad, 1805) 388 ff.

79. Ibid., p. 388.

80. Ibid., p. 390.

81. These observations are to be found in Hooker's following works: *Dissertation* (see note 60), *Lessons* (see note 12), and "The Present Mental Attitude and Tendencies of the Medical Profession," *The New Englander*, 10 (November 1852): 548-568.

82. Paul F. Eve, *The Present Position of the Medical Profession in Society*. An introductory lecture delivered in the Medical College of Georgia, November 5, 1849 (Augusta, GA: J. McCafferty, 1849), p. 11.

83. Louis G. Caldwell, "Early Legislation Regulating the Practice of Medicine," *Illinois Law Review* 18 (December 1923): 225 ff. Caldwell states that "modern medical practice acts date back only to 1873."

84. Cited by C.B. Coventry, "History of Medical Legislation in the State of New York," *New York Journal of Medicine* 4 (1845): 160.

Chapter 3

1. The concept of wonder as a catalyst to scientific inquiry is explored in Lorrain Daston and Katharine Park, *Wonders and the Order of Nature, 1150-1750* (New York: Zone Books, distributed by The MIT Press, 1998); on the New World, see especially pp. 146-149.

2. Translated in 1577 and reprinted as Nicholas Monardes, *Joyfull Newes Out of the Newe Founde Worlde*, translated by John Frampton, with an introduction by Stephen Gaselle, Volumes 1 and 2 (New York: Alfred A. Knopf, 1925).

3. See Arthur Aiton, "The Impact of the Flora and Fauna of the New World Upon the Old World During the Sixteenth Century," *Biologia* 2 (1950/1951): 121-125; and J. Worth Estes, "The European Reception of the First Drugs from the New World," *Pharmacy in History* 37 (1995): 3-23.

4. An interesting discussion of botanical medicine in colonial Massachusetts is given in George E. Gifford Jr., "Botanic Remedies in Colonial Massachusetts, 1620-1820," in *Medicine in Colonial Massachusetts, 1620-1820,* Volume 57 (Boston: The Colonial Society of Massachusetts, 1980), pp. 263-288. For a discussion of herbals and herbalists (including Culpeper), see J. Worth Estes, " 'To the Courteous and Well Willing Reader': Herbals and Their Audiences," *The Watermark* 18 (1995): 63-70; and Elanour Sinclair Rohde, *The Old English Herbals* (1922), Reprint Edition (New York: Dover Publications, 1971).

5. Gifford, "Botanic Remedies," p. 268. This idea of therapeutic specificity was eventually adapted to American conditions, where it persisted into the nineteenth century. See John Harley Warner, "From Specificity to Universalism in Medical Therapeutics: Transformation in the 19th-Century United States," in

Sickness and Health in America: Readings in the History of Medicine and Public Health, edited by Judith Walzer Leavitt and Ronald L. Numbers, Third Edition (Madison, WI: University of Wisconsin Press, 1997), pp. 87-101.

6.   David L. Cowen, "The Impact of the Materia Medica of the North American Indians on Professional Practice," in *Botanical Drugs of the Americas in the Old and New Worlds, Veröffentlichungen der Internationalen Gesellschaft für Geschichte der Pharmazie e. V.,* bd. 53 (Stuttgart, Germany: Wissenschaftliche Verlag. MBH, 1984), p. 55.

7.   On the contributions of each, see Gifford, "Botanic Remedies," pp. 271-282; and Christopher Hobbs, "The Medical Botany of John Bartram," *Pharmacy in History* 33 (1991): 181-189.

8.   " . . . not infrequently," wrote E.D. Merrill, "one finds runs of these magazines in botanical libraries, because trusting and not too well-informed librarians and even directors of botanical institutions have been beguiled into purchasing such sets from the titles." *American Philosophical Society Proceedings* 86 (1942): 80. As a typical example, one might cite the *Thomsonian Botanic Watchman* (Albany, NY, 1834-1835), which regularly featured on its masthead a picture of trees and flowers, accompanied by the caption "The Sun of Science Arising upon the Flora of North America." Some botanic practitioners, however, did try to produce a serious and scientific body of literature dealing with plant medicinals. Such an attempt was made by a number of prominent botanics, e.g., Elisha Smith, Wooster Beach, John Kost, Morris Mattson, Horton Howard, John Thomson, John King, and William H. Cook, whose work is the subject of this chapter.

9.   Benjamin Rush, "Observations on the Duties of a Physician and the Methods of Improving Medicine. Accommodated to the Present State of Society and Manners in the United States," in *Medical Inquiries and Observations,* Volume 1, Second Edition (Philadelphia: J. Conrad, 1805), pp. 406-407.

10.   George B. Wood, "Introductory Lecture to the Course of Materia Medica in the University of Pennsylvania Delivered Nov. 3, 1840," *American Journal of Pharmacy,* New Series, 6 (1841): 298-322. Wood listed the following indigenous plants as meriting special attention: (a) Astringents: different species of oak; roots of blackberry, dewberry, *Geranium maculatum, Heuchera americana* (alumroot); leaves of pipsissewa and *Uva ursi.* (b) Tonics: barks of different species of *Cornus* (dogwood). (c) Simple bitters: sabbatia, coptis, and xanthorriza. (d) Aromatics: angelica, calamus, sassafras, hedeoma (pennyroyal), marjoram, partridgeberry, *Laurus benzoin* (spicebush). (e) Stimulants: turpentine. (f) Narcotics: stramonium and dulcamara. (g) Antispasmodics: dracontium and cimifuga. (h) Emetics: lobelia. (i) Cathartics: *Cassia marilandica,* butternut, and podophyllum. (j) Expectorants: seneca *(Polygala senega).* (k) Anthelmintics: spigelia and chenopodium. (l) Miscellaneous: serpentaria, hops, wild cherry bark, boneset, slippery elm bark, sanguinaria.

11.   For excellent discussions of this Swedish botanist, see the collected essays in *Linnaeus: The Man and His Work,* edited by Tore Fränsmyr (Canton, MA: Science History Publications, 1994).

12.   An excellent history of American botany is available in James L. Reveal, *Gentle Conquest: The Botanical Discovery of North America with Illustra-*

tions from the Library of Congress (Washington, DC: Starwood Publishing, 1992).

13. Major Stephen H. Long's expedition was one of the first to be thus sponsored by the U.S. government in 1819-1820. Starting at Pittsburgh, Major Long's party journeyed to the Rocky Mountains. The physician-botanists of the expedition were Drs. W. Baldwin and E. James, and the party also included the naturalist Thomas Say. See Howard Ensign Evans, *The Natural History of the Long Expedition to the Rocky Mountains, 1819-1820* (New York: Oxford University Press, 1997).

14. See Andrew Denny Rodgers, *John Torrey: A Story of North American Botany* (Princeton, NJ: Princeton University Press, 1942), p. 38.

15. Glenn Sonnedecker, *Kremers and Urdang's History of Pharmacy,* Fourth Edition, Revised and reprinted (Madison, WI: American Institute of the History of Pharmacy, 1986), pp. 172-173.

16. Frederick Pursh, *Flora Americae Septentrionalis*, Second Edition (London: James Black and Son, 1816), p. v.

17. Manassah Cutler, "An Account of Some of the Vegetable Productions, Naturally Growing in this Part of America," *Memoirs American Academy of Arts and Sciences* I (1785): 396-493.

18. For an interesting account of Cutler's botanical and scientific activities, see Dirk J. Struik's *Yankee Science in the Making* (Boston: Little, Brown and Company, 1948), pp. 47-49.

19. Originally published in Philadelphia in two parts, it has since been reprinted. See Benjamin Smith Barton, *Collections for an Essay Towards a Materia Medica of the United States*, Bulletin of the Lloyd Library of Botany, Pharmacy and Materia Medica, no. 1 (1798-1804) (Cincinnati, OH: Lloyd Library, 1900).

20. Sonnedecker, *History of Pharmacy,* p. 173.

21. George B. Wood wrote, in 1840, "His book has been a storehouse of materials for subsequent authors, and will probably continue to be at the fountainhead of inquiry," in "Introductory Lecture," p. 308.

22. Ibid.

23. Rodgers, *John Torrey,* p. 41.

24. Pursh, *Flora Americae Septentrionalis,* p. ix.

25. For a detailed overview, see Ronald L. Stuckey, "Medical Botany in the Ohio Valley (1800-1850)," *Transactions & Studies of the College of Physicians of Philadelphia*, 45 (1978): 262-279; and Michael A. Flannery, "For 'a Voluptuous Glow of Health and Vigor': Medical Botany in Kentucky," *Journal of the Kentucky Academy of Science* 60 (1999): 33-48.

26. Many early medical botanists are discussed in the series of articles on nineteenth-century physicians by A.E. Waller in *Ohio Archæological & Historical Quarterly* 51-55 (1942-1946). For an interesting, but limited, discussion of some outstanding physician-botanists, see also Howard A. Kelly, *Some American Medical Botanists* (Troy, NY: Southworth, 1914); and also under individual biographies given in the *Dictionary of American Biography.*

27. See Alex Berman, "C. S. Rafinesque: A Challenge to the Historian of Pharmacy," *American Journal of Pharmaceutical Education,* 16 (1952): 409-418.

28. Reveal, *Gentle Conquest,* p. 121.

29. For a comprehensive and excellent paper dealing with this subject, see Martin I. Wilbert, "Some Early Botanical and Herb Gardens," *American Journal of Pharmacy* 80 (1908): 412-427.

30. Rodgers, *John Torrey,* p. 20. Unfortunately, Dr. Hosack's dream never came true. The garden was sold to New York State in 1811 and to Columbia University in 1814. The original garden was in the area of what is now Forty-eighth to Fifty-first Streets, from Fifth to Sixth Avenue (Avenue of the Americas). In 1929 this location was leased to John D. Rockefeller Jr., for three million dollars a year and now is the location of Rockefeller Center. See C. Stuart Gager, "Botanic Gardens of the World, Material for a History," *Brooklyn Botanic Garden Record,* 27 (1938): 387.

31. Wilbert, "Early Botanical and Herb Gardens," p. 424.

32. See Harvey Wickes Felter, *The Genesis of the American Materia Medica,* Bulletin of the Lloyd Library, no. 26 (Cincinnati, OH: Lloyd Library, 1927), p. 3. According to Wood, "plants resembling the simples with which they had been familiar received corresponding names and similar applications. Thus we have our Centaury, our Dittany, our Hellebore, our Pennyroyal, our Senna, our Wormseed, and numerous others so closely allied to the European plants by botanical affinities as to be entitled to the same generic designation" ("Introductory Lecture," p. 304).

33. Sonnedecker, *History of Pharmacy,* p. 153.

34. The vegetable materia medica of North American tribes was extensive. For a thorough compilation, see Daniel E. Moerman, *Native American Ethnobotany* (Portland, OR: Timber Press, 1998).

35. Benjamin Rush, "An Inquiry Into the Natural History of Medicine Among the Indians of North-America; And a Comparative View of their Diseases and Remedies with those of Civilized Nations" (Read before the American Philosophical Society, in Philadelphia, on February 4, 1774) in *Medical Inquiries and Observations,* Volume 1, Second Edition (Philadelphia: J. Conrad, 1805), pp. 28-29. Rush nevertheless very ably attacked the doctrine of plant teleology with respect to individual countries. Thus, he wrote, "We are taught to believe that every herb that grows in our woods is possessed of some medicinal virtue, and that Heaven would be lacking in benignity, if our country did not produce remedies for all the different diseases of its inhabitants. . . . I know not whether Heaven has provided every country with antidotes even to the *natural* diseases of its inhabitants. The intermitting fever is common in almost every corner of the globe; but a sovereign remedy for it has been discovered only in South-America" (p. 51).

36. Ibid., p. 52.

37. August C. Mahr, "Materia Medica and Therapy Among the North American Forest Indians," *Ohio Archæological & Historical Quarterly,* 60 (1951): 331-354, 334.

38. *History of Pharmacy,* p. 173. For an excellent collection of essays devoted to the nineteenth-century empirics, see *Medicine Without Doctors: Home Health Cure in American Medicine,* edited by Guenter B. Risse, Ronald L. Numbers, and Judith Walzer Leavitt (New York: Science History Publications, 1977).

39. Madge E. Pickard and R. Carlyle Buley, *The Midwest Pioneer: His Ills, Cures and Doctors* (New York: H. Schuman, 1946), pp. 89-90.

40. Philip D. Jordan, "The Eclectic of St. Clairsville," *Ohio Archæological & Historical Quarterly* 56 (1947): 388.

41. One Thomsonian, A.R. Porter, co-editor of *The Boston Thomsonian Medical Journal,* suddenly realizing that a scientific approach to the plant materia medica was desirable, informed his readers that "those who know nothing of botany may mistake a poisonous plant for an innocent one. . . . We have but little knowledge of the science of botany; we know but very few of the plants which grow in nature's extensive garden. We intend, however, to make ourself [sic] acquainted with more of them, and shall ere long go on a botanizing expedition, with as good a botanist as New England affords, and in a future number shall give our readers some of the results of our investigation" (*The Boston Thomsonian Medical Journal* 1 [1845]: 30).

42. Not to be confused with Elias Smith (1769-1846), the clergyman and early co-worker of Samuel Thomson. Only the barest facts are known about the life of Elisha Smith, who for a time functioned as the president of the New York Association of Botanic Physicians. Alexander Wilder mentions Smith's death as occurring a few months after the publication of his work in 1830; see his *History of Medicine* (Augusta, ME: Maine Farmer Publishing Company, 1904), p. 445.

43. The term *independent botanic* is used in this book to indicate highly individualistic practitioners who were not affiliated with Thomsonians or eclectic groups.

44. The full title of Elisha Smith's work is *The Botanic Physician: Being a Compendium of the Practice of Physic upon Botanical Principles; Containing All the Principal Branches Necessary to the Study of Medicine, as Anatomy; Physiology; Surgery; Causes, Symptoms and Cure of Diseases; Midwifery; Materia Medica; Pharmacy; Botany; &c. Together with a Great Variety of Useful Recipes* (New York: Murphy and Bingham, 1830).

45. Ibid., pp. iii-iv. It is interesting to note that three years later when Wooster Beach published the first edition of his influential *American Practice of Medicine* (see note 59), he quoted Smith's manifesto, without, however, having the common courtesy to mention Smith by name. Beach merely referred to Smith's declarations as "remarks of an author." See Wooster Beach, *The American Practice of Medicine,* Volume 1 (New York: Betts and Anstice, 1833), p. 9.

46. Smith, *The Botanic Physician,* p. v. The authorities referred to were two Englishmen: William Buchan, author of *Domestic Medicine; or, The Family Physician* (1769 and other editions), and Robert Thomas, whose *Treatise on Domestic Medicine* first appeared in this country in a revised edition by David Hosack, in 1822.

47. See Samuel Henry, *A New and Complete American Medical Family Herbal* (New York: Samuel Henry, 1814). Henry's work contained a description of some 160 indigenous plants, with crude black-and-white illustrations. Only the common names of plant medicinals were given. There was no attempt at botanical taxonomy, despite the fact that the author styled himself a "botanist." According to Henry, he was "one of the members of the late College of Physicians and Surgeons and of the Medical Society of the city and county of New-York." The work, in the author's words, was "the result of more than thirty years . . . practice" and "while a prisoner, towards the close of the last war [War of 1812] among the Creek Indians: and his travels through the Southern States, whilst making botanic discoveries on the real medicinal virtues of our indigenous plants, wherein he has made known all his new discoveries . . . in the cure of most diseases incident to the human body. Adapted for the benefit of Masters and Mistresses of families, and for the community at large, of our United, Free, and Independent States of America."

48. Smith, *The Botanic Physician*, p. v.

49. See the introduction to the first volume of C.S. Rafinesque's *Medical Flora, or, Manual of the Medical Botany of the United States of North America* (Philadelphia: Atkinson and Alexander, 1828).

50. "Bleeding may be useful in some cases," wrote Smith in *The Botanic Physician,* "but the extent to which it is generally carried appears to me to be an extravagant waste of the fountain of life" (p. vii). In his treatment of mental disease, however, Smith abandoned all restraint: "bleeding would be often repeated, for no persons can bear the loss of blood so well as maniacs, nor is there any case in which it is so necessary to draw it off, and so many times" (Ibid., p. 194).

51. See, for example, Smith's treatment of "inflammation of the liver," in *The Botanic Physician*, p. 219.

52. Ibid., pp. 84-149.

53. The full title of Horton Howard's book is *An Improved System of Botanic Medicine Founded Upon Correct Physiological Principles; Embracing a Concise View of Anatomy and Physiology; Together with an Illustration of the New Theory of Medicine. To Which Is Added a Treatise on Female Complaints, Midwifery, and the Diseases of Children,* Volumes 1 and 2 (Columbus, OH: Author, 1832).

54. For a detailed discussion of the Howard-Thomson controversy see John S. Haller Jr., *The People's Doctors: Samuel Thomson and the American Botanical Movement, 1790-1860* (Carbondale, IL: Southern Illinois University Press, 2000), pp. 67-73.

55. Howard, *An Improved System of Botanic Medicine,* Volume 2, p. 281.

56. Ibid., Volume 1, Preface.

57. Published twice a month, *The Eclectic, and Medical Botanist; Devoted Principally to Improvements in the Botanic Practice of Medicine* (Columbus, OH 1832-1834?), was one of the many ephemeral journals of the botanic movement and the organ of the abortive "Improved Botanic" faction (a thorough listing of such journals is given in Haller, *The People's Doctors,* Appendix "United States: Botanic Medical Journals from 1823-1860"). The term *eclectic* in the title of the

periodical antedates by a number of years the similar appellation taken on by the "Beachites."

58. Howard, *An Improved System of Botanic Medicine*, Volume 1, p. 56.

59. Wooster Beach, *The American Practice of Medicine; Being a Treatise on the Character, Causes, Symptoms, Morbid Appearances and Treatment of the Diseases of Men, Women, and Children of all Climates on Vegetable or Botanical Principles: As Taught at the Reformed Medical Colleges in the United States: Containing also a Treatise on Materia Medica and Pharmacy, or the Various Articles Prescribed, Their Description, History, Properties, Preparation, and Uses; with an Appendix on the Cholera, etc.*, Volumes 1, 2, and 3 (New York: Betts and Anstice, 1833).

60. Later this three-volume treatise was condensed and published as *The Family Physician*, which sold well and was published in many editions.

61. According to Beach, "Many of the plants have been drawn from nature, and a number from the excellent work of Professor Rafinesque, called the *Medical Flora*. Others have been reduced from Barton, Bigelow, &c. The foreign ones have been principally taken from the *British Flora*, and Thornton's *Family Herbal*" (*The American Practice of Medicine*, Volume 1, p. 19).

62. As was not uncommon for publishers of the period, many so-called "editions" were actually reprintings.

63. Wooster Beach, *The American Practice Condensed, or The Family Physician*, Fifty-sixth Edition (Cincinnati, OH: Moore, Wilstach, and Moore, 1879), p. 769 ff.

64. Morris Mattson, *The American Vegetable Practice of a New and Improved Guide to Health Designed For the Use of Families. In Six Parts. Part I. Concise View of the Human Body with Engraved and Wood-Cut Illustrations. Part II. Glance at the Old School Practice of Physic. Part III. Vegetable Materia Medica with Colored Illustrations. Part IV. Compounds. Part V. Practice of Medicine, Based upon What Are Deemed Correct Physiological and Pathological Principles. Part VI. Guide for Women, Containing a Simplified Treatise on Childbirth, with a Description of the Diseases Peculiar to Females and Infants.* (Boston: D.L. Hale, 1841). A second 1845 "edition" of this work was issued from the Bostonian press of William Johnson.

65. Published under the name of Samuel Thomson, the book was actually written by his son, John Thomson. The two "editions" (Twelfth and Thirteenth), printed in Albany in 1841, were identical, except for a portrait of Thomson and colored illustrations.

66. Mattson, *The American Vegetable Practice*, p. xi.

67. *The Botanic Medical Reformer and Home Physician* 2 (1842): 211.

68. Samuel Thomson, *The Thomsonian Materia Medica, or Botanic Family Physician*, Twelfth and Thirteenth Editions (Albany, NY: J. Munsell, 1841), pp. 654-655.

69. Ibid., Thirteenth Edition, p. 831.

70. William Procter Jr., *American Journal of Pharmacy* 30 (1858): 186-189.

71. William Procter Jr., "Eclectic Pharmacy," *American Journal of Pharmacy* 26 (1854): 569-575; an "Eclectic Pharmacy," *American Journal of Pharmacy* 31 (1859): 285-287, 384-391.

72. Procter's critique is also discussed in Gregory J. Higby, *In Service to American Pharmacy: The Professional Life of William Procter, Jr.* (Tuscaloosa, AL: University of Alabama Press, 1992), pp. 7-8.

73. In 1859, Kost's treatise was actually approved for study at the Eclectic Medical Institute in Cincinnati; see Harvey Wickes Felter, *History of the Eclectic Medical Institute* (Cincinnati, OH: Alumnal Association, 1902), p. 46.

74. Procter correctly pointed out that Kost "is evidently a disciple of Thompson [sic] when he treats of lobelia and capsicum, and in his repudiation of the very word narcotic; yet unlike that noted individual, he is a strong advocate for cathartics and anodynes" (*American Journal of Pharmacy* 30, p. 187). This was an approach taken by many neo-Thomsonians.

75. Ibid.

76. Ibid.

77. Ibid., p. 189.

78. Ibid. It is interesting to note that Procter's "inaugural essay" was on *Lobelia inflata* ("Lobelia Inflata [An Inaugural Essay]," *American Journal of Pharmacy* 9 [1837]: 98-108). Five years later, Procter published an outstanding article on the pharmaceutical preparations of lobelia (*American Journal of Pharmacy* 14 [1842]: 108).

79. Procter, *American Journal of Pharmacy* 30, p. 189.

80. Ibid.

81. Procter, "Eclectic Pharmacy," *American Journal of Pharmacy* 26, p. 569.

82. Ibid., p. 570.

83. Ibid., p. 573.

84. Ibid.

85. Procter, "Eclectic Pharmacy," *American Journal of Pharmacy* 31, p. 385.

86. Ibid., p. 386. It is interesting to note that of the thirty-four plants listed by Procter as being especially relied upon by the eclectics, by the 1860 decennial edition of the USP, twenty had past or present pharmacopoeial status; compare with the listing in Wade Boyle, *Official Herbs: Botanical Substances in the United States Pharmacopoeias, 1820-1990* (East Palestine, OH: Buckeye Naturopathic Press, 1991), pp. 14-51.

87. John Uri Lloyd, *A Treatise on the American Alkaloids, Resins, Oleo-Resins and Concentrated Principles (so-called Eclectic Concentrations),* Drug Treatise No. XXIV (Cincinnati, OH: Lloyd Brothers, 1909), p. 15.

88. Fortunately, this work has been made readily available through a high-quality and complete reprinting of the 1869 edition; see William Cook, *The Physio-Medical Dispensatory: A Treatise on Therapeutics, Materia Medica, and Pharmacy* (Cincinnati, OH: William. H. Cook, 1869/Sandy, OR: Eclectic Medical Publications, 1998).

89. This is not surprising, since Lloyd owned an original copy that is still available at the Lloyd Library and Museum, 917 Plum Street, Cincinnati, Ohio

(call number RM121.C66). See the *Western Druggist* 21 (1899): 19-20. Lloyd merely stated that "this work is authority with the followers of Samuel Thomson, and is a very interesting publication. This school of medicine (physio-medical) excludes poison from its materia medica, and has many advocates in the middle west."

90.   Cook, *The Physio-Medical Dispensatory,* p. 4.

91.   Ibid.

92.   Ibid., p. 8.

93.   Ibid., pp. 253-254. Interestingly, Cook pays considerable attention to *Apocynum androsaemifolium* for its action "upon the gall-ducts, gall-cyst, and tubuli of the liver" and calls it "one of the powerful and reliable articles of a harmless materia medica" (Ibid., pp. 253-254). Cook's faith notwithstanding, the action of this plant is not so innocuous. Today *A. androsaemifolium* is known to contain cardioactive glycosides similar to those of digitalis and has been used occasionally in the treatment of congestive heart failure (see Varro E. Tyler, *Herbs of Choice: The Therapeutic Use of Phytomedicinals* ([Binghamton, NY: Pharmaceutical Products Press, 1994], pp. 101-102). Because of its powerful action on the heart, *A. androsaemifolium* is considered a class 3 herb for safety—"To be used only under the supervision of an expert qualified in the appropriate use of this substance" (see *American Herbal Products Association's Botanical Safety Handbook* [Boca Raton, FL: CRC Press, 1997], p. 12). One can only speculate upon the "bedside observations" obtained at the "expert" hands of the physio-medicals looking for an entirely different set of actions from the plant.

94.   Cook, *The Physio-Medical Dispensatory,* p. 346.

95.   It should be pointed out, in passing, that a number of plant drugs employed exclusively in botanic practice eventually entered the official pharmaceutical compendia (the *United States Pharmacopeia* and, later, the *National Formulary*).

96.   See Berman, "C. S. Rafinesque," pp. 409-418; and Michael A. Flannery, "The Medicine and Medicinal Plants of C. S. Rafinesque," *Economic Botany* 52 (1998): 27-43.

97.   Francis R. Packard, *History of Medicine in the United States,* Volume 2 (New York: P.B. Hoeber, 1931), p. 1229.

98.   See *The Botanico-Medical Recorder* 6 (1837-1838). Numerous references are interspersed throughout the volume regarding Rafinesque and the *Medical Flora.*

99.   Thomas Cooke announced the purchase of these plates in the *Botanic Medical Reformer* 1 (1841): 105. He purchased them on December 19, 1840.

100.   Wilder, *History of Medicine,* pp. 421-422.

101.   R. Egelsfeld Griffith, "On Fraseri Walteri," *Journal of the Philadelphia College of Pharmacy* 3 (1832): 269-273. Griffith wrote, "In the *Medical Flora* of Mr. Rafinesque, a work we are induced to quote, from its containing much valuable information on our native plants; though unfortunately so mingled with wild hypotheses and unsubstantiated assertions, as to render it an unsafe guide" (pp. 272-273).

102.   Asahel Clapp, *A Synopsis or Systematic Catalogue of the Medicinal Plants of the United States* (Philadelphia: P.G. Collins, 1852), p. 8. Clapp referred to Rafinesque as "an ingenious but injudicious botanist (who created many new species out of the slightest variation of plants, which have not received the sanction of other botanists) [who] was not a physician, and is not entitled much confidence in regard to the properties of plants, when unsupported by other authorities; yet, as his account of them in his *Medical Flora* was mostly compiled from preceding writers—mostly from Schoepf, Thacher, Bigelow, Ives, and the two Bartons—it is therefore worthy of more credit than it could otherwise claim" (p. 8).

103.   Otto Juettner, *Daniel Drake and His Followers* (Cincinnati, OH: Harvey Publishing Company, 1909), pp. 110-111.

104.   See David L. Cowen and William H. Helfand, *Pharmacy: An Illustrated History* (New York: Harry N. Abrams, 1990), p. 135.

105.   *Eclectic Medical Journal* 55 (1895): 50.

106.   Alexander Wilder, "The Earlier Period of Eclectic Medicine," *Eclectic Medical Journal* 61 (1901): 68.

107.   See, for example, Wooster Beach, *The American Practice Condensed,* Twelfth Edition, p. xi.

108.   Quoted in an editorial by H.T. Webster, *California Medical Journal* 19 (1898): 284. A blow-by-blow citation of the editorial comments of this controversy can be found in the following: John King Scudder, "Rafinesque, the Eclectic," *Eclectic Medical Journal* 58 (1898): 669; William E. Bloyer, *Eclectic Medical Gleaner* 3 (1898): 378; H.T. Webster, *California Medical Journal* 19 (1899): 334-345; and H.T. Webster, "B. and His Tribulations," *California Medical Journal* 19 (1898): 345-346.

109.   Rafinesque, in his classification of physicians given in the introduction to the *Medical Flora,* defined eclectic practitioners as "those who select and adopt in practice, whatever is found most beneficial, and who change their prescriptions according to emergencies, circumstances and acquired knowledge" (see his *Medical Flora,* Volume 1 [Philadelphia: Samuel C. Atkinson, 1828] p. iv). There is no evidence that this designation was intended to apply to the followers of Wooster Beach. Later eclectic physicians simply appropriated this characterization and name as applying to their mode of practice.

110.   This is an extremely scarce tract; see Constantine S. Rafinesque, *The Pulmist; or, Introduction to the Art of Curing and Preventing the Consumption or Chronic Phthisis* (Philadelphia: Author, 1829).

111.   Ibid., p. 67.

112.   Mabel Clare Weaks, "Medical Consultation on the Case of Daniel Vanslyke. By C. S. Rafinesque, Pulmist, &c. Philadelphia 10th Septr. 1830," *Bulletin of the History of Medicine* 18 (1945): 425-437.

113.   Daniel Drake, "The People's Doctors," *The Western Journal of Medicine and Physical Sciences* 3 (1829): 395.

114.   See Ronald L. Stuckey and James S. Pringle, "Common Names of Vascular Plants Reported by C. S. Rafinesque in an 1819 Descriptive Outline of Four Vegetation Regions of Kentucky," *Transactions of the Kentucky Academy of Sci-*

ence 58 (1997): 9-19; and Ronald L. Stuckey, "Rafinesque's Botanical Pursuits in the Ohio Valley (1818-1826)," *Journal of the Kentucky Academy of Science* 59 (1998): 111-157.

115. Stuckey, "Rafinesque's Botanical Pursuits," pp. 147-148.

116. Flannery, "Medicinal Plants of C. S. Rafinesque," pp. 41-42.

117. John S. Haller Jr., *Kindly Medicine: Physio-Medicalism in America, 1836-1911* (Kent, OH: Kent State University Press, 1997), pp. 29-35.

118. See, for example, John Uri Lloyd, "To What Do Our Medicinal Plants Owe Their Value?" *Eclectic Medical Journal* 34 (1874): 551-553; and Lloyd's nine serialized articles under the title "Pharmaceutical Chemistry," appearing over a nineteen-month period, in the *Eclectic Medical Journal* 35 and 36 (1875-1876).

119. Sonnedecker, *History of Pharmacy*, p. 175.

120. *Eclectic Medical Journal* 58 (1898): 686-687.

121. Samuel Robinson, *A Course of Fifteen Lectures on Medical Botany* (Columbus, OH: H. Howard, 1829), pp. 18-19.

Chapter 4

1. Several organized groups of botanic physicians unaffiliated with the Thomsonians and eclectics are known to have sprung up locally before 1840, the most important of which were the New York Association of Botanic Physicians, localized in western New York, and the Pennsylvania Associate Medical Society of Botanic Physicians, active in Philadelphia and its environs.

2. The authors wrote that: "the period of the 1840's and 50's was one of flux and transition. It is impossible to keep track of the schisms, mergings, and crossings-over. Thomsonians not only became Eclectics, Physiomedicals, and Botanics; some joined the regulars. . . . Others went over to the water-cure system, and a number took up homeopathy" (see Madge E. Pickard and R. Carlyle Buley, *The Midwest Pioneer: His Ills, Cures and Doctors* [New York: H. Schuman, 1946], p. 198).

3. See, for example, Peter Smith's *The Indian Doctor's Dispensatory, Being Father Smith's Advice Respecting Diseases and Their Cure*, The Bulletin of the Lloyd Library, no. 2 (1813) (reprinted, Cincinnati, OH: Lloyd Library, 1901); S.H. Selman, *The Indian Guide to Health; or a Valuable Vegetable Medical Prescription for the Cure of All Disorders Incident to this Climate* (Columbus, IN: James M'Call, 1836); Robert D. Foster, *The North American Indian Doctor, or Nature's Method of Curing and Preventing Disease According to the Indians* (Canton, OH: Smith and Berin, 1838); William Daily, *The Indian Doctor's Practice of Medicine; or Daily's Family Physician* (Louisville, KY: Hull, 1848); and James Cooper, *The Indian Doctor's Receipt Book* (Uniontown, OH: np, 1855).

4. Samuel Thomson, *New Guide to Health; or, Botanic Family Physician, to which is Prefixed the Life and Medical Discoveries of the Author* (Boston: J.Q. Adams, 1835), pp. 19, 23, 25.

5. Beach wrote, "I have spared neither pains nor expense to acquire a knowledge of the most noted botanical physicians, retaining from each everything

which I have proved by experience to be useful. I have not thought it beneath me to converse with Root and Indian Doctors" (Wooster Beach, *The American Practice of Medicine*, Volume 1 [New York: Betts and Anstice, 1833], p. 7).

6.   Thomson, *New Guide to Health*, p. 40 ff.

7.   The Baltimore Platform was an important statement of principles that the neo-Thomsonians hoped would clearly spell out their basic medical tenets and weld their practitioners into a cohesive group. In brief, this manifesto reiterated their belief in the unity of disease as against the concept of diversity of disease entertained by the regulars; the nonpathological and beneficial character of inflammation, fever, and suppuration, as opposed to the pathological nature of these conditions taught by orthodox physicians; and, finally, the rejection of "poisons," as defined in the third paragraph from the end in Appendix 2. The implications of this significant document are discussed fully in Chapter 5.

8.   No records could be found to indicate whether the American Association of Physio-Medical Physicians and Surgeons was active after 1907. Its journal, the *Physio-Medical Recorder*, appears to have ceased publication in 1907. No other physio-medical periodicals are listed after this date in the *Union List of Serials*, or in the *Index-Catalogue of the Library of the Surgeon General's Office*. The last physio-medical medical school, The College of Medicine and Surgery, was absorbed by the eclectic Chicago College of Medicine and Surgery in 1911. For details, see John S. Haller Jr., *Kindly Medicine: Physio-Medicalism in America, 1836-1911* (Kent, OH: Kent State University Press, 1997), pp. 139-147.

9.   See A.I. Coffin, *Botanic Guide to Health and the Natural Pathology of Disease* (Manchester, England: William Irwin, 1846); and R. Swinburne Clymer, *The Thomsonian System of Medicine* (Allentown, PA: The Philosophical Publishing Company, 1905).

10.   Frederick C. Waite makes the following undocumented assertion: "In 1826 a group of the followers of botanicism in New York became tired of the personal domination of Samuel Thomson and his sons. Under the leadership of Wooster Beach (1794-1868), a native of Connecticut, they seceded and organized under the caption of the Reformed Medical Society" (*New England Journal of Medicine*, 207 [1932]: 984 ff).

11.   The designation "Reform" was used at different times by other botanics, e.g., the independent and neo-Thomsonian groups. It was also not uncommon for other sectarian physicians, viz., hydropaths or homeopaths, to be referred to as "Reform Physicians."

12.   For example, they differed in the employment of many mineral preparations, and such substances as opium, belladonna, cantharides, and digitalis, which were proscribed by the Thomsonians, and in the adoption of many elements inherent in the practice of the regulars. The pronouncement, published by the early followers of Beach, that their system "originated even before Thomson was known; and during its progress it was gradually improved and developed, without the least reference to his system, and for the most part, without even the knowledge that such a system as the Thompsonian [sic], or such a being as Samuel Thomson, was

in existence," was clearly false and propagandistic (see the *Western Medical Reformer* 1 [1836]: 5).

13. John S. Haller Jr., *Medical Protestants: The Eclectics in American Medicine, 1825-1939* (Carbondale, IL: Southern Illinois University Press, 1994), p. 71.

14. C.S. Rafinesque, *Medical Flora, or, Manual of the Medical Botany of the United States of North America*, Volume 1 (Philadelphia: Atkinson and Alexander, 1828), p. iv.

15. For a thorough treatment of the Eclectic Medical Institute (after 1910, the Eclectic Medical College), see John S. Haller Jr., *A Profile in Alternative Medicine: The Eclectic Medical College of Cincinnati, 1845-1942* (Kent, OH: Kent State University Press, 1999).

16. Alexander Wilder, *History of Medicine* (Augusta, ME: Maine Farmer Publishing Company, 1904), pp. 444-445. Wilder points out that a small cluster of independent botanic societies sprang up in western New York to combat the state medical regulatory act of 1827 (Ibid., pp. 482-483).

17. Wilder credits Smith's son with founding this school (Ibid., p. 446), but Waite attributes the organization of the school ("Medical College, Botanic") to Elisha Smith himself (see Frederick C. Waite, "American Sectarian Medical Colleges Before the Civil War," *Bulletin of the History of Medicine* 19 [1946]: 152).

18. *The Botanic Medical Reformer and Home Physician* 2 (1842): 201-202.

19. *The Botanic Medical Reformer and Home Physician* 1 (1840): 1.

20. Ibid., pp. 2-3.

21. Ibid., p. 11.

22. Wilder, *History of Medicine*, p. 592.

23. There were numerous medical sects in the United States during the nineteenth century: homeopathy, eclecticism, Thomsonianism, various hygiene cults, hydropathy, electrotherapy, Christian science, osteopathy, and chiropractic to name but a few. For some insights into nineteenth-century sectarian medicine, see the essays collected in *Other Healers: Unorthodox Medicine in America*, edited by Norman Gevitz (Baltimore, MD: Johns Hopkins University Press, 1988); and William G. Rothstein, *American Physicians in the Nineteenth Century: From Sects to Science* (Baltimore, MD: Johns Hopkins University Press, 1972).

In 1836, *The Boston Medical and Surgical Journal* took cognizance of a charge that "Irregulars, Broussaisians, Sangradorians, Brandethians, Beechitarians, Botanics, Regular Botanics, Thomsonians, Reformed Thomsonians, Theoretical, Practical, Experimental, Dogmatical, Emblematical, Electrical, Magnetical, Diplomatical, Homeopathians, Rootists, Herbists, Florists, and Quacks" were rampant in New York. It admitted that "[t]here are troops of quacks, foreign pretenders of all grades, from pill makers to magicians" and that "they abound in Boston, also, and are quite as successful in their knaveries as in other cities," but added that "the citizens of New York may well be proud of the great amount of talent, learning and skill of the regular physicians" (see *The Boston Medical and Surgical Journal* 15 [1836]: 241-242).

24. John Thomson, "General Introduction," in Samuel Thomson, *The Thomsonian Materia Medica; or Botanic Family Physician,* Thirteenth Edition (Albany, NY: J. Munsell, 1841), p. 11.

25. Coffinism is discussed in detail in Barbara Griggs' *Green Pharmacy: The History and Evolution of Western Herbal Medicine,* Second Edition (Rochester, VT: Healing Arts Press, 1997), pp. 188-216.

26. Griggs, *Green Pharmacy,* p. 190.

27. Coffin, *Botanic Guide,* p. iii.

28. Ibid., p. xi.

29. Griggs, *Green Pharmacy,* p. 191.

30. Ibid., p. 193.

31. Thomson, *New Guide to Health,* p. 26.

32. Ibid., p. 40.

33. Ibid., p. 43. The resemblance of this theory of disease to Galen's humoral pathology has been discussed in Edward Kremers and George Urdang's *History of Pharmacy,* Second Edition (Philadelphia: J.B. Lippincott, 1951), p. 225; and, most recently, in Haller's *Medical Protestants,* p. 41.

34. Thomson, *New Guide to Health,* p. 44.

35. Reprinted in John Uri Lloyd, *Life and Medical Discoveries of Samuel Thomson and a History of the Thomsonian Materia Medica,* Bulletin of the Lloyd Library of Botany, Pharmacy and Materia Medica, no. 11 (Cincinnati, OH: Lloyd Library, 1909), pp. 76-77.

Another list of seventy plant drugs was published by *The Thomsonian Recorder* 2 (1834) as comprising the materia medica of Thomson. See Appendix 1.

36. Lloyd, *Life of Samuel Thomson,* p. 86.

37. Lyman F. Kebler, "United States Patents Granted for Medicines During the Pioneer Years of the Patent Office," *Journal of the American Pharmaceutical Association* 24 (1935): 485 ff.

38. Ibid., p. 485.

39. Ibid., p. 489.

40. Citizens of the young republic were undoubtedly familiar with a host of English proprietary medicines with names (both descriptive and fanciful) such as Hooper's Female Pills, Dalby's Carminative, Godfrey's Cordial, Bateman's Pectoral Drops, and Turlington's Balsam of Life. For a complete description, see George B. Griffenhagen and James Harvey Young, "Old English Patent Medicines in America," *Pharmacy in History* 34 (1992): 200-228.

41. Kelber, "Patents Granted for Medicines," pp. 487, 489. Kebler wrote, "a disastrous fire in 1836 destroyed the entire office [Patent Office]. . . fortunately Congress published Indexes from time to time, copies of which were filed elsewhere and saved. In these documents were preserved the titles of the patents issued" (p. 487). Prior to 1836, patents were issued unnumbered. On July 13, 1836, the first numbered patent was issued. New quarters were built to house the Patent Office. Congress made attempts to restore some of the old records. Kebler adds that "[t]he old patents actually restored are extremely fragmentary but they con-

tain practically all the available data on the subject excepting that found in the Patent Indexes referred to above" (p. 487).

42. Ibid., p. 489.

43. Thomson, *Narrative of the Life and Medical Discoveries of Samuel Thomson* (Columbus, OH: J. Pike, 1835), p. 166.

44. Ibid., p. 122.

45. Reproduced in Lucius H. Zeuch, *History of Medical Practice in Illinois*, Volume 1 (Chicago: Book Press, 1927), p. 122.

46. Issued to the purchasers of the seventh edition of Thomson's *New Guide to Health*.

47. John S. Haller Jr., *The People's Doctors: Samuel Thomson and the American Botanical Movement, 1790-1860* (Carbondale, IL: Southern Illinois University Press, 2000), p. 83.

48. *The Thomsonian Recorder* 2 (1833): 43; Wilder, *History of Medicine*, p. 493; *The Thomsonian Recorder* 3 (1834): 65 ff.

49. Wilder, *History of Medicine*, p. 494. For a savage attack against the seceding Curtis faction made by Morris Mattson, then editor of *The Boston Thomsonian Manual and Lady's Companion* (see Appendix 6). This outburst is the richest piece of nineteenth-century invective we have encountered in the polemical literature of the period.

50. Ibid., pp. 497-498.

51. Frederick C. Waite, "Thomsonianism in Ohio," *Ohio Archæological & Historical Quarterly* 49 (1940): 325.

52. Ibid.

53. *The Thomsonian Recorder* 4 (1836): 103.

54. Ibid., pp. 98-101.

55. Ibid., p. 117.

56. Ibid., p. 187.

57. Ibid., p. 238.

58. Ibid., p. 413.

59. *The Thomsonian Recorder* 5 (1837): 30.

60. *The Western Medical Reformer* 3 (1838), edited by the medical professors of Worthington College, Worthington, Ohio. The Worthington College, chartered in 1830, was the first sectarian medical school chartered in this country.

61. Haller, *The People's Doctors*, p. 188.

62. Ibid., p. 184.

63. *The Botanic Medical Reformer and Home Physician* 2 (1841): 2.

64. Ibid., p. 3.

65. *The Botanic Medical Reformer and Home Physician* 2 (1842): 7.

66. Benjamin Colby, *A Guide to Health*, Third Edition (Milford, NH: J. Burns, 1846), p. viii.

67. Cited by Wyndham B. Blanton, *Medicine in Virginia in the Nineteenth Century* (Richmond, VA: Garrett and Massie, 1933), p. 196.

68. After stating that the "friends of the Botanic system would do well to shun Apothecary and Drug stores, as they would a contaminated district where the

Plague raged in all its malignant force," the editor of *The Botanic Medical Reformer and Home Physician* announced, "We have been informed that a number of those retailers of poisons, in this city [Philadelphia], have made up spurious articles of our medicines, with a view to injure the fame of the system. We say again—beware the assassin" (*The Botanic Medical Reformer and Home Physician* 2 [1842]: 144).

69.   Elias Smith is principally remembered today as a controversial religious figure and editor of the first religious newspaper in the United States, *The Herald of Gospel Liberty* (1808). His vehement antifederalist diatribes, along with his polemical attacks against the conventional theological attitudes of the time, nearly resulted in his being lynched on several occasions. He was the author of many sermons, hymns, and other religious works. In 1816, Smith became a disciple of Thomson and assisted him in his business. Subsequently, however, the two men quarreled bitterly, with Smith incurring the lifelong enmity of his mentor, who proceeded to put Smith's name at the head of his published list of "mongrel" agents. This did not prevent the clergyman from carrying on a lucrative botanic practice in Boston, or from publishing several editions of his *American Physician and Family Assistant* (see *Dictionary of American Biography,* Volume 17, p. 259).

70.   Elias Smith, *The American Physician and Family Assistant,* Fourth Edition (Boston: B. True, 1837), p. xvii.

71.   Ibid., p. xvi.

72.   Ibid., p. xviii.

73.   Ibid., pp. 201-211.

74.   John Uri Lloyd, *Concerning Lobelia,* Bulletin of the Lloyd Library, no. 11 (Cincinnati, OH: Lloyd Library, 1909), p. 78.

75.   *New York Daily Tribune* 3, no. 300, March 25 (1844).

76.   Samuel B. Emmons, *The Vegetable Family Physician* (Boston: np, 1842), p. 178.

77.   *Report of the Trial of Dr. Samuel Thomson, the Founder of the Thomsonian Practice for an Alleged Libel in Warning the Public against the Impositions of Paine D. Badger, as a Thomsonian Physician Sailing Under False Colors . . . etc.* (Boston: np, 1839), p. 51.

78.   Ibid., pp. 3-4.

79.   Ibid., p. 12 ff.

80.   David L. Cowen, "America's First Pharmacy Laws," *Journal of the American Pharmaceutical Association* 3 (1942): 162-169, 214-221.

81.   Ibid., p. 168.

82.   It is known, however, that in 1837 the Georgia State Legislature voted to protect botanic practice (see Haller, *The People's Doctors,* p. 133). If enforced, the net effect of such legislation was not to eliminate botanic apothecaries but to restrict those in operation to those finding favor with the botanico-medical board of physicians of that state.

83.   See Thomson's *New Guide to Health,* pp. 42-48.

84.   Ibid., pp. 48-54.

85.   Ibid., p. 55.

86. Ibid., pp. 59-62.
87. Ibid., pp. 62-63.
88. Ibid., p. 63.
89. Ibid., p. 164.
90. Ibid., p. 88.
91. Ibid., p. 186.
92. See, for example, the work of botanist John Riddell in his *Synopsis of the Flora of the Western States* (Cincinnati, OH: E. Deming, 1834-1835); and Drs. George B. Wood and Franklin Bache's *Dispensatory of the United States of America,* Second Edition (Philadelphia: Grigg and Elliot, 1834).
93. William Procter Jr., "Lobelia Inflata (An Inaugural Essay)," *American Journal of Pharmacy* 9 (1837): 98-108.
94. John Uri Lloyd, "Lobelia," *Drugs and Medicines of North America* 2 (1887): 74.
95. William Procter Jr., "Remarks on Some Pharmaceutical Preparations of Lobelia," *American Journal of Pharmacy* 14 (1842): 108.
96. Ibid., pp. 108-109.
97. Lloyd, "Lobelia," pp. 73-74.
98. Edward Parrish, "An Inaugural Essay on Statice Caroliniana, with a Chemical Analysis of the Root of This Plant," *American Journal of Pharmacy* 14 (1842): 111.
99. Lawrence Turnbull, "On *Populus Tremuloides,*" *American Journal of Pharmacy* 14 (1842): 275.
100. "Report of the Massachusetts College of Pharmacy," *Proceedings of the American Pharmaceutical Association* 3 (1853): 25.

Chapter 5

1. Clymer patented the name "Natura System" in 1908 as a term combining Thomsonian, physio-medical, and eclectic systems. In practice, however, the term seems little more than a replacement for physio-medicalism. See R. Swinburne Clymer, *Nature's Healing Agents: The Medicines of Nature (or The Natura System)* (1926) (reprinted, Philadelphia: Dorrance, 1963). Earlier, Clymer had written a medical text simply titled *The Thomsonian System of Medicine* (1905). Apparently, Clymer had attempted to steer an independent course and thus refused to identify openly with the physios, preferring to skirt this issue by first clinging to the term Thomsonian and later simply inventing a new one, Natura, to describe his practice.
2. Worthington Hooker, *Dissertation on the Respect Due to the Medical Profession and the Reasons That It Is Not Awarded by the Community* (Norwich: J.G. Cooley, 1844), p. 15.
3. Worthington Hooker, *Physician and Patient* (New York: Baker and Scribner, 1849) p. 119.
4. This occurred with an absorption of the last remaining physio-medical school with the eclectic Chicago College of Medicine and Surgery. See John S.

Haller Jr., *Kindly Medicine: Physio-Medicalism in America, 1836-1911* (Kent, OH: Kent State University Press, 1999), p. 147. Undoubtedly, some physio-medical physicians were still practicing after this date, but neither our research nor Haller's uncovered any data that would indicate organizational activity after 1911.

5. William H. Cook, *The Physio-Medical Dispensatory: A Treatise on Therapeutics, Materia Medica, and Pharmacy* (Cincinnati, OH: William H. Cook, 1869/Sandy, OR: Eclectic Medial Publications, 1998), pp. 5-6.

6. *Physio-Medical Recorder* 29 (1865): 189 ff. Cook wrote, "These lists I have prepared with the utmost care from the latest editions of the several Eclectic textbooks" (p. 189). The following is Cook's list of "poisons" used by the eclectics:

Fowler's Solution	Hyoscyamus
Antimony chloride	Stramonium
Litharge and lead acetate	Digitalis
Copper sulphate	Veratrum
Iodine	Aconite
Zinc salts	Conium
Silver nitrate	Cannabis sativa
Bismuth salts	Bitter almond
Gold chloride	Strychnine
Opium and derivatives	Prussic acid
Belladonna	Ergot

7. Cited by the *Cincinnati Medical Recorder* 51 (1883): 133.

8. "Illinois P-M Association. Report of Proceedings of Its Eighth Annual Convention" in *Physio-Medical Recorder* 29 (1865): 197 ff.

9. *Physio-Medical Recorder* 32 (1868): 126.

10. *The Southern Botanic Journal, Devoted to the Dissemination and Support of the Thomsonian System of Medical Practice* 1 (1837-1838): 197 ff. This is the earliest example of the use of quinine by a Thomsonian that we have discovered.

11. Ibid., p. 402.

12. Ibid., p. 403.

13. Ibid., p. 404.

14. *Physio-Medical Recorder* 29 (1865): 200.

15. Cook, *The Physio-Medical Dispensatory*, p. 346.

16. *The Botanic Medical Reformer and Home Physician* 1 (1841): 121.

17. *Physio-Medical Recorder* 29 (1865): 73.

18. *Physio-Medical Record* 10 (1907): 127.

19. Clymer, *Nature's Healing Agents*, p. 4.

20. Ibid., p. 205.

21. "Letter to Dr. Haggard, editor. From Dr. Th. Rimmelin, Schiltigheim.—Strassburg, Elsass, Germany, Dec. 12, 1906," in *Physio-Medical Record* 10 (1907): 42-45.

22. Ibid., p. 45.

23. *The Botanico-Medical Recorder* 7 (1838-1839): preface, vii.

24. Such names as the following had been suggested: "Thomsonian, Physiological Medical, Physio-Medical, Physiopathic, Anti-Pathic, Physio-American." See *Physio-Medical Recorder* 18 (1852): 97-99.

25. Alex Berman, "Neo-Thomsonianism in the United States," *Journal of the History of Medicine and Allied Sciences* 11 (1956): 138.

26. *The Middle States Medical Reformer and Advocate of Innocuous Medication* 1 (1854): 17.

27. Alexander Wilder, *History of Medicine* (Augusta, ME: Maine Farmer Publishing Company, 1904), pp. 589-590. This southern group was composed of members residing in Virginia, Alabama, Mississippi, Arkansas, Tennessee, and Kentucky.

28. Cited in the *Physio-Medical Recorder* 18 (1852): 101.

29. "Synopsis of Minutes of the Proceedings of the Reformed Medical Association of the United States . . . ," in *Physio-Medical Recorder* 18 (1852): 97 ff.

30. These were the Southern Botanico-Medical College at Macon, Georgia; the Physio-Medical College in Cincinnati, Ohio; and the Metropolitan Medical College in New York City.

31. These included *The Southern Medical Reformer* (organ of the Southern Botanico-Medical College); the *Physio-Medical Recorder* (organ of the Physio-Medical College); and a "journal to be established in New York." The New York journal appeared in 1854 under the name of *The Journal of Medical Reform* and represented the views of the Metropolitan Medical College.

32. Cited in the *Physio-Medical Recorder* 18 (1852): 100.

33. This dispensatory was finally written and published on the individual initiative of William H. Cook in 1869, under the title of *The Physio-Medical Dispensatory*.

34. We are in substantial agreement with Wilder, who points out that the botanic practitioners of this period, feeling secure in the absence of restrictive medical legislation, became indifferent to the need for organization (see Wilder, *History of Medicine,* pp. 670-671). Another factor to be considered in this connection was the constant bickering and feuding that went on between the physio-medicals and eclectics. In 1859, the editor of the *Physio-Medical Recorder* vainly chided the faithful because of their indifference to national organization: "It seems high time now . . . for the staunch advocates of sanative medication to meet again and compare notes. Many have fallen off from the ranks since 1852; many have supposed that the Baltimore Platform was a thing of moonshine, to be altered and set aside at pleasure." (*Physio-Medical Recorder* 24 [1859]: 162).

35. *The Middle States Medical Reformer and Advocate of Innocuous Medication* 1 (1854): 28.

36. Ibid., p. 28.

37. Ibid., p. 52. As indicated earlier, the prevailing duration of study at the medical schools of this period consisted usually of two sixteen-week terms of repetitive course work.

38. *Physio-Medical Recorder* 19 (1854): 118.

39. *The Middle States Medical Reformer and Advocate of Innocuous Medication* 1 (1854): 54.

40. *The Middle States Medical Reformer and Advocate of Innocuous Medication* 2 (1855): 52.

41. Wilder, *History of Medicine,* p. 592.

42. *Physio-Medical Recorder* 31 (1867): 228.

43. *The Botanico-Medical Recorder* 18 (1851): 26.

44. *The Botanico-Medical Recorder* 19 (1852): 1.

45. *Cincinnati Medical Recorder* 61 (1883): 63. The circular letter defined "true and genuine" physio-medicals as "those whose practice conforms to the great Physio-Medical doctrine of rejecting all poisons. And those who are not *true and genuine* in this sense, as also those who have diplomas procured by money or otherwise fraudulently, and those who sell or issue such fraudulent diplomas, and all who procure abortion, or otherwise are guilty of criminal practices, shall be debarred from the deliberations of this meeting" (p. 63).

46. Ibid., pp. 61-62.

47. Ibid., p. 72.

48. Ibid.

49. *The Boston Thomsonian Manual and Lady's Companion* 5 (1839): 171.

50. Wilder, *History of Medicine,* pp. 500, 525.

51. Each school is discussed at length in Haller, *Kindly Medicine,* pp. 45-78.

52. See James A. Pittman Jr., "Mobile Wasn't First Medical School," *Alabama Medicine* 63 (1993): 23; and Howard L. Holley, *A History of Medicine in Alabama* (1982) (reprinted, Birmingham, AL: University of Alabama School of Medicine, 1997), p. 244.

53. For example, in 1848, one of the professors of the school announced, "We are pleased to find all our students to be fully established in the fundamental doctrines of Thomsonism [sic]. There are no mongrels amongst us; none that advocate the peculiar notions of the Beachites. . . . We are all very far from confounding the *name* of an Institution with the doctrines taught therein. Although our college is called the Eclectic Institute of Virginia, yet our students will all bear witness, that the doctrines herein taught, are in perfect accordance with the fundamentals of Samuel Thomson. They wish it fully understood that our Institute is not the advocate of the peculiar notions of these termed Eclectics in the West, but that we are Eclectics in the broad sense of the word, which leads us to

    Seize upon the truth wherever found
    On Christian, or on heathen ground—
to select, from the accumulated wisdom of the past" (*New England Botanic Medical and Surgical Journal,* 2 [1848]: 14).

54. See Haller, *Kindly Medicine,* pp. 52-60.

55. Calvin Newton (1800-1853) graduated from Union College in 1826 and from Newton Theological Institute in 1829. He served as Baptist minister (1828-1831); Professor of Rhetoric and Hebrew at Waterville (now Colby) College, Maine (1831-1838); and Professor and President of the Theological Institute at Thomaston, Maine. He entered Berkshire Medical Institution in 1842 and re-

ceived MD degrees in 1844. He became a Fellow of the Massachusetts Medical Society (1845); he embraced neo-Thomsonianism and founded Worcester Medical School (1846); he was President of the National Eclectic Medical Association (1852) and editor of the *New England Eclectic and Guide to Health,* Worcester, 1846 (title later changed to *New England Botanic Medical and Surgical Journal*).

56. The *Journal of Medical Reform,* organ of the Metropolitan Medical College, ran an announcement describing the aims of the college as follows: "The teachings of the Metropolitan will be strictly based upon the doctrines contained in the Platform of Principles of Medical Reform, adopted by the National Reform Convention in the city of Baltimore in 1852 . . . for this Reform we claim Dr. Samuel Thomson of New Hampshire, the father and founder . . . we think to Samuel Thomson belongs the honor of being considered the father of this Reform, and to whom the world is indebted" (*Journal of Medical Reform* 1 [1854]: 251).

57. William G. Rothstein, *American Physicians in the Nineteenth Century* (Baltimore, MD: Johns Hopkins University Press, 1972), pp. 88-89.

58. Haller, *Kindly Medicine,* pp. 83-84.

59. *Journal of the American Medical Association* 51 (1908): 607.

60. For a brief period, the name "Physo-Medical" was used but was subsequently dropped for "Physio-Medical."

61. *Physo-Medical Recorder and Surgical Journal* 18 (1850): 167, edited and published by E.H. Stockwell, MD, Professor of Anatomy and Physiology, in the Physo-Medical College.

62. *Physio-Medical Recorder* 18 (1850): 165.

63. Ibid., p. 167.

64. Ibid., p. 168.

65. *The Botanico-Medical Recorder* 18 (1852): 191.

66. *The Middle States Medical Reformer and Advocate of Innocuous Medication* 3 (1856): 49 ff.

67. This journal was long-running and changed its official title over time: from 1857-1865, *American Druggists' Circular and Chemical Gazette;* from 1866 to 1906, *Druggists Circular and Chemical Gazette;* after 1906, *Druggists Circular.* Examples of advertisements are William S. Merrell and Company of Cincinnati, on p. 119; B. Keith and Company of New York, on p. 85; and Jacob S. Merrell of St. Louis, on p. 57, in *American Druggists' Circular and Chemical Gazette* 1 (1857). For a detailed discussion of concentrated remedies, see John Uri Lloyd, *The Eclectic Alkaloids . . . etc.* Bulletin of the Lloyd Library, no. 12 (Cincinnati, OH: Lloyd Library, 1910); and Alex Berman, "The Eclectic 'Concentrations' and American Pharmacy (1847-1861)," *Pharmacy in History* 22 (1980): 91-103.

68. *The Middle States Medical Reformer and Advocate of Innocuous Medication* 3 (1856): 60.

69. *Physio-Medical Recorder* 24 (1859): 83.

70. *Physio-Medical Journal* 21 (1895): 174.

71. Ibid.

72. *American Journal of Pharmacy* 30 (1858): 189.

Chapter 6

1.   Alexander Wilder, an authoritative spokesman and historian of the eclectic movement, has gone so far as to say that "their [the eclectics] existence as a distinct school was its permanency to their achievement in the field of pharmacy," and in another passage, he speaks of William S. Merrell's pioneer work in eclectic pharmacy, beginning in 1847-1848, as having "imparted new energy to the Eclectic cause. The practitioners now felt confident that the trite designation of 'unscientific' could no longer be applied" (*History of Medicine,* pp. 655, 660).

2.   Sources: Alexander Wilder, "Wooster Beach," *Eclectic Medical Journal* 53 (1893): 113, 121; Harvey Wickes Felter, "Wooster Beach M.D.," *Eclectic Medical Journal* 68 (1908): 9-13; Alexander Wilder, *History of Medicine* (Augusta, ME: Maine Farmer Publishing Company, 1904), pp. 432-439, 468, 484, 762; Harvey Wickes Felter, *History of the Eclectic Medical Institute* (Cincinnati, OH: Alumnal Association, 1902), pp. 5-10, 81-83; Obituary in the *New York Herald,* Jan. 30, 1868; *The Telescope,* 1-4 (1825-1828), edited by Wooster Beach; and John Haller Jr., *Medical Protestants: The Eclectics in American Medicine, 1825-1939* (Carbondale, IL: Southern Illinois University Press, 1994), pp. 66-75 passim.

3.   Quoted by Felter, *History of the Eclectic Medical Institute,* p. 82.

4.   Samuel Thomson, *New Guide to Health; or Botanic Family Physician, to which is Prefixed the Life and Medical Discoveries of the Author* (Boston: J.Q. Adams, 1835), p. 182.

5.   *The Western Medical Reformer* 3 (1838): 43, edited by the medical professors of Worthington College, Worthington, Ohio.

6.   Wilder, *History of Medicine,* p. 517.

7.   Felter, *History of the Eclectic Medical Institute,* p. 17.

8.   Ibid., p. 146. See also Jonathon Forman, "The Worthington School and Thomsonianism," *Bulletin of the History of Medicine* 21 (1947): 772-787; and Haller, *Medical Protestants,* pp. 75-82.

9.   Felter, *History of the Eclectic Medical Institute,* p. 27.

10.   Ibid.

11.   Ibid., p. 30.

12.   Madge E. Pickard, and R. Carlyle Buley, *The Midwest Pioneer: His Ills, Cures and Doctors* (New York: H. Schuman, 1946), p. 193.

13.   John S. Haller Jr., *A Profile in Alternative Medicine: The Eclectic Medical College of Cincinnati* (Kent, OH: Kent State University Press, 1999), p. 28.

14.   Alva Curtis, *A Fair Examination of All the Medical Systems in Vogue* (Cincinnati, OH: Printed for the proprietor, 1855), p. 128.

15.   Ibid., p. 129.

16.   Quoted in *Eclectic Medical Journal* 10 (1851): 581.

17.   *The Medical and Surgical Reporter* 2 (1859): 27.

18.   Felter, *History of the Eclectic Medical Institute,* p. 38.

19. Ronald L. Numbers, "The Making of an Eclectic Physician: Joseph M. McElhinney and the Eclectic Medical Institute of Cincinnati," *Bulletin of the History of Medicine* 47 (1973): 159-160.

20. John Milton Scudder, "A Brief History of Eclectic Medicine," *Eclectic Medical Journal* 39 (1879): 305.

21. Felter, *History of the Eclectic Medical Institute,* p. 118.

22. See John Uri Lloyd, *Biographies of John King, Andrew Jackson Howe and John Milton Scudder, . . . etc.* Bulletin of the Lloyd Library and Museum, no. 19 (Cincinnati, OH: Lloyd Library, 1912).

23. John Milton Scudder, "On Specific Action of Medicines," *Eclectic Medical Journal* 29 (1869): 393. He later expanded this into book form as *Specific Medication and Specific Medicines* (Cincinnati, OH: Wilstach, Baldwin and Company, 1870).

24. Scudder, "On Specific Action of Medicines," p. 393.

25. Wilder, *History of Medicine,* p. 680.

26. Herbert Tracey Webster, "How About a Coalition?" *Eclectic Medical Journal* 75 (1915): 405.

27. *Eclectic Medical Journal* 39 (1879): 305.

28. Edwin S. Wayne, "Criticism of the Value of Concentrated Preparations," *College Journal of Medical Science* 1 (1856): 45-48.

29. John King, "Concentrated Medicines Adulterated," *Worcester Journal of Medicine* 10 (1855): 225-227.

30. For an exhaustive account of eclectic organizational activity, see Haller's *Medical Protestants.*

31. Cited in the *Eclectic Medical Journal* 39 (1879): 301-302; and *Electic Medical Journal* 53 (1893): 210.

32. This last graduating class consisted of thirty-six students, bringing the total number of EMI graduates to 4,666, which included 440 women. See Haller, *Medical Protestants,* p. 246.

33. Wilder, *History of Medicine,* p. 741.

34. John Hughes Bennett (1812-1875) was a Fellow of the Royal Society of Edinburgh and the Edinburgh College of Physicians. He was also physician to the Royal Dispensary and pathologist to the Royal Infirmary, with international fame as a teacher, clinician, and physiologist. He is credited with demonstrating "the injuriousness of the antiphlogistic treatment which had ruled the best minds of the civilized world for ages" (*Lancet* 2 [1875]: 533-534). See also the *Dictionary of National Biography,* Volume 4 (London: Smith, Elder, and Company, 1885), p. 244 ff.

35. *Eclectic Medical Journal* 39 (1879): 302.

36. Ibid., p. 302.

37. *Eclectic Medical Journal* 54 (1894): 396.

38. John Milton Scudder, "A Brief History of Eclecticism," *Eclectic Medical Journal* 46 (1886): 92.

39. William Osler, *License to Practice* (Chicago: American Medical Association, 1889), p. 3.

40.   William G. Rothstein, *American Physicians in the Nineteenth Century* (Baltimore, MD: Johns Hopkins University Press, 1972), p. 229.

41.   *Antiphlogistic* simply means against inflammation, but the concept itself formed a prominent and powerful part of nineteenth-century therapeutics. As William S. Haubrich explains, "phlogiston is an archaic term once used to designate the supposed component that produced fire in whatever was combustible. The term was first used in the 17th century, being taken from the Greek *phlogistos,* 'set on fire.' Later, this dubious idea was adopted to explain the origin of inflammation in body tissues, especially that externally visible. Within living memory there was a concoction of glycerin, kaolin, and aromatics called Antiphlogistine which was purveyed as an anodyne and antiseptic preparation puported to suppress inflammation in skin lesions" (see his *Medical Meanings: A Glossary of Word Origins* (Philadelphia: American College of Physicians, 1997), pp. 168-169.

42.   For example, in "Remittent Fever," Beach prescribed vegetable emetics (e.g., lobelia, ipecac, etc.) and purgatives (e.g. jalap, senna, cream of tartar mixture). In addition, Beach was fond of diaphoretics. In this particular case, he suggested a dram each of Virginia snakeroot (*Serpentaria virginiana,* today known as *Aristolochia sepentaria*), saffron, ipecac, camphor, opium, added to eight ounces of "best gin" (Wooster Beach, *The American Practice of Medicine,* Volume 1 [New York: Betts and Anstice, 1833], p. 279). A similar treatment was advocated by Beach for "Inflammatory Fever." Of this disease, he wrote, "It is necessary to deplete the system, not by bloodletting, which will often bring on typhus and other serious consequences, but by promoting all the secretions and excretions" (Ibid., p. 287).

43.   Beach, *The American Practice of Medicine,* Volume 3, pp. 205-211, and later versions of this work list the following typical chemicals:

    (a) Sulfuric acid (diluted for internal use)
    (b) Ether (diluted for internal use)
    (c) Lime (to make lime water)
    (d) Copper sulfate (externally as an astringent, and for piles)
    (e) Corrosive sublimate [sic!] ("We use it only as a caustic, and as an external application.")
    (f) Ammonium chloride (for external application in solution for inflammation)
    (g) Potassium nitrate (as a diuretic)
    (h) Red oxide of lead (for external use in ointments and plasters)
    (i) Lead acetate (externally as an astringent)
    (j) Cream of tartar (laxative and diuretic)
    (k) Potassium bicarbonate (internal use)
    (l) Borax (used externally as astringent)
    (m) Flowers of sulfur (internal and external use)
    (n) Ammonium carbonate (internal use)
    (o) Zinc sulfate (externally in astringent eye wash)

44.   *Catalogue of Shaker Herbs, Roots, and Medicinal Plants . . . Raised, Manufactured and Put Up By the Shakers of New Lebanon . . . etc.* (New York:

A. Warner, 1848), p. 8. This catalog is in the library of the New York Academy of Medicine.

45. Beach, *The American Practice of Medicine;* and Wooster Beach, *Beach's Family Physician and Home Guide* (Cincinnati, OH: Moore, Wilstach, Keys, 1859).

46. John Uri Lloyd, "New Medicines and Old Eclectic Compounds," *Druggists Circular,* 63 (1919): 7.

47. Ibid. Lloyd wrote that "formulas of Beach have furnished numberless opportunities for advertisers of liniments, of cough syrups, and of cathartics, to such an extent that one would be astonished over the financial returns that have come to the advertisers" (p. 7).

48. John Uri Lloyd, *The Eclectic Alkaloids . . . etc.,* Bulletin of the Lloyd Library and Museum, no. 12 (Cincinnati, OH: Lloyd Library, 1910), pp. 8-9; and the condensed version of this work, *A Treatise on the American Alkaloids, Resins, Resinoids, Oleo-Resins and Concentrated Principles (so-called Eclectic Concentrations),* Drug Treatise No. XXIV (Cincinnati, OH: Lloyd Brothers, 1909), p. 9. It is impossible to write about the history of eclectic "concentrations" without drawing heavily on these two authoritative studies of Lloyd.

49. Lloyd, *A Treatise,* p. 9.

50. Hodgson's assay of podophyllum rhizome was published in the *American Journal of Pharmacy* 14 (1832): 273-275; Lewis's article appeared in the *American Journal of Pharmacy* 29 (1847): 165-172.

51. *American Journal Pharmacy,* 30 (1848): 510.

52. Lloyd, *The Eclectic Alkaloids,* p. 7.

53. Meaning "resembling resins" or "resinlike," this term was first introduced by William S. Merrell; see Lloyd, *The Eclectic Alkaloids,* p. 26.

54. Quoted in *Eclectic Medical Journal* 9 (1850): 297.

55. King had published in the *Western Medical Reformer* (April 1846, pp. 175-176), processes for preparing resins of iris, cimicifuga, podophyllum, etc.

56. Lloyd, *The Eclectic Alkaloids,* p. 11.

57. Ibid., p. 12.

58. *Eclectic Medical Journal* 12 (1853).

59. These included Podophyllin, Leptandrin, Macrotys, Caulophylline, Cornine, Geranine, Myricin, Prunine, Sanguinarin (Resin), Sanguinarina (Alkaloid), Diosorine, Irisine, Hydrastine, and Corydalia. It will be noted that, in several instances, Merrell affixed other terminations than *in* to his products but does not mention the reasons in the advertisement, except in the case of Sanguinarina, which he considered the alkaloid of sanguinaria.

60. These included Apocynin, Asclepedin, Aletrin, Cypripedin, Eupatorin, Eupurpurin, Iridin, Xanthoxylin, Lobeline or Oil of Lobelia, Ptelein or Oil of Ptelea, Capsicine or Oil of Stillingia, and Ethereal Oil of Male Fern. As with the "powdered resinoids," no explanation was given for the ending *line*.

61. Wilder, *History of Medicine,* p. 660.

62. *Eclectic Medical Journal* 15 (1856): 456.

63. "What is the use of our having to swallow half an ounce of the crude material, while the whole of the real active medicinal principle is contained in a single grain?" queried the editor of the *Eclectic Medical Journal* 18 (1858): 192.

64. Within a very few years, the following more important concerns were flooding the country with concentrated remedies: in Cincinnati, F. D. Hill and Co., T. C. Thorp, Geo. M. Dixon, H. H. Hill and Co., and T. L. A. Greve; in St. Louis, Wm. H. Baker and Co.; in New Lebanon, NY, Tilden and Company; and in New York City, B. Keith and Co. See Lloyd, *The Eclectic Alkaloids*, p. 22.

65. *Eclectic Medical Journal* 16 (1857): 220.

66. Rothstein, *American Physicians in the Nineteenth Century*, p. 228.

67. Merrell did not confine himself to botanic supplies, as Phillip D. Jordan states in his paper "Purveyors to the Profession: Cincinnati Drug Houses, 1850-60," *Ohio Archaeological and Historical Quarterly* 54 (1945): 374.

68. Wilder credited William S. Merrell with "creating and establishing the new [eclectic] pharmacy" (*History of Medicine*, p. 657). Merrell was, for a number of years, a trustee and president of the Eclectic Medical Institute (see Felter, *History of the Eclectic Medical Institute*, p. 78).

69. Wilder, *History of Medicine*, p. 660.

70. *Proceedings of the American Pharmaceutical Association* 7 (1858): 434-440.

71. Lloyd, *A Treatise*, p. 15.

72. Lloyd, *The Eclectic Alkaloids*, p. 43. The alkaloids of sanguinaria and hydrastis, along with the resins of cimicifuga and podophyllum, were the only eclectic concentrated products that Lloyd endorsed as being therapeutically established. (*A Treatise*, p. 26). Lloyd gave credit to William S. Merrell for introducing "the alkaloidal American preparations of sanguinaria and hydrastis canadensis" (*Eclectic Alkaloids*, biographical sketch of Merrell, p. viii).

73. Wilder, *History of Medicine*, p. 657.

74. *Eclectic Medical Journal* 14 (1855): 248.

75. Ibid., pp. 248-249.

76. *American Journal of Pharmacy* 27 (1855): 93-94.

77. Ibid., p. 93.

78. Ibid.

79. Edward S. Wayne, "Examination of the Preparations Made by the American Chemical Institute, New York," *American Journal of Pharmacy* 27 (1855): 388-391.

80. Ibid., p. 391.

81. See Wayne, "Criticism of Concentrated Preparations."

82. Wayne, "Examination of Preparations," p. 389.

83. *Eclectic Medical Journal* 15 (1856): 92-96, and 206-209.

84. *Eclectic Medical Journal*, 206 ff.

85. *Eclectic Medical Journal*, 350 ff.

86. Edward S. Wayne, "Examination of Keith and Co.'s Preparations—No. 2," *The College Journal of Medical Science* 1 (1856): 23.

87. *Eclectic Medical Journal* 15 (1856): 468.

88. Wayne, "Criticism of Concentrated Preparations," pp. 45-48.

89. Ibid., p. 45.

90. Ibid., p. 47.

91. William S. Merrell, "Reply of Mr. Merrell," *College Journal of Medical Science* 1 (1856): 48-49.

92. Ibid., p. 49.

93. John King, "Concentrated Medicines Adulterated," p. 227.

94. Grover Coe, *Concentrated Organic Medicines . . . etc.* (New York: B. Keith and Company, 1858), p. 8.

95. *American Journal of Pharmacy* 30 (1858): 578.

96. Wilder, *History of Medicine,* p. 657.

97. Lloyd Brothers Manufacturing Pharmacists, *Condensed Price List of Select Pharmaceutical Preparations* (Cincinnati, OH: Lloyd Brothers, 1921), pp. 31-32.

98. Ibid., p. 32.

99. Edward Parrish, "Eclectic Pharmacy," *American Journal of Pharmacy* 23 (1851): 329-335.

100. Ibid., p. 331.

101. Ibid.

102. Edward Parrish, *An Introduction to Practical Pharmacy* (Philadelphia: Blanchard and Lea, 1856), pp. 163-164.

103. Ibid., p. 164.

104. Parrish, *An Introduction to Practical Pharmacy,* Second Edition (Philadelphia: Blanchard and Lea, 1859), pp. 189-194.

105. Ibid., p. 189.

106. Ibid., p. 194.

107. Edward Parrish, *A Treatise on Pharmacy,* Third Edition (Philadelphia: Blanchard and Lea, 1864), pp. 280-296.

108. Ibid., p. 280.

109. Ibid., p. 281.

110. Ibid., pp. 285-295.

111. Ibid., pp. 282-283.

112. See Procter's review in the *American Journal of Pharmacy* 26 (1854): 572; and *American Journal of Pharmacy* 31 (1859): 286, 388, 390.

113. Merrell was elected to membership in the American Pharmaceutical Association in 1854. See *Proceedings American Pharmaceutical Association* 3 (1854): 3.

114. John Uri Lloyd, "American Pharmacopoeias and Dispensatories," *Western Druggist* 21 (1899): 19-20.

115. Authority to comment on the USP was finally granted to the authors of the *American Dispensatory,* beginning with the USP (1890) Seventh decennial revision.

116. The literature on Shaker pharmacy is extensive. See E.D. Andrews, *The Community Industries of the Shakers,* New York State Museum Handbook 15 (Albany: New York State Museum, 1933), pp. 87-109; Procter's illuminating articles in the *American Journal of Pharmacy* (22 [1850]: 205-209; 23 [1851]:

93-95, 386-388; 24 [1852]: 88-91, 187-188; and 27 [1855]: 568-570); Charles O. Lee, "The Shakers As Pioneers in the American Herb and Drug Industry," *American Journal of Pharmacy* 132 (1960): 178-193; J. Worth Estes, " 'Shaker-Made' Remedies," *Pharmacy in History* 34 (1992): 63-73; Galen Beale and Mary Rose Boswell, *The Earth Shall Blossom: Shaker Herbs and Gardening* (Woodstock, VT: Countryman Press, 1991); and Amy Bess Miller, *Shaker Medicinal Herbs: A Compendium of History, Lore, and Uses* (Pownal, VT: Storey Publications, 1998). Of the seventeen Shaker societies located in New England, New York, Ohio, and Kentucky during the nineteenth century, the New York society at New Lebanon was the most important pharmaceutically. In addition to cultivating and selling large quantities of herbs, roots, and medicinal plants, this remarkable people also manufactured extracts, ointments, "double distilled fragrant waters," household remedies of various kinds, etc.

117.   Andrews cites one source to the effect that "the sale of Shaker herbs was prompted by the popularity of the so-called Thomsonian medical system" (*Community Industries of the Shakers*, p. 100). It should be strongly emphasized that the Shakers were also important suppliers of plant medicinals to the regular physicians and drug trade, as well as large producers of such household remedies as Corbett's Shaker Syrup of Sarsaparilla, Dr. White's Curative Syrup, Shaker Digestive Cordial, and many others. For statistics on Shaker pharmaceutical production and related data, see Lee, "Shakers As Pioneers," p. 188, and, especially, the extensive discussion in Miller, *Shaker Medicinal Herbs*, pp. 37-75 passim.

118.   Alex Berman performed primary source research on Shaker pharmaceutical and medical materials at the Western Reserve Historical Society Library in Cleveland. This collection consisted of letters, bills, advertising circulars, and catalogs of medicinals, ledgers, and recipe books. In addition, the society had microfilmed the extensive collection of Shaker manuscript materials in the New York State Museum, Albany. Michael Flannery consulted the extensive holdings (both original and on microfilm) at Shaker Village of Pleasant Hill, located in Harrodsburg, Kentucky. Although Pleasant Hill did not have any considerable herb trade, the Shaker archives located there contain material related to this group beyond the immediate Pleasant Hill community.

119.   Beale and Boswell, *The Earth Shall Blossom*, p. 107.

120.   William Procter, "Eclectic Remedies As Prepared by the Shakers," *American Journal of Pharmacy* 28 (1856): 91.

121.   *Eclectic Medical Journal* 39 (1879): 308. In 1869, Scudder wrote, "Many persons are in error in regard to *our* use of the term *specific*. They think of a specific medicine as one that will cure all cases of a certain disease according to our present nosology. . . . A disease according to our present nosology may be formed of one, or of a half-dozen or more distinct pathological changes, bearing a determinate relation to one another. We do not propose to reach all of these by one remedy, except in those cases in which one lesion is primary, and the others result from it. But on the contrary, we propose a remedy for each pathological feature, using the remedy for the first which is first in the chain of morbid action, and the

second which stands second, and so on" (*Eclectic Medical Journal* 29 [1869]: 393.

122. *Eclectic Medical Journal* 39 (1879): 306.

123. Ibid.

124. Ibid.

125. Ibid.

126. Lloyd Brothers Pharmacists, Inc., *Dose Book* (Cincinnati, OH: Lloyd Brothers, 1932).

127. Ibid., p. 6.

128. Cited in the *California Medical Journal* 19 (1898): 310.

129. Albert Merrell, *A Digest of Materia Medica and Pharmacy: Forming a Complete Pharmacopoeia for the Use of Physicians, Druggists, and Students* (Philadelphia: Blakiston, 1883), p. 17. Merrell announced himself on the title page as "Professor of Chemistry, Pharmacy and Toxicology in the American Medical College, St. Louis." The book was dedicated to "My Father and Preceptor, Wm. S. Merrell, A.M., M.D., whose laborious . . . investigations have contributed so extensively to existing knowledge of American Materia Medica and Pharmacy."

130. Wilder, *History of Medicine*, p. 662.

131. Ibid., p. 705.

132. Ibid., p. 859.

133. Ibid., p. 703.

134. For details on the life and legacy of John Uri Lloyd, see Michael A. Flannery, *John Uri Lloyd: The Great American Eclectic* (Carbondale, IL: Southern Illinois University Press, 1998).

135. Will H. Blackwell and Martha J. Powell, "An Analysis of Works of, and Upon, Curtis Gates Lloyd," *Mycotaxon* 58 (1996): 353-374.

136. Quoted in Alex Berman, "The Eclectic 'Concentrations' and American Pharmacy (1847-1861)," *Pharmacy in History* 22 (1980): 92.

137. George Urdang, *The Scope of Pharmacy* (Madison, WI: American Institute of the History of Pharmacy, 1946), p. 25.

138. For a complete English translation of Ostwald's comments, see Flannery, *John Uri Lloyd*, pp. 185-187.

139. Lloyd's contribution has been recognized in the *National Formulary* ever since its first "Historical Introduction" in the fourth edition (1916), and it is still carried today; see *National Formulary*, Volume 18 (1995), p. 2196.

140. For a complete discussion of the role of elixirs in spawning the *National Formulary*, see Gregory J. Higby, "Publication of the National Formulary: A Turning Point for American Pharmacy," in *One Hundred Years of the National Formulary: A Symposium*, edited by Gregory J. Higby (Madison, WI: American Institute of the History of Pharmacy, 1989), pp. 3-19.

141. For the disposition of the Lloyd Brothers firm, see *Pharmaceutical Company Histories*, edited by Gary L. Nelson (Bismark, ND: Woodbine Publishing, 1983), pp. 1, 43. There were some legal difficulties involving S.B. Penick and Lloyd's son, John Thomas. See the discussion in Flannery, *John Uri Lloyd*, p. 164.

142. John King wrote of E.S. Wayne as one "who ranks among the best theoretical and practical Pharmaceutists and chemists in our country, and to him I am particularly indebted for aid in his special department" (*The American Dispensatory,* Eighth Edition [Cincinnati, OH: Wilstach and Baldwin, 1870], p. xii).

143. *Eclectic Medical Journal* 24 (1864): 133.

144. Cited in the *American Journal of Pharmacy* 35 (1863): 568.

145. John Uri Lloyd, "Eclectic Pharmacy," *Eclectic Medical Journal* 84 (1924): 519-524.

146. Some examples are the following articles: W. Procter, "On the Volatile Oil of Erigeron Philadelphicum," *American Journal of Pharmacy* 27 (1855): 105-106; W. Procter, "On Gelsemium Sempervirens or Yellow Jassamin," *American Journal of Pharmacy* 24 (1852): 307-310; by E.S. Wayne: "On Jeffersonia Diphylla," *American Journal of Pharmacy* 27 (1855): 1-7; R.H. Stabler, "On Podophyllin," *American Journal of Pharmacy* 30 (1858): 502-512; and an inaugural essay by J.M. Abernathy, "On the Resinoids," *American Journal of Pharmacy* 33 (1861): 299-303.

147. See, for example, the theses of graduating students published in the *American Journal of Pharmacy* 30 (1858): 270. Five of the topics out of a total of thirty-one were devoted to plant remedies publicized by the eclectics; three were on podophyllum, one on leptandra, and another on gelsemium.

148. John Uri Lloyd, *Origin and History of All the Pharmacopoeial Vegetable Drugs* (Cincinnati, OH: The Caxton Press, 1929), pp. 31, 132, 263; see also Wade Boyle, *Official Herbs: Botanical Substances in the United States Pharmacopoeias, 1820-1990* (East Palestine, OH: Buckeye Naturopathic Press, 1991), pp. 14-51.

149. Cited by Lloyd in *A Treatise,* p. 22 and in *Eclectic Alkaloids,* p. 43. Rice's statement occurs in an article titled "Note sur certains médicaments végétaux americains et sur leur formes pharmaceutiques," which was published in the *Journal de Pharmacie,* Anvers, 35 (1879).

Chapter 7

1. John Uri Lloyd, "Vegetable Drugs Employed by American Physicians," *Journal of the American Pharmaceutical Association* 1 (1917): 1228-1241.

2. Ibid., p. 1234.

3. Ibid., p. 1241.

4. In 1900, the percentage of botanicals was 54; by 1910, the number had fallen to 47 percent, or 367 botanical substances out of a total of 773. See Wade Boyle, *Official Herbs: Botanical Substances in the United States Pharmacopoeias, 1820-1990* (East Palestine, OH: Buckeye Naturopathic Press, 1991), p. 57; and Benjamin Hershenson, "A Botanical Comparison of the United States Pharmacopoeias of 1820 and 1960," *Economic Botany* 18 (1964): 342-356.

5. Glenn Sonnedecker, *Kremer's and Urdang's History of Pharmacy,* Fourth Edition, Revised and reprinted (Madison, WI: American Institute of the History of Pharmacy, 1986), p. 50. See also Ernst Bäumler, *In Search of the Magic Bullet:*

Great Adventures in Modern Drug Research (London: Thames and Hudson, 1965), pp. 15-39.

6. See *Dictionary of Scientific Biography*, edited by Charles Coulston Gillispie, Volume 4 (New York: Charles Scribner's Sons, 1972), p. 298.

7. Abraham Flexner, *Medical Education in the United States and Canada: A Report to the Carnegie Foundation for the Advancement of Teaching*, Bulletin no. 4 (New York: The Carnegie Foundation, 1910).

8. Paul Starr, *The Social Transformation of American Medicine* (New York: Basic Books, 1982), p. 121. Others have looked past the elitist and restrictive effects of the Flexner Report and offered a more benevolent appraisal. See, for example, Kenneth M. Ludmerer, *Time to Heal: American Medical Education from the Turn of the Century to the Era of Managed Care* (New York: Oxford University Press, 1999), pp. 4-6, 22-26, 370.

9. Flexner, *Medical Education*, p. 163.

10. Varro E. Tyler, "The Recent History of Pharmacognosy," in *The Inside Story of Medicines*, edited by Gregory J. Higby and Elaine Stroud (Madison, WI: American Institute of the History of Pharmacy, 1997), pp. 161-162.

11. Ibid., p. 163.

12. *The Cambridge Illustrated History of Medicine*, edited by Roy Porter (Cambridge: Cambridge University Press, 1996), p. 264.

13. Robert Kanigel, *Apprentice to Genius: The Making of a Scientific Dynasty* (1986) (reprinted, Baltimore, MD: Johns Hopkins University Press, 1993), p. 45.

14. Its last meeting was held in Hot Springs, Arkansas, June 15-17, 1965.

15. Joseph F. Kett, *The Formation of the American Medical Profession: The Role of Institutions, 1780-1860* (New Haven, CT: Yale University Press, 1968), pp. 178-179.

16. Daniel J. Wallace, "Thomsonians: The People's Doctors," *Clio Medica* 14 (1980): 176.

17. Richard L. Bushman, *The Refinement of America: Persons, Houses, Cities* (New York: Vintage Books, 1992), p. 279.

18. Kett, *Formation of the American Medical Profession*, p. 180.

19. Richard H. Shryock, *The Development of Modern Medicine: An Interpretation of the Social and Scientific Factors Involved*, Reprint Edition (Madison, WI: University of Wisconsin Press, 1979), p. 314.

20. William G. Rothstein, *American Physicians in the Nineteenth Century* (Baltimore, MD: Johns Hopkins University Press, 1972), p. 323.

21. John S. Haller Jr., *Kindly Medicine: Physio-Medicalism in America, 1836-1911* (Kent, OH: Kent State University Press, 1997), pp. 147-151.

22. John S. Haller Jr., *Medical Protestants: The Eclectics in American Medicine, 1825-1939* (Carbondale, IL: Southern Illinois University Press, 1994), p. 251.

23. Lynn Payer, *Medicine and Culture* (New York: Henry Holt, 1993), p. 24.

24. Ibid., p. 22.

25. Francis Brinker, "The Role of Botanical Medicine in 100 Years of American Naturopathy," *HerbalGram* 42 (1998): 49-59.

26. Ibid., p. 54.

27. *Naturae Medicina and Naturopathic Dispensatory,* edited by A.W. Kuts-Cheraux (Des Moines, IA: American Naturopathic Physicians and Surgeons Association, 1953).

28. Brinker, "The Role of Botanical Medicine," p. 54.

29. Ibid., p. 58.

30. For a full discussion, see Donald J. Brown, *Herbal Prescriptions for Better Health* (Rocklin, CA: Prima Publishing, 1996), pp. 2-3.

31. See Barbara Griggs' chapter, "The Green People," in *Green Pharmacy: The History and Evolution of Western Herbal Medicine,* Second Edition (Rochester, VT: Healing Arts Press, 1997), pp. 331-345.

32. Richard Schulze was one of the early "Green People." His mentor, Dr. John Christopher, adopted a philosophy closely allied to Samuel Thomson and made lobelia his therapeutic cornerstone (see Griggs, "The Green People," p. 334). Today Mark Blumenthal, Steven Foster, Dan Gagnon, Rosemary Gladstar, Christopher Hobbs, David Hoffman, Michael Moore, Jeanne Rose, Ed Smith, Michael Tierra, Roy Upton, and David Winston would head any list of who's who in the current American herb scene.

33. For an exhaustive account of this legislation, see I. Scott Bass and Anthony L. Young, *Dietary Supplement Health and Education Act: A Legislative History and Analysis* (Washington, DC: The Food and Drug Law Institute, 1996).

34. See, for example, Dixie Farley, "Dietary Supplements: Making Sure Hype Doesn't Overwhelm Science," *FDA Consumer* 27 (November 1993): 9-13.

35. Bass and Young, *Dietary Supplement Health and Education Act,* p. 167.

36. Varro E. Tyler, *Herbs of Choice: The Therapeutic Use of Phytomedicinals* (Binghamton, NY: Pharmaceutical Products Press, 1994), p. 10.

37. Mark Blumenthal, "Congress Passes Dietary Supplement Health and Education Act of 1994," *HerbalGram* 32 (1994): 18. The NLEA amended the Food, Drug, and Cosmetic Act to make special provisions for vitamins, minerals, and herbs as "dietary supplements." It specifically exempted dietary supplements from legal standards for conventional foods and permitted manufacturers to make limited health claims. Despite these provisions, the American Herb Products Association (AHPA) became concerned over how the FDA might respond to the act. For specifics, see "The Complete Text of the AHPA Botanical Ingredient Review Proposal to the Food and Drug Administration," *HerbalGram* 25 (1991): 32-37. See also Bass and Young, *Dietary Supplement Health and Education Act,* pp. 271-293.

38. Mark Blumenthal, "Harvard Study Estimates Consumers Spend $5.1 Billion on Herbal Products?" *HerbalGram* 45 (1999): 68.

39. Ibid.

40. American Association of Colleges of Pharmacy, *Examples of Alternative Therapy Programs,* Pamphlet distributed at the 1999 Annual Meeting, July 3-7, Boston, Massachusetts.

41. An excellent historical review of antibiotic therapy is available in Donna Hoel and David N. Williams, "Antibiotics: Past, Present, and Future," *Postgraduate Medicine* 101 (January 1997): 114-122.

42. Some plants, most notably *Echinacea* spp. (purple coneflower) and *Astragalus membranaceus,* have received attention not for their antibiotic properties but for their ability to boost the body's own immune system. In particular, the high molecular weight heteroglycan polysaccharides of echinacea have been found to have "profound immuno-stimulatory effects" due to the binding of these constituents to carbohydrate receptors on macrophages and T-lymphocytes. Others, such as *Hydrastis canadensis* (goldenseal), contain berberine, which has been shown to be a bacteriostatic agent against streptococci and to possess antifungal properties. For an abstracted review of hundreds of in vitro and clinical studies on medicinal plants, see Melvyn R. Werbach and Michael T. Murray's *Botanical Influences on Illness: A Sourcebook of Clinical Research* (Second edition) (Tarzana, CA: Third Line Press, 2000). On the immunostimulant properties of echinacea, see especially pp. 381-382; on the bacteriostatic and antifungal properties of goldenseal, see especially pp. 376-377.

43. Bass and Young, *Dietary Supplement Health and Education Act,* p. 227.

44. "Status of USP-NF and USP-DI Botanical Monograph Development," available at the United States Pharmacopeial Convention Web site <www.usp.org/dietary/availability.htm>.

45. "AMA Recognizes USP's Role in Off-Label Uses and Dietary Supplement Standards," *The Standard* (July 1999), full text available at <www.usp.org/aboutusp/standard/9907/9907_06.htm>.

46. U.S. Food and Drug Administration Center for Food Safety and Applied Nutrition, "Dietary Supplement Strategy (Ten Year Plan)" (January 2000), available at <http://vm.cfsan.fda.gov/~dms/ds-strat.html>.

47. James A. Duke and Mary Jo Bogenschutz-Godwin offer an emphatic, but admittedly speculative, defense of plant synergy in "The Synergy Principle at Work in Plants, Pathogens, Insects, Herbivores, and Humans," in *Natural Products from Plants*, edited by Peter B. Kaufman, Leland J. Cseke, Sara Warber, James A. Duke, and Harry L. Brielmann (Boca Raton, FL: CRC Press, 1999), pp. 183-205.

Bibliography

Abbott, Simon B. *The Southern Botanic Physician.* Charleston, SC: Abbott, 1844.

Abernathy, J.M. "On the Resinoids." *American Journal of Pharmacy* 33 (1861): 299-303.

Ackerknecht, Erwin H. "Elisha Bartlett and the Philosophy of the Paris Clinical School." *Bulletin of the History of Medicine* 24 (1950): 43-60.

_____. *Malaria in the Upper Mississippi Valley, 1760-1900.* Baltimore, MD: Johns Hopkins University Press, 1945.

_____. *Medicine at the Paris Hospital, 1794-1848.* Baltimore, MD: Johns Hopkins University Press, 1967.

_____. *A Short History of Medicine,* Revised Edition. Baltimore, MD: Johns Hopkins University Press, 1982.

Acosta, Joseph De. *The Natural and Moral History of the Indies,* Volumes 1 and 2. Reprinted from the English translated edition of Edward Grimston. London: Hakluyt Society, 1880.

Allen, Paul W. *Eclectic Medicine: The Lessons of Its Past and the Duties of Its Future.* Annual Address before the Eclectic Medical Society of the State of New York. Delivered in Albany, January 15, 1868.

American Druggists' Circular and Chemical Gazette 1 (1857).

Andrews, Edward D. *The Community Industries of the Shakers,* New York State Museum Handbook 15. Albany, NY: New York State Museum, 1933.

Arber, Agnes. *Herbals. Their Origin and Evolution. A Chapter in the History of Botany, 1470-1670,* Second Edition. Cambridge: Cambridge University Press, 1938.

Arny, Henry Vinecome. "Seven Glimpses of John Uri Lloyd," *Journal of the American Pharmaceutical Association* 25 (1936): 885.

The Badianus Manuscript, Codex Barberini, Latin 241, Vatican Library. An Aztec Herbal of 1552. Introduction, translation, and annotations by Emily W. Emmart. Baltimore, MD: Johns Hopkins University Press, 1940.

Bagley, George K. *The Family Instructor or Guide to Health.* Vermont: np, 1848.

Bartholow, Roberts. *Annual Oration on the Degree of Certainty in Therapeutics.* Baltimore, MD: np, 1876.

Bartlett, Elisha. *An Essay on the Philosophy of Medical Science.* Philadelphia: Lea and Blanchard, 1844.

_____. *An Inquiry into the Degree of Certainty in Medicine; and into the Nature and Extent of Its Power over Disease.* Philadelphia: Lea and Blanchard, 1848.

Barton, Benjamin Smith. *Collections for an Essay Towards a Materia Medica of the United States,* Bulletin of the Lloyd Library of Botany, Pharmacy, and Materia Medica, no. 1 (1798-1804). Cincinnati, OH: Lloyd Library, 1900.

_____. *Collections for an Essay Towards a Materia Medica of the United States,* Third Edition. Philadelphia: Edward Earle and Company, Fry and Krammerer, 1810.

Barton, William P.C. *Vegetable Materia Medica of the United States.* Philadelphia: M. Carey and Son, 1817-1819.

Bass, I. Scott and Anthony L. Young. *Dietary Supplement Health and Education Act: A Legislative History and Analysis.* Washington, DC: The Food and Drug Law Institute, 1996.

Bäumler, Ernst. *In Search of the Magic Bullet: Great Adventures in Modern Drug Research.* London: Thames and Hudson, 1965.

Beach, Wooster. *The American Practice of Medicine,* Volumes 1-3. New York: Betts and Anstice, 1833.

_____. *A Treatise on Pulmonary Consumption . . . etc.* New York: J.B. Allee, Printers, 1840.

_____. *The American Practice Condensed, or The Family Physician,* Fifty-sixth Edition. Cincinnati, OH: Moore, Wilstach, and Baldwin, 1865.

Beale, Galen and Mary Rose Boswell. *The Earth Shall Blossom: Shaker Herbs and Gardening.* Woodstock, VT: Countryman Press, 1991.

Benton, Joel. "A Dead Medical System." *New York Times* 21 (September 22, 1901): 133.

Berman, Alex. "The Thomsonian Movement and Its Relation to American Pharmacy and Medicine." *Bulletin of the History of Medicine* 25 (1951): 405-428; 519-538.

_____. "C. S. Rafinesque: A Challenge to the Historian of Pharmacy." *American Journal of Pharmaceutical Education* 16 (1952): 314.

_____. "The Heroic Approach in 19th Century Therapeutics." *Bulletin of the American Society of Hospital Pharmacists* 11 (1954): 320-327.

_____. "Neo-Thomsonianism in the United States." *Journal of the History of Medicine and Allied Sciences* 11 (1956): 133-155.

_____. "Social Roots of the 19th Century Botanico-Medical Movement in the United States," *Actes du VIIIe Congrès International d'Histoire des Sciences,* Florence (September 3-9, 1956): 561-565.

_____. "A Striving for Scientific Respectability: Some American Botanics and the Nineteenth-Century Plant Materia Medica." *Bulletin of the History of Medicine* 30 (1956): 7-29.

_____. "Wooster Beach and the Early Eclectics." *University of Michigan Medical Bulletin* 24 (1958): 277-286.

_____. "An Unpublished Letter from G. K. Lawrence to C. S. Rafinesque, October 8, 1828." *Bulletin of the History of Medicine* 34 (1960): 461-470.

_____. "The Eclectic 'Concentrations' and American Pharmacy." *Pharmacy in History* 22 (1980): 91-103.

Bigelow, Jacob. *American Medical Botany,* Volumes 1-3. Boston: Cummings and Hilliard, 1817-1820.

_____. "Discourse on Self-Limited Disease," in *Medical Communications of the Massachusetts Medical Society.* Boston: H. Hale, 1835.

Blackwell, Will H. *Poisonous and Medicinal Plants.* Englewood Cliffs, NJ: Prentice Hall, 1990.

Blackwell, Will H., and Martha J. Powell. "An Analysis of Works of, and Upon, Curtis Gates Lloyd." *Mycotaxon* 58 (1996): 353-374.

Blanton, Wyandham Bolling. *Medicine in Virginia in the Nineteenth Century.* Richmond, VA: Garrett and Massie, 1933.

The Boston Medical and Surgical Journal 15 (1836): 158-159, 241-242; 11 (1834): 214-215; 49 (1854): 96-97.

Boston Patriot and Daily Mercantile Advertiser (January 28, 1823).

Boston Thomsonian Manual and Lady's Companion 5 (1838-1839).

The Boston Thomsonian Medical Journal 1 (1845).

Boston True Thomsonian 1-2 (1841-1842).

The Botanic Medical Reformer and Home Physician 1-2 (1841-1842).

Botanico-Medical Recorder 6-17 (1837-1852).

Bowditch, Henry I. "Venesection, Its Former Abuse and Present Neglect," *Publications of the Massachusetts Medical Society* 3.3 (1871): 223-249.

Boyle, Wade. *Official Herbs: Botanical Substances in the United States Pharmacopoeias, 1820-1990.* East Palestine, OH: Buckeye Naturopathic Press, 1991.

Brinker, Francis. "The Role of Botanical Medicine in 100 Years of American Naturopathy." *HerbalGram* 42 (1998): 49-59.

The British and Foreign Medical Review 21 (1846): 262-265.

Buchan, William. *Domestic Medicine; or, The Family Physician . . . etc.* Philadelphia: R. Aitken, 1771, and later editions.

Buckner, P.J. "Address," in *Constitution, By-Laws and Proceedings of the Medical Association of Adams, Brown, and Clermont Counties,* Ohio, May, 1847.

Bushman, Richard L. *The Refinement of America: Persons, Houses, Cities.* New York: Vintage Books, 1992.

Caldwell, L.G. "Early Legislation Regulating the Practice of Medicine." *Illinois Law Review,* 18 (1923): 225-244.

California Medical Journal 19 (1898).

Catalogue of Shaker Herbs, Roots, and Medicinal Plants . . . Raised, Manufactured and Put Up by the Shakers of New Lebanon . . . etc. New York: A. Warner, 1848.

Chambers, John Sharpe. *The Conquest of Cholera: America's Greatest Scourge.* New York: Macmillan, 1938.

Chambers, Reuben. *The Thomsonian Practice of Medicine.* Bethania, PA: np, 1842.

Cincinnati Medical Recorder 51-52 (1883-1884).

Clapp, Asahel. *A Synopsis or Systematic Catalogue of the Medicinal Plants of the United States.* Philadelphia: T.K. and P.G. Collins, 1852.

Clymer, R. Swinburne. *The Thomsonian System of Medicine.* Allentown, PA: The Philosophical Pub. Co., 1905.

_____. *Nature's Healing Agents: The Medicines of Nature (or The Natura System)* (1926) Reprint Edition. Philadelphia: Dorrance, 1963.

Coe, Grover. *Positive Medical Agents.* New York: C.B. Norton, 1855.

_____. *Concentrated Organic Medicines,* Sixth Edition. New York: B. Keith and Company, 1858.

Coffin, A.I. *Botanic Guide to Health and the Natural Pathology of Disease.* Manchester, England: William Irwin, 1846.

Colby, Benjamin. *A Guide to Health,* Third Edition. Milford, NH: J. Burns, 1846.

College Journal of Medical Sciences 1-4 (1856-1859).

Comfort, Aaron. *Thomsonian Medical Instructor.* Philadelphia: Comfort, 1855.

Cook, William. H. "Leaving First Principles." *Physio-Medical Recorder* 29 (1865): 69-75.

_____. *Physio-Medical Dispensatory.* Cincinnati, OH: William H. Cook, 1869.

Cooper, J.W. *The Experienced Botanist or Indian Physician.* Lancaster, PA: J. Bear, Printer, 1840.

Cooper, James. *The Indian Doctor's Receipt Book.* Uniontown, OH: np, 1855.

Coventry, C.B. "History of Medical Legislation in the State of New York," *New York Journal of Medicine* 4 (1845): 152.

Cowen, David L. "America's First Pharmacy Laws." *Journal of the American Pharmaceutical Association,* Practical Pharmacy Edition, 3 (1942): 162-169, 214-221.

_____. *America's Pre-pharmacopoeial Literature.* Madison, WI: American Institute of the History of Pharmacy, 1961.

_____. "The Impact of the Materia Medica of the North American Indians on Professional Pharmacy," in *Botanical Drugs of the Americas in the Old and New Worlds: Invitational Symposium at the Washington-Congress 1983.* Edited by Wolfgang-Hagen Hein. Veröffentlichungen der Internationalen Gesellschaft für Geschichte der Pharmazie e. V., Band 53. Stuttgart, Germany: Wissenschaftliche Verlagsgesellschaft, 1984, pp. 51-63.

Cowen, David L. and William H. Helfand. *Pharmacy: An Illustrated History.* New York: Harry N. Abrams, 1990.

Cowen, David L. and Donald F. Kent. "Medical and Pharmaceutical Practice in 1854." *Pharmacy in History* 39 (1997): 91-100.

Curtis, Alva. *Discussions Between Several Members of the Regular Medical Faculty and the Thomsonian Botanic Physicians on the Comparative Merits of Their Respective Systems.* Columbus, OH: A. Curtis, 1836.

_____. *Synopsis of a Course of Lectures on Medical Science Delivered to the Students of the Botanico-Medical College of Ohio.* Cincinnati, OH: Edwin Shepard, 1846.

_____. *A Fair Examination and Criticism of All the Medical Systems in Vogue.* Cincinnati, OH: Printed for the proprietor, 1855.

Cutler, Manasseh. *An Account of Some of the Vegetable Productions, Naturally Growing in This Part of America.* Bulletin of the Lloyd Library and Museum, no. 7. Cincinnati, OH: Lloyd Library, 1903.

Daily, William. *The Indian Doctor's Practice of Medicine; or Daily's Family Physician.* Louisville, KY: Hull, 1848.

Daston, Lorraine and Katharine Park. *Wonders and the Order of Nature, 1150-1750.* New York: Zone Books, 1998.

Davis, Nathan Smith. *Contributions to the History of Medical Education and Medical Institutions in the United States of America, 1776-1876.* Special Report prepared for the United States Bureau of Education. Washington, DC: Government Printing Office, 1877.

Dawson, John. "Dr. Dawson's Address," in *Proceedings of the Medical Convention of Ohio Held at Columbus on the 5th, 6th, and 7th of May, 1841,* pp. 80-84.

Densmore, Frances. "Uses of Plants by the Chippewa Indians," *Annual Report,* Bureau of American Ethnology, no. 44. Washington, DC: Government Printing Office, 1928, pp. 275-397.

Downey, William. *An Investigation of the Properties of the Sanguinaria Canadensis; or Puccoon.* Bulletin of the Lloyd Library and Museum, no. 9. Reprinted, Cincinnati, OH: Lloyd Library, 1907.

Drake, Daniel. "The People's Doctors," *The Western Journal of the Medical and Physical Sciences* 3 (1829): 455-462.

_____. *Practical Essays on Medical Education and the Medical Profession in the United States* (1832). Introduction by David A. Tucker Jr. Baltimore, MD: Johns Hopkins University Press, 1952.

Duffy, John. *From Humors to Medical Science: A History of American Medicine,* Second Edition. Urbana, IL: University of Illinois Press, 1993.

The Eclectic and Medical Botanist: Devoted Principally to Improvements in the Botanic Practice of Medicine, Columbus, Ohio, 1832-1834.

Eclectic Medical Journal 1-84 (1849-1924).

Edwards, Linden F. "Resurrection Riots During the Heroic Age of Anatomy in America." *Bulletin of the History of Medicine* 25 (1951): 178-184.

Emmons, Samuel B. *The Vegetable Family Physician.* Boston: np, 1842.

Estes, J. Worth. " 'Shaker-Made' Remedies." *Pharmacy in History* 34 (1992): 63-73.

_____. "The European Reception of the First Drugs from the New World. *Pharmacy in History* 37 (1995): 3-23.

Evans, Howard Ensign. *The Natural History of the Long Expedition to the Rocky Mountains, 1819-1820.* New York: Oxford University Press, 1997.

Eve, Paul F. *Present Position of the Medical Profession in Society.* Augusta, GA: J. McCafferty, 1849.

Felter, Harvey Wickes. *A History of the Eclectic Medical Institute, 1845-1903.* Cincinnati, OH: Alumnal Association, 1902.

_____. "Wooster Beach, M.D." *Eclectic Medical Journal* 68 (1908): 9-13.

_____. *The Genesis of the American Materia Medica.* Bulletin of the Lloyd Library and Museum, no. 26. Cincinnati, OH: Lloyd Library, 1927.

Fenton, William N. "Contacts Between Iroquois Herbalism and Colonial Medicine." *Smithsonian Report for 1941.* Washington, DC: Government Printing Office, 1941, pp. 503-526.

Fernald, Merritt Lyndon. *Gray's Manual of Botany,* Eighth Edition. Reprinted, Portland, OR: Dioscorides Press, 1987.

Fillmore, Susan E. "Samuel Thomson and His Effect on the American Health Care System." *Pharmacy in History* 28 (1986): 188-191.

Flannery, Michael A. "Thomas Vaughan Morrow, 1804-1850: The Apostle of Eclecticism." *Transactions of the Kentucky Academy of Science* 57 (1996): 113-119.

_____. *John Uri Lloyd: The Great American Eclectic.* Carbondale, IL: Southern Illinois University Press, 1998.

_____. "The Medicine and Medicinal Plants of C. S. Rafinesque." *Economic Botany* 52 (1998): 27-43.

_____. "Medicine's Remarkable Brothers: Simon and Abraham Flexner of Louisville, Kentucky." *Journal of the Kentucky Academy of Science* 59 (1998): 158-167.

_____. "What Did Doctors Really Do? In Search of a Therapeutic Perspective of American Medicine." *Journal of Clinical Pharmacy and Therapeutics* 24 (1999): 151-156.

_____ "Another House Divided: Sectarians and Union Medical Service During the Civil War." *Journal of the History of Medicine and Allied Science.* 54 (1999): 478-510.

Flexner, Abraham. *Medical Education in the United States and Canada: A Report to the Carnegie Foundation for the Advancement of Teaching.* Bulletin no. 4. New York: The Carnegie Foundation, 1910.

Fonerden, William Henry. *Institutes of Thomsonianism.* Philadelphia: Botanic Sentinel, 1837.

Forbes, John. "Homeopathy, Allopathy, and 'Young Physic'." *British and Foreign Medical Review* 21 (1846): 225-265.

Forman, Jonathan. "Dr. Alva Curtis in Columbus: The Thomsonian Recorder and Columbus' First Medical School." *The Ohio State Archæological and Historical Quarterly* 51 (1942): 332-340.

_____. "The Worthington School and Thomsonianism." *Bulletin of the History of Medicine* 21 (1947): 772-787.

Foster, Robert D. *The North American Indian Doctor, or Nature's Method of Curing and Preventing Disease According to the Indians.* Canton, OH: np, 1838.

Foster, Steve. *Forest Pharmacy: Medicinal Plants in American Forests.* Durham, NC: Forest History Society, 1995.

Fyfe, John William. *Specific Diagnosis and Specific Medication.* Cincinnati, OH: Scudder, 1909.

Gager, C.S. "Botanic Gardens of the World, Material for a History." *Brooklyn Botanic Garden Record* 27.3 (1938): 387.

Gathercoal, E.N. *The Prescription Ingredient Survey.* Washington, DC: American Pharmaceutical Association, 1933.

Gevitz, Norman, ed. *Other Healers: Unorthodox Medicine in America.* Baltimore, MD: Johns Hopkins University Press, 1988.

Gifford, George E. Jr. "Botanic Remedies in Colonial Massachusetts, 1620-1820." In *Medicine in Colonial Massachusetts.* Publications of the Colonial Society of Massachusetts, Volume 57. Boston: The Society, 1980, pp. 263-288.

Gould, A.A. *Search Out the Secrets of Nature.* Paper read at the Annual Meeting of the Massachusetts Medical Society, 1855.

Griffith, R. Egelsfeld. "On Fraseri Walteri." *Journal of the Philadelphia College of Pharmacy* 3 (1832): 269-273.

_____. *Medical Botany.* Philadelphia: Lea and Blanchard, 1847.

Griggs, Barbara. *Green Pharmacy: The History and Evolution of Western Herbal Medicine,* Second Edition. Rochester, VT: Healing Arts Press, 1997.

Gross, Samuel D. "A Discourse on Bloodletting Considered As a Therapeutic Agent." *Transactions of the American Medical Association* 26 (1875): 421-433.

_____. *Autobiography of Samuel Gross, M.D.,* Volume 1, Philadelphia: G. Baine, 1887.

Gunn, John C. *Domestic Medicine, or, Poor Man's Friend in the Hours of Affliction, Pain and Sickness,* Tenth Edition. Xenia, OH: J.H. Purdy, 1838.

Haller, John S., Jr. "Samson of the Materia Medica: Medical Theory and the Use and Abuse of Calomel." *Pharmacy in History* 13 (1971): 27-34, 67-76.

_____. "The Use and Abuse of Tartar Emetic in the 19th-Century Materia Medica." *Bulletin of the History of Medicine* 49 (1975): 235-257.

_____. *Medical Protestants: The Eclectics in American Medicine, 1825-1939.* Carbondale, IL: Southern Illinois University Press, 1994.

_____. *Kindly Medicine: Physio-Medicalism in America, 1836-1911.* Kent, OH: Kent State University Press, 1997.

_____. *A Profile in Alternative Medicine: The Eclectic Medical College of Cincinnati, 1845-1942.* Kent, OH: Kent State University Press, 1999.

_____. *The People's Doctors: Samuel Thomson and the American Botanical Movement, 1790-1860.* Carbondale, IL: Southern Illinois University Press, 2000.

Halstead, Frank G. "A First-Hand Account of a Treatment by Thomsonian Medicine in the 1830s." *Bulletin of the History of Medicine* 10 (1941): 680-687.

Hamilton, James. *Observations on the Use and Abuse of Mercurial Medicines in Various Diseases.* Notes and an appendix by Ansel W. Ives, M.D. New York: Bliss and White, 1821.

Henry, Samuel. *A New and Complete American Family Herbal.* New York: S. Henry, 1814.

Hershenson, Benjamin. "A Botanical Comparison of the United States Pharmacopoeias of 1820 and 1960." *Economic Botany* 18 (1964): 342-356.

Higby, Gregory J. "Publication of the National Formulary: A Turning Point for American Pharmacy." In *One Hundred Years of the National Formulary: A*

Symposium, edited by Gregory J. Higby. Madison, WI: American Institute of the History of Pharmacy, 1989, pp. 3-19.

_____. *In Service to American Pharmacy: The Professional Life of William Procter, Jr.* Tuscaloosa, AL: University of Alabama Press, 1992.

Hobbs, Christopher. "The Medical Botany of John Bartram." *Pharmacy in History* 33 (1991): 181-185.

Holmes, Oliver Wendell. *Currents and Counter-Currents in Medical Science.* Boston: Ticknor and Fields, 1861.

Hooker, Worthington. *Dissertation on the Respect Due to the Medical Profession and the Reasons That It Is Not Awarded by the Community.* Norwich, CT: J.G. Cooley, 1844.

_____. *Physician and Patient; or, A Practical View of the Mutual Duties, Relations, and Interests of the Medical Profession and the Community.* New York: Baker and Scribner, 1849.

_____. *Lessons from the History of Medical Delusions.* New York: Baker and Scribner, 1850.

_____. "The Present Mental Attitude and Tendencies of the Medical Profession." *New Englander* 10 (1852): 557-568.

_____. "Rational Therapeutics: A Prize Essay." *Publications of the Massachusetts Medical Society* 1:2. Boston: J. Wilson and Son, 1857.

Howard, Horton. *An Improved System of Botanic Medicine.* Columbus, OH: Author, 1832.

Jeffries, Theodore W. "Barton's Unpublished Materia Medica." *Pharmacy in History* 17 (1978): 69-71.

Jordan, Philip D. "The Secret Six: An Inquiry into the Basic Materia Medica of the Thomsonian System of Botanic Medicine." *Ohio Archæological and Historical Quarterly* 52 (1943): 347-355.

_____. "Purveyors to the Profession: Cincinnati Drug Houses, 1850-1860." *Ohio Archæological and Historical Quarterly* 54 (1945): 371-380.

_____. "The Eclectic of St. Clairsville." *Ohio Archæological and Historical Quarterly* 56 (1947): 388.

Journal of Medical Reform 1 (1854).

The Journal of the Franklin Institute 3, New Series (1829): 130-134.

Juettner, Otto. *Daniel Drake and His Followers: Historical and Biographical Sketches.* Cincinnati, OH: Harvey Publishing Company, 1909.

Kanigle, Robert. *Apprentice to Genius: The Making of a Scientific Dynasty.* Baltimore, MD: Johns Hopkins University Press, 1993.

Kaufman, Martin. *Homeopathy in America: The Rise and Fall of a Medical Heresy.* Baltimore, MD: Johns Hopkins University Press, 1971.

Kebler, Lyman F. "United States Patents Granted for Medicines during the Pioneer Years of the Patent Office." *Journal of the American Pharmaceutical Association* 24 (1935): 485.

Kelly, Howard A. *Some American Medical Botanists Commemorated in Our Botanical Nomenclature.* New York: Southworth, 1914.

Kett, Joseph F. *The Formation of the American Medical Profession: The Role of Institutions, 1780-1860.* New Haven, CT: Yale University Press, 1968.

King, John and Newton, Robert S. *The Eclectic Dispensatory of the United States.* Cincinnati, OH: Derby, 1852, and other editions.

Kloss, Jethro. *Back to Eden: A Human Interest Story of Health and Restoration to Be Found in Herb, Root, and Bark.* Coalmont, TN: Longview Publishing House, 1939.

Kost, John. *Elements of Materia Medica and Therapeutics.* Cincinnati, OH: Kost and Pool, 1849; and the Second Edition. Cincinnati, OH: Moore, Wilstach, Keys, 1858.

Krantz, John C. and C. Jelleff Carr. *The Pharmacologic Principles of Medical Practice.* Baltimore, MD: Williams and Wilkins, 1951.

Kuts-Cheraux, A.W., ed. *Naturae Medicina and Naturopathic Dispensatory.* Des Moines, IA: American Naturopathic Physicians and Surgeons Association, 1953.

Larson, Cedric. "Patent-Medicine Advertising and the Early American Press." *Journalism Quarterly* 14 (1937): 333-341.

Lee, Charles O. "The Shakers As Pioneers in the American Herb and Drug Industry." *American Journal of Pharmacy* 132 (1960): 178-193.

Lloyd, John Uri. *Elixirs and Flavoring Extracts: Their History, Formulæ, and Methods of Preparation.* New York: William Wood, 1892.

_____. "American Pharmacopoeias and Dispensatories." *Western Druggist* 21 (1899): 19-20.

_____. *A Treatise on the American Alkaloids, Resins, Oleo-Resins and Concentrated Principles (so-called Eclectic Concentrations).* Drug Treatise no. 24. Cincinnati, OH: Lloyd Brothers, 1909.

_____. *The Eclectic Alkaloids.* Bulletin of the Lloyd Library, no. 12. Cincinnati, OH: Lloyd Library, 1910.

_____. *Biographies of John King, Andrew Jackson Howe and John Milton Scudder.* Bulletin of the Lloyd Library and Museum, no. 19. Cincinnati, OH: Lloyd Library, 1912.

_____. "Vegetable Drugs Employed by American Physicians." *The Journal of the American Pharmaceutical Association* 1 (1912): 1228-1241.

_____. "New Medicines and Old Eclectic Compounds." *Druggists' Circular* 63 (1919): 7-8.

_____. "Fragments from an Autobiography: My Entrance into Eclectic Pharmacy." *Eclectic Medical Journal* 87 (1927): 303-311.

_____. *Origin and History of All the Pharmacopeial Vegetable Drugs.* Cincinnati, OH: The Caxton Press, 1929.

Lloyd Brothers Pharmacists, Inc. *Dose Book* (Concise Presentation of the Principal Uses and Usual Doses of All Specific Medicines). Cincinnati, OH: Lloyd Brothers, Inc., 1932.

Lloyd, John Uri and Lloyd, Curtis Gates. *Drugs and Medicines of North America.* Cincinnati, OH: Lloyd Brothers, Inc., 1884-1887.

Louis, P.C.A. *Researches on the Effects of Bloodletting in Some Inflammatory Diseases and on the Influence of Tartatized Antimony and Vesication in Pneumonitis,* translated by C.G. Putnam, MD. Preface and Appendix by James Jackson, MD. Boston: Hilliard, Gray and Company, 1836.

Ludmerer, Kenneth M. *Time to Heal: American Medical Education from the Turn of the Century to the Era of Managed Care.* New York: Oxford University Press, 1999.

Lukens, I. *The Sick Man's Guide or Family Director.* Bridgeton, NJ: G.S. Harris, 1845.

Magner, Lois. *A History of Medicine.* New York: Marcel Dekker, 1992.

Mahr, August C. "Materia Medica and Therapy Among the North American Forest Indians." *Ohio Archæological and Historical Quarterly* 60 (1951): 331-354.

Mattson, Morris. *The American Vegetable Practice, or, A New and Improved Guide to Health.* Boston: D.L. Hale, 1841.

Mayo, Caswell A. *The Lloyd Library and Its Makers.* Bulletin of the Lloyd Library and Its Makers, no. 28. Cincinnati, OH: Lloyd Library, 1928.

McCarl, Mary Rhinelander. "Publishing the Works of Nicholas Culpeper, Astrological Herbalist and Translator of Latin Medical Works in Seventeenth-Century London." *Canadian Bulletin of Medical History* 13 (1996): 225-276.

Means, Alexander. "Calomel—Its Chemical Characteristics and Mineral Origin Considered, in View of Its Curative Claims." *Southern Medical & Surgical Journal* (March 1845), cited in the *New Orleans Medical Journal* 1 (1845): 588.

The Medical and Surgical Reporter 3-5 (1859-1860).

Merrell, Albert. *A Digest of Materia Medica and Pharmacy: Forming a Complete Pharmacopoeia for the Use of Physicians, Druggists, and Students.* Philadelphia: P. Blakiston, 1883.

Merrell, William S. "Eclectic Pharmacy." *Eclectic Medical Journal* 2 (1850): 297-305.

Merrill, E.D. "A Generally Overlooked Rafinesque Paper." *American Philosophical Society Proceedings* 86 (1942): 72-90.

The Middle States Medical Reformer and Advocate of Innocuous Medication 1-3 (1854-1856).

Miller, Amy Bess. *Shaker Medicinal Herbs: A Compendium of History, Lore, and Uses.* Pownal, VT: Storey Books, 1998.

Mitchell, T.D. "Calomel Considered As a Poison." *New Orleans Medical & Surgical Journal* 1 (1844-1845): 28.

Moerman, Daniel E. *Native America Ethnobotany.* Portland, OR: Timber Press, 1998.

Monardes, Nicolas. *Joyfull Newes Out of the Newe Founde Worlde,* Volumes 1 and 2, translated by John Frampton, Tudor translations. New York: A.A. Knopf, 1925.

The New England Botanic Medical and Surgical Journal 1-2 (1847-1848).

Norwood, William Frederick. *Medical Education in the United States Before the Civil War.* Philadelphia: University of Pennsylvania Press, 1944.

Numbers, Ronald L. "The Making of an Eclectic Physician: Joseph M. McElhinney and the Eclectic Medical Institute of Cincinnati." *Bulletin of the History of Medicine* 47 (1973): 155-166.

Olmsted, J.M.D. *Francois Magendie: Pioneer in Experimental Physiology and Scientific Medicine in XIX Century France.* New York: Schuman's, 1944.

Packard, Francis R. *History of Medicine in the United States,* Volumes 1 and 2. New York: P.B. Hoeber, 1931.

Parascandola, John. *The Development of American Pharmacology: John J. Abel and the Shaping of a Discipline.* Baltimore, MD: Johns Hopkins University Press, 1992.

Parrish, Edward. "An Inaugural Essay on *Statice caroliniana* with a Chemical Analysis of the Root of This Plant." *American Journal of Pharmacy* 14 (1842): 111.

_____. "Eclectic Pharmacy." *American Journal of Pharmacy* 23 (1851): 329-335.

_____. *An Introduction to Practical Pharmacy.* Philadelphia: Blanchard and Lea, 1856, and other editions.

Payer, Lynn. *Medicine and Culture.* New York: Henry Holt, 1996.

Peaslee, E.R. *Comparative Intellectual Standing of the Medical Profession.* Concord, NH: McFarland and Jenks, 1851.

Peirce, Andrea. *The American Pharmaceutical Association Practical Guide to Natural Medicines.* New York: William Morrow, 1999.

The Philadelphia Botanic Sentinel and Thomsonian Medical Revolutionist, Volumes 1-4. Philadelphia, PA: J. Coates 1837-1839.

The Physio-Medical Journal 21 (1895).

Physio-Medical Record 10 (1907).

Physio-Medical Recorder 18-43 (1852-1880).

The Physio-Medical Recorder and Surgical Journal 18 (1850).

Pickard, Madge E. and Buley, R. Carlyle. *The Midwest Pioneer: His Ills, Cures and Doctors.* New York: H. Schuman, 1946.

Porcher, Francis Peyre. *Resources of the Southern Fields and Forests.* Richmond, VA: West and Johnson, 1863.

Porter, Roy. *The Greatest Benefit to Mankind: A Medical History of Humanity* New York: W.W. Norton, 1997.

Proceedings of the American Pharmaceutical Association 2 (1853).

Procter, William Jr. "On Lobelia Inflata, (An Inaugural Essay)." *American Journal of Pharmacy* 9 (1837): 98-108.

_____. "Remarks on Some Pharmaceutical Preparations of Lobelia inflata." *American Journal of Pharmacy* 14 (1842): 108.

_____. "On Gelsemium Sempervirens or Yellow Jassamin." *American Journal of Pharmacy* 24 (1852): 307-310.

_____. "On the Volatile Oil of Erigeron philadelphicum." *American Journal of Pharmacy* 27 (1855): 105-106.

_____. "Eclectic Remedies As Prepared by the Shakers." *American Journal of Pharmacy* 28 (1856): 91.

Pursh, Frederick. *Flora Americae Septentrionalis, or, A Systematic Arrangement and Description of the Plants of North America,* Second Edition. London: James Black and Son, 1816.

Rafinesque, Constantine S. *Medical Flora, or, Manual of the Medical Botany of the United States of North America,* Volumes 1 and 2. Philadelphia: Atkinson and Alexander, 1828-1830.

_____. *The Pulmist; or, the Art of Curing and Preventing the Consumption or Chronic Phthisis.* Philadelphia: Author, 1829.

The Reformed Practice of Medicine, As Taught at the Reformed Medical Colleges of New York, at Worthington, Ohio and all the Reformed Schools in the United States. Boston: np, 1831.

Report of the Trial of Dr. Samuel Thomson, the Founder of the Thomsonian Practice, for an Alleged Libel in Warning the Public Against the Impositions of Paine D. Badger, As a Thomsonian Physician Sailing Under False Colors, . . . etc. Boston: Henry P. Lewis, 1839.

Reveal, James L. *Gentle Conquest: The Botanical Discovery of North America with Illustrations from the Library of Congress.* Washington, DC: Starwood Publishing, 1992.

Risse, Guenter B., Ronald L. Numbers, and Judith Walzer Leavitt, eds. *Medicine Without Doctors: Home Health Care in American History.* New York: Science History Publications, 1977.

Robinson, Samuel. *A Course of Fifteen Lectures on Medical Botany.* Columbus, OH: Horton Howard, 1829, and later editions.

Rodgers, Andrew Denny. *John Torrey: A Story of North American Botany.* Princeton, NJ: Princeton University Press, 1942.

Rosenberg, Charles E. *The Cholera Years: The United States in 1832, 1849, and 1866.* Chicago: University of Chicago Press, 1962.

Rothstein, William G. *American Physicians in the Nineteenth Century: From Sects to Science.* Baltimore, MD: Johns Hopkins University Press, 1972.

Rush, Benjamin. "A Defense of Blood-letting As a Remedy for Certain Diseases." *Medical Inquiries and Observations.* Philadelphia: Thomas Dobson, 1796, pp. 244-255.

_____. "An Inquiry into the Natural History of Medicine Among the Indians of North-America; and a Comparative View of Their Diseases and Remedies with Those of Civilized Nations," in *Medical Inquiries and Observations,* Second Edition, Volumes 1-4. Philadelphia: J. Conrad and Company, T. & G. Palmer, 1805.

_____. "Observations on the Duties of a Physician and the Methods of Improving Medicine. Accommodated to the Present State of Society and Manners in the United States," in *Medical Inquiries and Observations,* Second Edition, Volumes 1-4. Philadelphia: Matthew Carey, Brown and Merritt, 1809, pp. 1, 388 ff.

Sanborn, Peter E. *The Sick Man's Friend.* Boston: W. Johnson, 1840.

Schoepf, Johann David. *Materia Medica Americana Potissimum Regni Vegetabilis.* Bulletin of the Lloyd Library and Museum, no. 6. Reprinted, Cincinnati, OH: Lloyd Library, 1903.

Scudder, John Milton. "On Specific Action of Medicines." *Eclectic Medical Journal* 29 (1869): 393.

_____. *Specific Medication and Specific Medicines.* Cincinnati, OH. Wilstach, Baldwin, and Company, 1870, and other editions.

_____. "A Brief History of Eclectic Medicine." *The Eclectic Medical Journal* 39 (1879): 297-308.

Selman, S.H. *The Indian Guide to Health or a Valuable Vegetable Medical Prescription for the Cure of All Disorders Incident to this Climate.* Columbus, IN: James M'Call, 1836.

Shafer, Henry Burnell. *The American Medical Profession (1783-1850).* New York: Columbia University Press, 1936.

Shryock, Richard H. "Public Relations of the Medical Profession in Great Britain and the United States." *Annals of Medical History* 2 (1930): 315-322.

_____. *American Medical Research, Past and Present.* New York: Columbia University Press, 1947.

_____. "Empiricism versus Rationalism in American Medicine, 1650-1950." *Proceedings of the American Antiquarian Society* (April 1969): 99-150.

_____. *The Development of Modern Medicine: An Interpretation of the Social and Scientific Factors Involved.* Reprinted, Madison, WI: University of Wisconsin Press, 1979.

Skelton, John. *Family Medical Adviser.* Leeds, England: np, 1852.

_____. *A Plea for the Botanic Practice of Medicine.* London: np , 1853.

Smith, Elias. *The Life, Conversion, Preaching, Travels and Sufferings of Elias Smith.* Portsmouth, NH: Beck and Foster, 1816.

_____. *The American Physician and Family Assistant,* Fourth Edition. Boston: B. True, 1837.

Smith, Elisha. *The Botanic Physician.* New York: Murphy and Bingham, 1830.

Smith, Peter. *The Indian Doctor's Dispensatory Being Father Smith's Advice Respecting Diseases and Their Cure.* Bulletin of the Lloyd Library and Museum, no. 2. Cincinnati, OH: Lloyd Library, 1901.

Sonnedecker, Glenn. *Kremers and Urdang's History of Pharmacy,* Fourth Edition. Reprinted and revised, Madison, WI: American Institute of the History of Pharmacy, 1986.

The Southern Botanic Journal, Devoted to the Dissemination and Support of the Thomsonian System of Medical Practice 1 (1837-1838).

Stabler, R.H. "On Podophyllin." *American Journal of Pharmacy* 30 (1858): 508-512.

Starr, Paul. *The Social Transformation of American Medicine.* New York: Basic Books, 1982.

Stebbins, Sumner. *Address in Refutation of the Thomsonian System of Medical Practice.* West Chester, PA: np, 1837.

Steele, I.K. "A London Trader and the Atlantic Empire: Joseph Cruttenden, Apothecary, 1710 to 1717," *William and Mary Quarterly* 34 (1977): 281-297.

Stern, Bernhard J. *Society and Medical Progress.* Princeton, NJ: Princeton University Press, 1941.

_____. *American Medical Practice.* New York: Commonwealth Fund, 1945.

Stillé, Alfred. *Therapeutics and Materia Medica,* Volumes 1 and 2. Philadelphia: H.C. Lea, 1874.

Struik, Dirk J. *Yankee Science in the Making.* Boston: Little, Brown, 1948.

Stuckey, Ronald L. "Medical Botany in the Ohio Valley (1800-1850)." *Transactions & Studies of the College of Physicians of Philadelphia* 45 (1978): 262-278.

_____. "Rafinesque's Botanical Pursuits in the Ohio Valley (1818-1829)." *Journal of the Kentucky Academy of Science* 59 (1998): 111-157.

Stuckey, Ronald L. and James S. Pringle. "Common Names of Vascular Plants Reported by C. S. Rafinesque in an 1819 Descriptive Outline of Four Vegetation Regions of Kentucky." *Transactions of the Kentucky Academy of Science* 58 (1997): 9-19.

The Telescope 1-4 (1825-1828).

Thacher, James. *The American New Dispensatory.* Boston: T.B. Wait, 1810.

Thomson, John. *A Vindication of the Thomsonian System of the Practice of Medicine on Botanical Principles.* Albany, NY: Webster and Wood, 1825.

_____. *A Historical Sketch of the Thomsonian System of the Practice of Medicine on Botanical Principles As Originated by Samuel Thomson and Continued by His Coadjutors.* Albany, NY: B.D. Packard and Company, 1830.

_____. *A View of Science and Quackery Compared Theoretically; or the Difference Between Vegetable and Mineral Medicines, etc.* Albany, NY: Printed for the author, 1831.

_____. *A Philosophical Theory of an "Empiric" Proved Practically.* Albany, NY: Printed for the author, 1833.

Thomson, Samuel. *Family Botanic Medicine with the Preparation and System of Practice Under the Nature and Operation of the Four Elements.* Boston: T.G. Bangs, 1819.

_____. *New Guide to Health; or, Botanic Family Physician.* Boston: J.Q. Adams, 1835.

_____. *A Portrait of the Character and Conduct of Aaron Dow & Nathaniel S. Magoon.* Compiled from the Thomsonian Manual. Boston: George A. Chapman, 1837.

_____. *The Thomsonian Materia Medica; or Botanic Family Physician,* Twelfth and Thirteenth Editions. Albany, NY: J. Munsell, 1841.

_____. *Life and Medical Discoveries of Samuel Thomson.* Bulletin of the Lloyd Library and Museum, no. 7. Reprinted, Cincinnati, OH: Lloyd Library, 1909.

The Thomsonian Botanic Watchman 1.1 (January 1, 1834).

The Thomsonian Manual and Vade Mecum. Philadelphia: Philadelphia Branch of the U.S. Botanic Society, 1835.

Thomsonian Messenger 1.1 (1841).

The Thomsonian Recorder 1-4 (1832-1837).

Tilden & Co. Catalogue of Pure Medicinal Extracts, Prepared in Vacuo. New York: Tilden, 1852-1859.

Transactions of the American Medical Association 14 (1864): 29-33.

Tschirch, Alexander. *Handbuch der Pharmakognosie,* Volumes 1-3. Leipzig, Germany: Bernhard Tauchnitz, 1930-1933 (see especially Volume 1, pp. 1541-1558).

Turnbull, Laurence. "On Populus Tremuloides." *American Journal of Pharmacy* 14 (1842): 275.

Tyler, Varro E. *Herbs of Choice: The Therapeutic Use of Phytomedicinals.* Binghamton, NY: Pharmaceutical Products Press, 1994.

_____. "The Recent History of Pharmacognosy," in *The Inside Story of Medicines: A Symposium,* edited by Gregory J. Higby and Elaine C. Stroud. Madison, WI: American Institute of the History of Pharmacy, 1997, pp. 161-170.

Urdang, George. *The Scope of Pharmacy.* Madison, WI: American Institute of the History of Pharmacy, 1946.

Utah Historical Bulletin 10.4 (1942).

Waite, Frederick C. "The First Sectarian Medical School in New England, at Worcester (1846-1859) and Its Relation to Thomsonianism." *New England Journal of Medicine* 207 (1932): 984.

_____. "Thomsonianism in Ohio." *Ohio Archæological and Historical Quarterly* 49 (1940): 322-331.

_____. "American Sectarian Medical Colleges before the Civil War." *Bulletin of the History of Medicine* 19 (1946): 148-166.

Wallace, Daniel J. "Thomsonians: The People's Doctors." *Clio Medica* 14 (1980): 169-186.

Ward, John William. *Andrew Jackson: Symbol for an Age.* New York: Oxford University Press, 1955.

Warner, John Harley. *The Therapeutic Perspective: Medical Practice, Knowledge, and Identity in America, 1820-1885.* Cambridge, MA: Harvard University Press, 1986. Reprinted, Princeton, NJ: Princeton University Press, 1997.

Warren, Charles. "Medical Education in the United States," in *Annual Report of the Commissioner of Education Made to the Secretary of the Interior for the Year 1870.* Washington, DC: Government Printing Office, 1871.

Wayne, E.S. "Examination of the Preparations Made by the American Chemical Institute, New York." *American Journal of Pharmacy* 27 (1855): 388, 391.

_____. "On Jeffersonia diphylla." *American Journal of Pharmacy* 27 (1855): 1-7.

_____. "Criticism on the Value of Concentrated Preparations." *College Journal of Medical Science* 1 (1856): 45-48.

_____. "Examination of Keith and Co.'s Preparations—No. 2." *The College Journal of Medical Science* 1 (1856): 23.

Weaks, Mabel Clare. "Medical Consultation on the Case of Daniel Vanslyke. By C. S. Rafinesque, Pulmist, &c. Philadelphia 10th Septr. 1830." *Bulletin of the History of Medicine* 18 (1945): 425-437.

Webb, William Henry. *Standard Guide to Non-Poisonous Herbal Medicine.* Southport, England: "Visitor" Printing Works, 1916.

Webster, H.T. "How About a Coalition?" *Eclectic Medical Journal* 75 (1915): 405.

Western Medical Reformer 1-3 (1836-1838).

Wilbert, Martin I. "Some Early Botanical and Herb Gardens." *American Journal of Pharmacy* 80 (1908): 412.

Wilder, Alexander. "Wooster Beach." *Eclectic Medical Journal* 53 (1893): 113-121.

_____. "The Earlier Period of Eclectic Medicine." *Eclectic Medical Journal* 61 (1901): 68.

_____. *History of Medicine.* Augusta, ME: Maine Farmer Publishing Company, 1904.

Wilder, Charles W. "Pulmonary Consumption, Its Causes, Symptoms & Treatment," *Medical Communications of the Massachusetts Medical Society,* 7, Second Series, Volume 3. Boston: The Society, 1848.

Wood, George B. "Introductory Lecture to the Course of Materia Medica in the University of Pennsylvania." *American Journal of Pharmacy* 6 (1841): 298-322.

Zeuch, Lucius H. *History of Medical Practice in Illinois.* Chicago: Book Press, 1927.

Zollickoffer, William. *Materia Medica of the United States.* Baltimore, MD: Lovegrove and Dell, 1819.

Index

Order Your Own Copy of
This Important Book for Your Personal Library!

AMERICA'S BOTANICO-MEDICAL MOVEMENTS
Vox Populi

_____in hardbound at $69.95 (ISBN: 0-7890-0899-8)

_____in softbound at $24.95 (ISBN: 0-7890-1235-9)

COST OF BOOKS_____

OUTSIDE USA/CANADA/
MEXICO: ADD 20%_____

POSTAGE & HANDLING_____
*(US: $4.00 for first book & $1.50
for each additional book
Outside US: $5.00 for first book
& $2.00 for each additional book)*

SUBTOTAL_____

IN CANADA: ADD 7% GST_____

STATE TAX_____
*(NY, OH & MN residents, please
add appropriate local sales tax)*

FINAL TOTAL_____
*(If paying in Canadian funds,
convert using the current
exchange rate. UNESCO
coupons welcome.)*

☐ **BILL ME LATER:** ($5 service charge will be added)
(Bill-me option is good on US/Canada/Mexico orders only;
not good to jobbers, wholesalers, or subscription agencies.)

☐ Check here if billing address is different from
shipping address and attach purchase order and
billing address information.

Signature_____

☐ **PAYMENT ENCLOSED: $**_____

☐ **PLEASE CHARGE TO MY CREDIT CARD.**

☐ Visa ☐ MasterCard ☐ AmEx ☐ Discover
☐ Diner's Club ☐ Eurocard ☐ JCB

Account #_____

Exp. Date_____

Signature_____

Prices in US dollars and subject to change without notice.

NAME_____

INSTITUTION_____

ADDRESS_____

CITY_____

STATE/ZIP_____

COUNTRY_____ COUNTY (NY residents only)_____

TEL_____ FAX_____

E-MAIL_____

May we use your e-mail address for confirmations and other types of information? ☐ Yes ☐ No
We appreciate receiving your e-mail address and fax number. Haworth would like to e-mail or fax special
discount offers to you, as a preferred customer. **We will never share, rent, or exchange your e-mail
address or fax number.** We regard such actions as an invasion of your privacy.

Order From Your Local Bookstore or Directly From
The Haworth Press, Inc.
10 Alice Street, Binghamton, New York 13904-1580 • USA
TELEPHONE: 1-800-HAWORTH (1-800-429-6784) / Outside US/Canada: (607) 722-5857
FAX: 1-800-895-0582 / Outside US/Canada: (607) 772-6362
E-mail: getinfo@haworthpressinc.com
PLEASE PHOTOCOPY THIS FORM FOR YOUR PERSONAL USE.
www.HaworthPress.com

BOF00